THERAPEUTIC STRATEGIES IN COPD

THERAPEUTIC STRATEGIES IN COPD

Edited by

Mario Cazzola, Bartolome Celli,
Ronald Dahl and Stephen Rennard

CLINICAL PUBLISHING

OXFORD

Distributed worldwide by
Taylor & Francis Ltd
Boca Raton · London · New York · Washington, DC

Clinical Publishing
an imprint of Atlas Medical Publishing Ltd

Oxford Centre for Innovation
Mill Street, Oxford OX2 0JX, UK

Tel: +44 1865 811116
Fax: +44 1865 251550
Web: www.clinicalpublishing.co.uk

Distributed by:

Taylor & Francis Ltd
6000 Broken Sound Parkway NW, Suite 300
Boca Raton, FL 33487, USA
E-mail: orders@crcpress.com

Taylor & Francis Ltd
23–25 Blades Court
Deodar Road
London SW15 2NU, UK
E-mail: uk.tandf@thomsonpublishingservices.co.uk

A catalogue record for this book is available from the British Library

ISBN 1 904392 42 3

The publisher makes no representation, express or implied, that the dosages in this
book are correct. Readers must therefore always check the product information and
clinical procedures with the most up-to-date published product information and data
sheets provided by the manufacturers and the most recent codes of conduct and safety
regulations. The authors and the publisher do not accept any liability for any errors in
the text or for the misuse or misapplication of material in this work

Project manager: Gavin Smith
Typeset by Mizpah Publishing Services Private Limited, Chennai, India
Printed in Spain by T G Hostench SA, Barcelona, Spain
Cover image provided by Dr Adam T. Hill, University of Edinburgh, Scotland

Contents

Contributors

IAN MICHAEL ADCOCK, PhD, Professor of Respiratory Cell and Molecular Biology, Airways Disease Section, National Heart & Lung Institute, Imperial College London, London, UK

LUIGI ALLEGRA, MD, Professor, Respiratory Diseases, University of Milan, Director, Cardiorespiratory Department, IRCCS, Policlinico Hospital, Milan, Italy

PETER J. BARNES, FMedSci, Professor of Thoracic Medicine, National Heart and Lung Institute, Imperial College, London, UK

MARIA G. BELVISI, BSc, PhD, Professor of Respiratory Pharmacology, Respiratory Pharmacology Group, Airway Disease Section, National Heart & Lung Institute, Imperial College School of Medicine, London, UK

VICTORIA BOSWELL-SMITH, BSc, Sackler Institute of Pulmonary Pharmacology, Guy's, King's and St Thomas' School of Biomedical Sciences, Kings College London, London, UK

PETER M. A. CALVERLEY, MB ChB, FRCP, FRCPE, Professor of Medicine (Pulmonary & Rehabilitation), Clinical Sciences Centre, University Hospital Aintree, Liverpool, UK

GAETANO CARAMORI, MD, PhD, Centro di Ricerca su Asma e BPCO, Università di Ferrara, Ferrara, Italy

MARIO CAZZOLA, MD, Consultant in Respiratory Medicine, Chief of Respiratory Medicine, Unit of Pneumology and Allergology, Department of Respiratory Medicine, A. Cardarelli Hospital, Naples, Italy

BARTOLOME R. CELLI, MD, Professor of Medicine, Tufts University, Chief, Pulmonary and Critical Care Medicine, Caritas St Elizabeth's Medical Center, Boston, MA, USA

RONALD DAHL, MD, Dr.med.sci. Professor of Respiratory Medicine, Department of Respiratory Diseases, Aarhus University Hospital, Aarhus, Denmark

LYNETTE B. FERNANDES, BSc, PhD, Lecturer in Pharmacology, Western Australian Institute for Medical Research, Pharmacology Unit, School of Medicine & Pharmacology, The University of Western Australia, Australia

ROY G. GOLDIE, BSc, PhD, Executive Dean, Faculty of Health Sciences, Western Australian Institute for Medical Research, Pharmacology Unit, School of Medicine & Pharmacology, The University of Western Australia, Australia

PETER J. HENRY, BSc, PhD, Senior Lecturer in Pharmacology, Western Australian Institute for Medical Research, Pharmacology Unit, School of Medicine & Pharmacology, The University of Western Australia, Australia

SONIA KHIRANI, PhD, Doctor in Biomedical Engineering, Ospedale Riuniti di Bergamo, Bergamo, Italy

ANDERS LINDÉN, MD, PhD, Associate Professor, Certified Specialist in Respiratory Medicine and Allergology, Lung Pharmacology Group, Department of Respiratory Medicine and Allergology, Göteborg, Sweden

JAN LÖTVALL, MD, PhD, Professor of Allergy, Head of Department, Department of Respiratory Medicine and Allergology, Göteborg University, Göteborg, Sweden

WILLIAM MACNEE, MBChB, MD(Hons), FRCP (Glas), FRCP (Edin), Professor of Respiratory and Environmental Medicine, ELEGI Colt Laboratory, MRC Centre for Inflammation Research, University of Edinburgh Medical School, Edinburgh, UK

MARIA GABRIELLA MATERA, MD, PhD, Researcher in Pharmacology and Consultant in Clinical Pharmacology, Unit of Pharmacology, Department of Experimental Medicine, School of Medicine, Second University, Naples, Italy

GIACOMO MORLINI, RRT, Respiratory Therapist, Ospedale Riuniti di Bergamo, Bergamo, Italy

CLIVE PETER PAGE, BSc, PhD, Professor of Pharmacology, Sackler Institute of Pulmonary Pharmacology, Guy's, King's and St Thomas' School of Biomedical Sciences, Kings College London, London, UK

HEMA J. PATEL, BSc, PhD, Respiratory Pharmacology Group, Airway Disease Section, Imperial College School of Medicine at the National Heart & Lung Institute, London, UK

GUIDO POLESE, MD, Pulmonary Division, Ospedale Riuniti di Bergamo, Bergamo, Italy

KLAUS F. RABE, MD, PhD, Leiden University Medical Centre, Leiden, The Netherlands

STEPHEN I. RENNARD, MD, Larson Professor of Medicine, University of Nebraska Medical Center, Omaha, Nebraska, USA

ANDREA ROSSI, MD, Director, Pulmonary Division, Ospedale Riuniti di Bergamo, Bergamo, Italy

TERESA D. TETLEY, BSc, PhD, Reader in Lung Cell Biology, National Heart & Lung Institute, Imperial College, London, UK

1

COPD: molecular and cellular mechanisms

P. J. Barnes

INTRODUCTION

COPD is a major and increasing global health problem, which is currently the 4th commonest cause of death and predicted to become the the 5th commonest cause of disability in the world by 2020. While there have been major advances in the understanding and management of asthma, COPD has been relatively neglected and there are no current therapies that reduce the inevitable progression of this disease. However, because of the enormous burden of disease and escalating health care costs, there is now renewed interest in the underlying cellular and molecular mechanisms [1] and a search for new therapies [2], resulting in a re-evaluation of this disease [3].

COPD is characterised by slowly progressive development of airflow limitation that is poorly reversible, in sharp contrast to asthma where there is variable airflow obstruction that is usually reversible spontaneously or with treatment. The definition of COPD adopted by the Global Initiative on Obstructive Lung Disease (GOLD) for the first time encompasses the idea that COPD is a chronic inflammatory disease and much of the recent research has focused on the nature of this inflammatory response [4].

COPD includes chronic obstructive bronchiolitis with fibrosis and obstruction of small airways, and emphysema with enlargement of airspaces and destruction of lung parenchyma, loss of lung elasticity and closure of small airways. Chronic bronchitis, by contrast, is defined by a productive cough of more than 3 months duration for more than 2 successive years; this reflects mucus hypersecretion and is not necessarily associated with airflow limitation. Most patients with COPD have all three pathological mechanisms (chronic obstructive bronchiolitis, emphysema and mucus plugging) as all are induced by smoking, but may differ in the proportion of emphysema and obstructive bronchiolitis [1]. In developed countries cigarette smoking is by far the commonest cause of COPD accounting for over 95% of cases, but there are several other risk factors, including air pollution (particularly indoor air pollution from burning fuels), poor diet, and occupational exposure. COPD is characterised by acceleration in the normal decline of lung function seen with age. The slowly progressive airflow limitation leads to disability and premature death and is quite different from the variable airway obstruction and symptoms in asthma, which rarely progresses in severity. While COPD and asthma both involve inflammation in the respiratory tract there are marked differences in the nature of the inflammatory process, with differences in inflammatory cells, mediators, response to inflammation, anatomical distribution and response to anti-inflammatory therapy [3, 5]. Some patients appear to share the

Peter J. Barnes, FMedSci, Professor of Thoracic Medicine, National Heart and Lung Institute, Imperial College, London, UK.

characteristics of COPD and asthma, however. Rather than this representing a graded spec-trum of disease, it is more likely that these patients have both of these common diseases at the same time.

DIFFERENCES FROM ASTHMA

Histopathological studies of COPD show a predominant involvement of peripheral airways (bronchioles) and lung parenchyma, whereas asthma involves inflammation in all airways but usually without involvement of the lung parenchyma [6]. There is obstruction of bronchioles, with fibrosis and infiltration with macrophages and T-lymphocytes. There is destruction of lung parenchyma and an increased number of macrophages and T-lymphocytes, with a greater increase in CD8$^+$ (cytotoxic) than CD4$^+$ (helper) cells [7] (Figure 1.1). Bronchial biopsies show similar changes with an infiltration of macrophages and CD8$^+$ cells and an increased number of neutrophils in patients with severe COPD [8]. Bronchoalveolar lavage (BAL) fluid and induced sputum demonstrate a marked increase in macrophages and neu-trophils [9, 10]. In contrast to asthma, eosinophils are not prominent except during exacer-bations or when patients have concomitant asthma [6, 11].

INFLAMMATORY CELLS

Although abnormal numbers of inflammatory cells have been documented in COPD, the relationship between these cell types and the sequence of their appearance and their persis-tence are largely unknown. Most studies have been cross-sectional based on selection of patients with different stages of the disease and comparisons have been made between smokers without airflow limitation (normal smokers) and those with COPD, who have

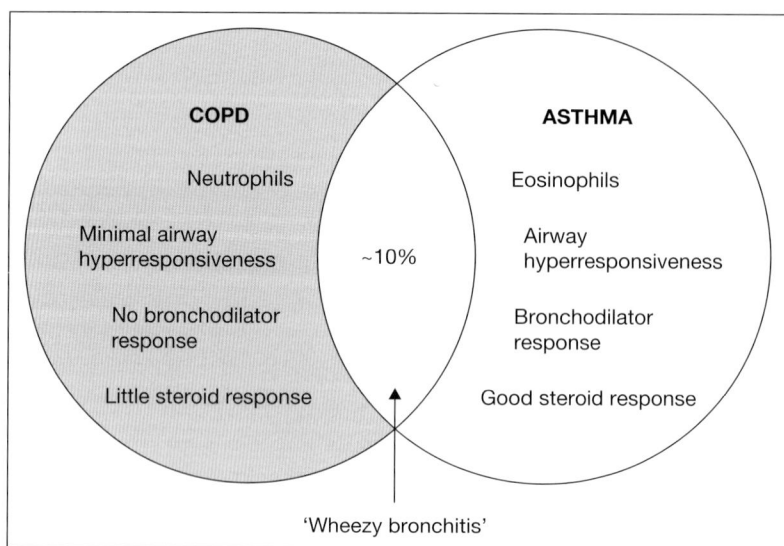

Figure 1.1   Overlap between COPD and asthma. Asthma and COPD are different diseases but some patients share features of both diseases which some have suggested represents a spectrum of a single disease (this is the essence of the 'Dutch hypothesis'). Approximately 10% of patients with COPD have asthma and will share inflammatory features between these diseases. This overlap group may be termed 'wheezy bronchitis'. It is important to recognise these patients as they may require treatment for both diseases to optimise symptom control.

smoked a similar amount. There are no serial studies and selection biases (such as selecting tissue from patients suitable for lung volume reduction surgery) may give misleading results. Analysis of the cell profile in alveoli and small airways shows an increase in all of the cell types implicated in COPD, including macrophages, T-lymphocytes, B-lymphocytes and neutrophils [12].

NEUTROPHILS

Increased numbers of activated neutrophils are found in sputum and BAL fluid of patients with COPD [10, 13], yet are relatively little increased in the airways or lung parenchyma [14]. This may reflect their rapid transit through the airways and parenchyma. Neutrophils secrete serine proteases, including neutrophil elastase (NE), cathepsin G and proteinase-3, as well as matrix metalloproteinase (MMP8 and MMP9), which may contribute to alveolar destruction (Figure 1.2). These serine proteases are also potent mucus stimulants. Neutrophil recruitment to the airways and parenchyma involves adhesion to endothelial cells and E-selectin is up-regulated on endothelial cells in the airways of COPD patients [15]. Adherent neutrophils then migrate into the respiratory tract under the direction of neutrophil chemotactic factors, which include interleukin (IL)-8 and leukotriene B_4 (LTB$_4$). Neutrophil survival in the respiratory tract may be increased by cytokines, such as granulocyte-macrophage colony stimulating factor (GM-CSF) and granulocyte colony stimulating factor (G-CSF).

The role of neutrophils in COPD is not yet clear. There is a correlation between the number of circulating neutrophils and fall in FEV$_1$ [16]. Neutrophil numbers in bronchial biopsies and induced sputum are correlated with COPD disease severity [8, 10] and with the rate of decline in lung function [17]. Smoking has a direct stimulatory effect on granulocyte production and release from the bone marrow, possibly mediated by GM-CSF and G-CSF released from lung macrophages [18]. Smoking may also increase neutrophil retention in the lung [19]. There is no doubt that the neutrophils recruited to the airways of COPD patients are activated as

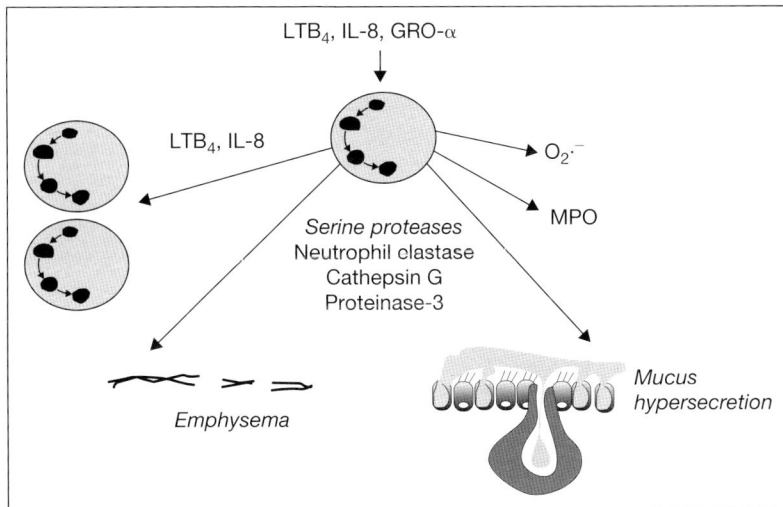

Figure 1.2 Neutrophils in COPD. Neutrophils recruited to the lungs by chemotactic factors such as leukotriene B$_4$ (LTB$_4$), interleukin-8 (IL-8) and growth-related oncogene-α (GRO-α) are activated and release superoxide anions (O$_2$·$^-$), myeloperoxidase (MPO), LTB$_4$ and IL-8, and serine proteases.

there is increased concentrations of granule proteins, such as myeloperoxidase (MPO) and human neutrophil lipocalin, in the sputum supernatant [20–22]. These neutrophils also show an increase in the respiratory burst response which correlates with the degree of airflow limitation [23].

Neutrophils have the capacity to induce tissue damage through the release of serine proteases and oxidants. Priming is a prerequisite for degranulation and superoxide anion generation in neutrophils [24]. Neutrophils in the peripheral circulation show evidence of priming in COPD [25], but this may result from rather than contribute to lung pathophysiology. There are several chemotactic signals that have the potential for neutrophil recruitment in COPD, including LTB$_4$, IL-8 and related CXC chemokines, including GRO-α (growth-related oncoprotein) and ENA-78 (epithelial neutrophil activating protein of 78 kDa) which are increased in COPD airways [26, 27]. These mediators may be derived from alveolar macrophages and epithelial cells, but the neutrophil itself may be a major source of IL-8 [28].

Neutrophils from the circulation marginate in the pulmonary circulation and adhere to endothelial cells in the alveolar wall before passing into the alveolar space [29]. The precise route for neutrophil migration in large airways is less certain, but it is more likely that they reach the airway from the tracheobronchial circulation and migrate across post-capillary venules [30]. The cellular mechanisms underlying neutrophil adhesion and transmigration differ between systemic and pulmonary circulations and this might confer different properties on the neutrophils arriving from the alveolar or bronchial compartments. There may be significant differences in neutrophil transit times in different areas of the lung that may account for differential distribution of emphysema, for example, the upper lobe predominance in centrilobular emphysema. Little is known about survival and apoptosis of neutrophils in COPD airways. Theoretically GM-CSF may prolong neutrophil survival but it has proved difficult to culture neutrophils from sputum samples.

However, while neutrophils have the capacity to cause elastolysis, this is not a prominent feature of other pulmonary diseases where chronic airway neutrophilia is even more prominent, including cystic fibrosis and bronchiectasis. This suggests that other factors are involved in the generation of emphysema. Indeed there is a *negative* association between the number of neutrophils and the amount of alveolar destruction in COPD [14] and neutrophils are not a prominent feature of parenchymal inflammation in COPD. It is likely that airway neutrophilia is linked to mucus hypersecretion in chronic bronchitis, however. Serine proteases from neutrophils, including NE, cathepsin G and proteinase-3 are all potent stimulants of mucus secretion from submucosal glands and goblet cells in the epithelium [31, 32].

MACROPHAGES

Macrophages appear to play a pivotal role in the pathophysiology of COPD and can account for most of the known features of the disease [33] (Figure 1.3). There is a marked increase (5–10-fold) in the numbers of macrophages in airways, lung parenchyma, BAL fluid and sputum in patients with COPD. A careful morphometric analysis of macrophage numbers in the parenchyma of patients with emphysema showed a 25-fold increase in the numbers of macrophages in the tissue and alveolar space compared with normal smokers [12]. Furthermore, macrophages are localised to sites of alveolar wall destruction in patients with emphysema [14, 34]. There is a correlation between macrophage numbers in the airways and the severity of COPD [8].

Macrophages may be activated by cigarette smoke extract to release inflammatory mediators, including TNF-α, IL-8, other CXC chemokines, MCP-1, LTB$_4$ and reactive oxygen species (ROS), providing a cellular mechanism that links smoking with inflammation in COPD. Alveolar macrophages also secrete elastolytic enzymes, including MMP2, MMP9,

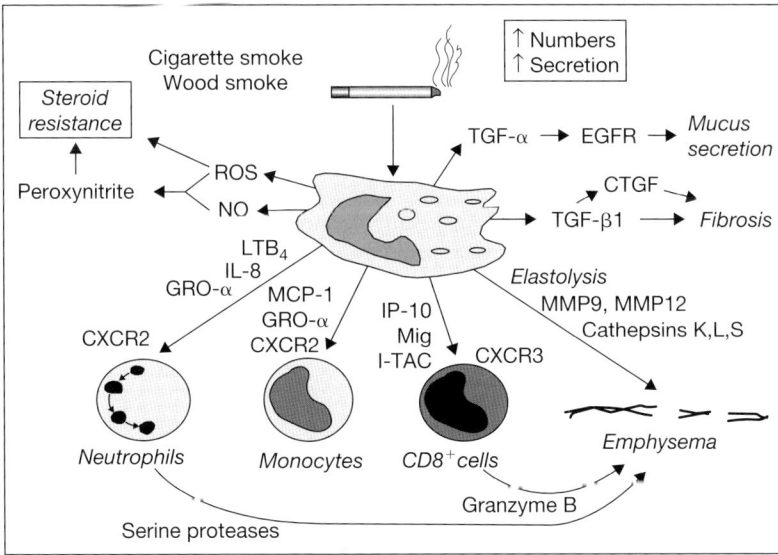

Figure 1.3 Macrophages may play a pivotal role in COPD as they are activated by cigarette smoke extract and secrete many inflammatory proteins that may orchestrate the inflammatory process in COPD. Neutrophils may be attracted by interleukin (IL)-8, growth-related oncogene-α (GRO-α) and leukotriene B_4 (LTB_4), monocytes by macrophage chemotactic protein-1 (MCP-1), and CD8$^+$ lymphocytes by interferon-γ-inducible protein (IP-10), monokine induced by interferon-γ (Mig) and interferon-inducible T-cell α-chemoattractant (I-TAC). Release of elastolytic enzymes including matrix metalloproteinases (MMP) and cathepsins cause elastolysis, and release of transforming growth factor (TGF)-β1 and connective tissue growth factor (CTGF). Macrophages also generate reactive oxygen species (ROS) and nitric oxide (NO) which together form peroxynitrite and may contribute to steroid resistance.

MMP12, cathepsins K, L and S and NE taken up from neutrophils [35, 36]. Alveolar macrophages from patients with COPD secrete more inflammatory proteins and have a greater elastolytic activity at baseline than those from normal smokers and this is further increased by exposure to cigarette smoke [36–38]. Macrophages demonstrate this difference even when maintained in culture for 3 days and therefore appear to be intrinsically different from the macrophages of normal smokers and non-smoking normal control subjects [36]. The predominant elastolytic enzyme secreted by alveolar macrophages in COPD patients is MMP9. Most of the inflammatory proteins that are up-regulated in COPD macrophages are regulated by the transcription factor nuclear factor-κB (NF-κB) which is activated in alveolar macrophages of COPD patients, particularly during exacerbations [39, 40].

The increased numbers of macrophages in smokers and COPD patients may be due to increased recruitment of monocytes from the circulation in response to monocyte-selective chemokines. The monocyte-selective chemokine MCP-1 is increased in sputum and BAL of patients with COPD [26, 41], with increased expression in macrophages [42]. CXC chemokines are also chemoattractant to monocytes acting *via* CXCR2 and the concentration of the CXC chemokine GRO-α is markedly increased in sputum and BAL of patients with COPD [26]. Monocytes from patients with COPD show a greater chemotactic response to GRO-α than cells from normal smokers and non-smokers, but this is not explained by an increase in CXCR2 [43]. Interestingly, while all monocytes express CCR2, the receptor for MIP1, only ~30% of monocytes express CXCR2. It is possible that these CXCR2-expressing monocytes transform into macrophages that behave differently – e.g., release more inflammatory proteins. Macrophages also have the capacity to release the chemokines IP-10, I-TAC and Mig, which are chemotactic for CD8$^+$ Tc1 cells *via* interaction with the CXCR3 receptor expressed on these cells [44].

The increased numbers of macrophages in COPD may be due to increased recruitment of monocytes, but may also be due to increased proliferation and prolonged survival in the lungs. Macrophages have a very low proliferation rate in the lungs, but we have demonstrated that there is some increase in cell proliferation measured by proliferative cell nuclear antigen (PCNA) [45]. Macrophages have a long survival time so this is difficult to measure directly. However, in macrophages from smokers, there is markedly increased expression of the anti-apoptotic protein Bcl-X$_L$ and increased expression of p21$^{CIP/WAF1}$ in the cytoplasm [45]. This suggests that macrophages may have a prolonged survival in smokers and patients with COPD.

Corticosteroids are ineffective in suppressing inflammation, including cytokines, chemokines and proteases, in patients with COPD [46, 47]. *In vitro* the release of IL-8, TNF-α and MMP9 macrophages from normal subjects and normal smokers are inhibited by corticosteroids, whereas corticosteroids are ineffective in macrophages from patients with COPD [48]. Curiously, this does not apply to GM-CSF which does not appear to have increased secretion in COPD, and is suppressed by corticosteroids, albeit to a lesser extent than in macrophages from normal smokers. The reasons for resistance to corticosteroids in COPD, and to a lesser extent macrophages from smokers, may be the marked reduction in activity of histone deacetylase (HDAC) [49], which is recruited to activated inflammatory genes by glucocorticoid receptors to switch off inflammatory genes [50]. The reduction in HDAC activity in macrophages is correlated with increased secretion of cytokines like TNF-α and IL-8 and reduced response to corticosteroids. The reduction of HDAC activity on COPD patients may be mediated through oxidative stress and peroxynitrite formation [51].

Although corticosteroids are not effective in inhibiting the secretion of cytokines and proteases from macrophages, other drugs may be beneficial. Theophylline in low concentrations increases HDAC activity in alveolar macrophages and *in vitro* reverses the steroid resistance induced by oxidative stress [52]. Resveratrol, a flavonoid found in red wine, is an effective inhibitor of cytokine expression from macrophages from COPD patients, but its molecular mechanisms of action have not yet been determined [53, 54].

T-LYMPHOCYTES

There is an increase in the total numbers of T-lymphocytes in lung parenchyma, peripheral and central airways of patients with COPD, with a greater increase in CD8$^+$ than CD4$^+$ cells [12, 14, 55–57]. There is a correlation between the numbers of T cells and the amount of alveolar destruction and the severity of airflow obstruction. There is also an increase in the absolute number of CD4$^+$ T cells, but the ratio of CD4$^+$:CD8$^+$ cells is reversed in COPD. This is mainly found in smokers with COPD rather than smokers without evidence of airflow limitation [55]. It is not known whether these cells are classified as Tc1 (interferon-γ producing) or Tc2 (IL-4 producing) subtypes [58], but there is evidence that the majority of T cells in COPD airways are of the Tc1 subtype [44]. CD8$^+$ and CD4$^+$ T cells show increased expression of activation markers compared to T cells in the circulation, although there is no clear difference between patients with COPD and normal controls [59].

The mechanisms by which CD8$^+$, and to a lesser extent CD4$^+$ cells, accumulate in the airways and lungs of patients with COPD is not yet understood. However, homing of T cells to the lung must depend upon some initial activation then adhesion and selective chemotaxis. T cells in peripheral airways of COPD patients show increased expression of CXCR3, a receptor activated by IP-10, Mig and I-TAC. There is increased expression of IP-10 by

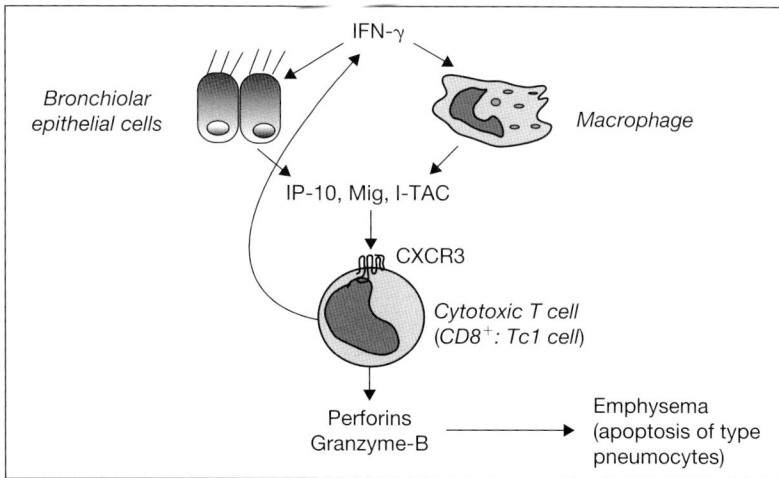

Figure 1.4 Chemotaxis of cytotoxic (CD8$^+$) T-lymphocytes *via* activation of CXCR3 by the CXC chemokines interferon-γ-inducible protein of 10 kDa (IP-10), monokine induced by interferon-γ (Mig) and interferon-inducible T cell-α chemoattractant (I-TAC). CD8$^+$ cells may release perforins and granzyme-B which may induce apoptosis in alveolar cells and release interferon-γ (IFN-γ) which in turn activates the release of these chemokines.

bronchiolar epithelial cells and this could contribute to the accumulation of CD8$^+$ cells, which preferentially express CXCR3 [44] (Figure 1.4).

There is also an increase in the numbers of CD8$^+$ cells in the circulation in COPD patients who do not smoke [60, 61] and an increase in Th1 type (IFN-γ producing) CD4$^+$ cells in COPD patients [62]. This indicates that there may be chronic immune stimulation *via* antigens presented *via* the HLA Class 1 pathway. Dendritic cells may migrate from the airways to regional lymph nodes and stimulate proliferation of CD8$^+$ and CD4$^+$ T cells. CD8$^+$ cells are typically increased in airway infections and it is possible that the chronic colonisation of the lower respiratory tract of COPD patients by bacterial and viral pathogens is responsible for this inflammatory response [63]. It is also possible that protease-induced lung injury may uncover previously sequestered autoantigens or that cigarette smoke itself may damage airway epithelial cells and make them antigenic [64]. There is a marked increase in T cells in the walls of small airways in patients with severe COPD and the T cells are formed into lymphoid follicles, surrounding B lymphocytes [65].

The role of increased numbers of CD4$^+$ cells in COPD, particularly in severe disease is also unknown [12]; it is possible that they have immunological memory and play a role in perpetuating the inflammatory process in the absence of cigarette smoking. Natural killer (NK, CD56$^+$) cells are the first line defence against viral infections. Circulating NK cells are reduced in patients with COPD and have reduced phagocytic activity [66] and similar findings are found in normal smokers [67], although no difference in NK cells was found in lung parenchyma of COPD patients [55]. There is an increase in γ/δ T cells in alveoli of smokers, whether they have airway obstruction or not [55].

The role of T cells in the pathophysiology of COPD is not yet certain. CD8$^+$ cells have the capacity to cause cytolysis and apoptosis of alveolar epithelial cells through release of perforins, granzyme-B and TNF-α [68]. There is an association between CD8$^+$ cells and apoptosis of alveolar cells in emphysema [55]. In a mouse model of cigarette-induced emphysema there is a predominance of T cells which are directly related to the severity of emphysema [69].

EOSINOPHILS

The role of eosinophils in COPD is uncertain. There are some reports of increased numbers of inactive eosinophils in the airways and lavage of patients with stable COPD, whereas others have not found increased numbers in airway biopsies, BAL or induced sputum [70]. The presence of eosinophils in patients with COPD predicts a response to corticosteroids and may indicate coexisting asthma [71, 72]. Increased numbers of eosinophils have been reported in bronchial biopsies and BAL fluid during acute exacerbations of chronic bronchitis [73, 74]. Surprisingly, the levels of eosinophil basic proteins in induced sputum are as elevated in COPD as in asthma, despite the absence of eosinophils, suggesting that they may have degranulated and are no longer recognisable by microscopy [20]. Perhaps this is due to the high levels of neutrophil elastase (NE) that have been shown to cause degranulation of eosinophils [75].

DENDRITIC CELLS

The dendritic cell plays a central role in the initiation of the innate and adaptive immune response [76]. The airways and lungs contain a rich network of dendritic cells that are localised near the surface, so that they are ideally located to signal the entry of foreign substances that are inhaled [77]. Dendritic cells can activate a variety of other inflammatory and immune cells, including macrophages, neutrophils, T- and B-lymphocytes [78]. It is, therefore, likely that the dendritic cell may play an important role in the pulmonary response to cigarette smoke and other inhaled noxious agents and may, therefore, be a key cellular element in COPD. The mechanism by which tobacco smoke activates the immune system is not yet understood, but a glycoprotein isolated from tobacco has powerful immunostimulatory actions [79]. There is an increase in the number of dendritic cells in rat lungs exposed to cigarette smoke [80] and in the airways and alveolar walls of smokers [81, 82]. Pulmonary histiocytosis is a disease caused by dendritic cell granulomata in the lung and is characterised by destruction of the lung parenchyma that resembles emphysema [83, 84]. The adult form of the disease occurs almost exclusively in smokers. In mice exposed to chronic cigarette smoke there is an increase in dendritic cells in the airways and lung parenchyma [85]. The role of dendritic cells in recruiting other effector cells in COPD deserves further study.

EPITHELIAL CELLS

Airway and alveolar epithelial cells may be an important source of inflammatory mediators and proteases in COPD. Epithelial cells are activated by cigarette smoke to produce inflammatory mediators, including TNF-α, IL-1β, GM-CSF and IL-8 [86–88]. Epithelial cells in small airways may be an important source of transforming growth factor (TGF)-β, which then induces local fibrosis [89]. Vascular endothelial growth factor (VEGF) appears to be necessary to maintain alveolar cell survival and blockade of VEGF receptors (VEGFR2) and in rats induces apoptosis of alveolar cells and an emphysema-like pathology [90]. The role of VEGF in the pathogenesis of human emphysema is not yet known, however.

Airway epithelial cells are also important in defence of the airways. Mucus produced from goblet cells protects and traps bacteria and inhaled particulates [91]. Epithelial cells secrete defensins and other cationic peptides with antimicrobial effects and is a part of the innate defence system, but is also involved in tissue repair processes [92]. They also secrete antioxidants as well as antiproteases, such as secretory leukoprotease inhibitor (SLPI). Epithelial cells also transport IgA and are therefore also involved in adaptive immunity [93]. It is possible that cigarette smoke and other noxious agents impair these innate and adaptive immune responses of the airway epithelium, increasing susceptibility to infection.

The airway epithelium in chronic bronchitis and COPD often shows squamous metaplasia, which may result from increased proliferation of airway epithelial cells. Proliferation in basal airway epithelial cells, measured by proliferating cell nuclear antigen (PCNA) is increased in some normal smokers, but is markedly increased in patients with chronic bronchitis and correlates with the degree of squamous metaplasia [94]. The nature of the growth factors involved in epithelial cell proliferation, cell cycle and differentiation in COPD are not yet known. Epithelial growth factor receptors show increased expression in airway epithelial cells of smokers and may contribute to basal cell proliferation, resulting in squamous metaplasia and an increased risk of bronchial carcinoma [95].

OXIDATIVE STRESS

Oxidative stress occurs when ROS are produced in excess of the antioxidant defence mechanisms and result in harmful effects, including damage to lipids, proteins and DNA. There is increasing evidence that oxidative stress is an important feature in COPD [96–98].

FORMATION

Inflammatory and structural cells that are activated in the airways of patients with COPD produce ROS, including neutrophils, eosinophils, macrophages, and epithelial cells [97]. Superoxide anions ($O_2 \cdot^-$) are generated by NADPH oxidase and this is converted to hydrogen peroxide (H_2O_2) by superoxide dismutases (SODs). H_2O_2 is then dismuted to water by catalase. $O_2 \cdot^-$ and H_2O_2 may interact in the presence of free iron to form the highly reactive hydroxyl radical ($\cdot$OH). $O_2 \cdot^-$ may also combine with NO to form peroxynitrite, which also generates $\cdot$OH [99]. Oxidative stress leads to the oxidation of arachidonic acid and the formation of a new series of prostanoid mediators called isoprostanes, which may exert significant functional effects [100], including bronchoconstriction and plasma exudation [101–103] (Figure 1.5).

Granulocyte peroxidases, such as MPO in neutrophils, play an important role on oxidative stress. In neutrophils H_2O_2 generated from $O_2 \cdot^-$ is metabolised by MPO in the presence of chloride ions to hypochlorous acid which is a strong oxidant. MPO is also able to nitrate tyrosine residues, as can peroxynitrite [104–106].

ANTIOXIDANTS

The normal production of oxidants is counteracted by several antioxidant mechanisms in the human respiratory tract [107]. The major intracellular antioxidants in the airways are catalase, SOD and glutathione, formed by the enzyme γ-glutamyl cysteine synthetase, and glutathione synthetase. Oxidant stress activates the inducible enzyme heme oxygenase-1 (HO-1), converting heme and hemin to biliverdin with the formation of carbon monoxide (CO) [108]. Biliverdin is converted via bilirubin reductase to bilirubin, which is a potential antioxidant. HO-1 is widely expressed in human airways [109] and CO production is increased in COPD [110]. In the lung intracellular antioxidants are expressed at relatively low levels and are not induced by oxidative stress, whereas the major antioxidants are extracellular [111]. Extracellular antioxidants, particularly glutathione peroxidase, are markedly up-regulated in response to cigarette smoke and oxidative stress. The glutathione system is the major antioxidant mechanism in the airways. There is a high concentration of reduced glutathione (GSH) in lung epithelial lining fluid [107] and concentrations are increased higher in cigarette smokers. Extracellular glutathione peroxidase (eGPx) is an important antioxidant in the lungs and may be secreted by epithelial cells and macrophages, particularly in response to cigarette smoke or oxidative stress [112]. eGPx inactivates H_2O_2 and $O_2 \cdot^-$, but may also inactivate reactive nitrogen species [111]. Extracellular antioxidants also include

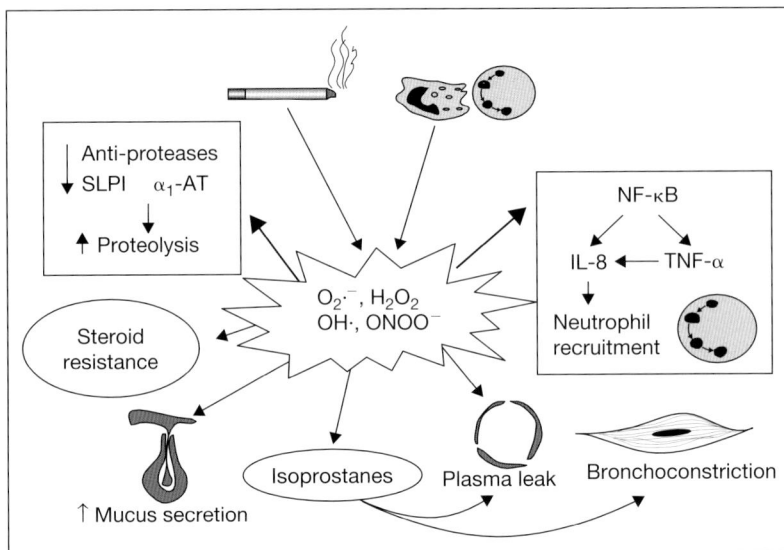

Figure 1.5 Oxidative stress in COPD. Oxidative stress plays a key role in the pathophysiology of COPD and amplifies the inflammatory and destructive process. Reactive oxygen species from cigarette smoke or from inflammatory cells (particularly macrophages and neutrophils) result in several damaging effects in COPD, including decreased anti-protease defences such as α_1-antitrypsin (AT) and secretory leukoprotease inhibitor (SLPI), activation of nuclear factor-κB (NF-κB) resulting in increased secretion of the cytokines interleukin-8 (IL-8) and tumour necrosis factor-α (TNF-α), increased production of isoprostanes and direct effects on airway function. In addition recent evidence suggests that oxidative stress induces steroid resistance.

the dietary antioxidants vitamin C (ascorbic acid) and vitamin E (α-tocopherol), uric acid, lactoferrin and extracellular SOD3. SOD3 is highly expressed in human lung, but its role in COPD is not yet clear [113].

EFFECTS ON AIRWAYS

ROS have several effects on the airways, which would have the effect of increasing the inflammatory response. These effects may be mediated by direct actions of ROS on target cells in the airways, but may also be mediated indirectly *via* activation of signal transduction pathways and transcription factors and *via* the formation of oxidised mediators such as isoprostanes and hydroxy-nonenal.

ROS activate NF-κB, which switches on multiple inflammatory genes resulting in amplification of the inflammatory response [114]. The molecular pathways by which oxidative stress activates NF-κB have not been fully elucidated, but there are several redox-sensitive steps in the activation pathway [115]. Many of the stimuli that activate NF-κB appear to do so *via* the formation of ROS, particularly H_2O_2. ROS activate NF-κB in an epithelial cell line [116] and increase the release of pro-inflammatory cytokines from cultured human airway epithelial cells [117]. Oxidative stress results in activation of histone acetyltransferase activity which opens up the chromatin structure and is associated with increased transcription of multiple inflammatory genes [118, 119].

Another transcription factor that activates inflammatory genes is activator protein-1 (AP-1), a heterodimer of Fos and Jun proteins. As with NF-κB there are several redox-sensitive steps in the activation pathway [120]. Exogenous oxidants may also be important in worsening airway disease. Cigarette smoke, ozone and, to a lesser extent, nitrogen dioxide, impose an oxidative stress on the airways [121].

Oxidants also activate mitogen-activated protein (MAP) kinase pathways. H_2O_2 is a potent activator of extracellular regulated kinases (ERK) and p38 MAP kinase pathways that regulate the expression of many inflammatory genes and survival in certain cells, and spreading of macrophages [122]. Indeed many aspects of macrophage function are regulated by oxidants through the activation of multiple kinase pathways [123].

EVIDENCE FOR INCREASED OXIDATIVE STRESS

There is considerable evidence for increased oxidative stress in COPD [96, 97]. Cigarette smoke itself contains a high concentration of ROS [124]. Inflammatory cells, such as activated macrophages and neutrophils, also generate ROS, as discussed above. Epidemiological evidence indicates that reduced dietary intake of antioxidants may be a determinant of COPD and population surveys have linked a low dietary intake of the antioxidant ascorbic acid (vitamin C) with worse lung function [125, 126].

There are several markers of oxidative stress that may be detected in the breath and several studies have demonstrated increased production of oxidants in exhaled air or breath condensates [127–129]. There is an increased concentration of H_2O_2 in exhaled breath condensate of patients with COPD, particularly during exacerbations [130, 131].

There is also an increase in the concentration of 8-iso prostaglandin $F_{2\alpha}$ (8-isoprostane) in exhaled breath condensate, which is found even in patients who are ex-smokers [132] and is increased further during acute exacerbations [133]. Isoprostane is also increased in the breath of normal smokers, but to a lesser extent than in COPD, suggesting that there is an exaggeration of oxidative stress in COPD. 8-Isoprostane is similarly increased in the urine of patients with COPD and further increased during exacerbations [134].

There is also evidence for increased systemic markers of oxidative stress in patients with COPD as measured by biochemical markers of lipid peroxidation [135]. A specific marker of lipid peroxidation, 4-hydroxy-2-nonenal, which forms adducts with basic amino acid residues in proteins, can be detected by immunocytochemistry and has been detected in lungs of patients with COPD [136]. This signature of oxidative stress is localised to airway and alveolar epithelial cells, endothelial cells and neutrophils.

ROLE OF OXIDATIVE STRESS

The increased oxidative stress in the airways of COPD patients may play an important pathophysiological role in the disease by amplifying the inflammatory response in COPD. This may reflect the activation of NF-κB and AP-1, which then induce a neutrophilic inflammation via increased expression of IL-8 and other CXC chemokines, TNF-α and MMP9. NF-κB is activated in airways and alveolar macrophages of patients with COPD and is further activated during exacerbations [39, 40]. It is likely that oxidative stress is an important activation of this transcription factor in COPD patients.

Oxidative stress may also impair the function of antiproteases such as α_1-antitrypsin (α_1-AT) and SLPI, and thereby accelerates the breakdown of elastin in lung parenchyma [137].

Corticosteroids are much less effective in COPD than in asthma and do not reduce the progression of the disease [138–141]. In contrast to patients with asthma, those with COPD do not show any significant anti-inflammatory response to corticosteroids [46, 47]. Alveolar macrophages from patients with COPD show a marked reduction in responsiveness to the anti-inflammatory effects of corticosteroids, compared to cells from normal smokers and non-smokers [48]. Recent studies suggest that there may be a link between oxidative stress and the poor response to corticosteroids in COPD. Oxidative stress impairs binding of glucocorticoid receptors to DNA and the translocation of these receptors from the cytoplasm to the nucleus [142, 143]. Corticosteroids switch off inflammatory genes by recruiting histone deacetylase-2 (HDAC2) to the active transcription site and by deacetylating the hyperacetylated histones of the actively transcribing inflammatory gene, they are able to switch off its transcription and thus suppress inflammation [50, 144]. In cigarette smokers and patients with COPD there is a marked reduction in activity of HDAC and reduced expression of HDAC2 in alveolar macrophages [49] and an even greater reduction in HDAC2 expression in peripheral lung tissue [145]. This reduction in HDAC activity is correlated with reduced expression of inflammatory cytokines and a reduced response to corticosteroids. This may result directly or indirectly from oxidative stress and is mimicked by the effects of H_2O_2 in cell lines [145].

Oxidative stress may also induce apoptosis in endothelial and epithelial cells. Apoptosis of type 1 pneumocytes may be contributory to the development of emphysema and this might be induced by cytotoxic T-lymphocytes or by inhibition of vascular-endothelial growth factor receptors [55, 90]. ROS may induce apoptosis by activating the NF-κB pathway, by direct DNA damage *via* activation of poly-ADP-ribose and *via* the generation of 4-hydroxy-nonenal. Apoptosis signal-regulating kinase-1 is held in an inactive conformation by thioredoxin and when oxidised by ROS this triggers apoptotic pathways [146].

PROTEASES

It has long been proposed that various proteases break down connective tissue components, particularly elastin, in lung parenchyma to produce emphysema and that there is an imbalance between proteases and endogenous antiproteases which should normally protect against protease-mediated effects. Elastin may be the most important target for these enzymes as there is a loss of elasticity in the lung parenchyma in patients with emphysema and elastin cannot be regenerated in an active form. Evidence for elastin degradation in COPD is provided by the increased excretion of desmosine, derived from elastin cross-links, in smokers with rapid decline in lung function compared to those with a normal decline [147]. Although early attention was focused on NE, many other proteases that have the capacity to degrade elastin have now been implicated [148].

NEUTROPHIL ELASTASE

There has been particular emphasis on the role of NE since patients with inherited α_1-AT deficiency were shown to develop early onset emphysema. Furthermore, the demonstration that α_1-AT may be inactivated by cigarette smoke exposure raised the possibility that NE may also be important in smokers with normal plasma α_1-AT concentrations. This was supported by animal models in which tracheal instillation of NE induces emphysema and infiltration of neutrophils [149] and immunocytochemical localisation of NE on elastin fibres in the lung parenchyma of patients with emphysema [150]. NE (E.C.3.4.21.37) is a serine protease which is inhibited by α_1-AT in the lung parenchyma. It is stored in azurophilic granules in neutrophils and in cells primed by cytokines; it may be expressed on the cell surface [151]

NE has subsequently been shown to have several other actions relevant to its potential role on COPD. It is a potent mucus secretagogue of submucosal gland cells and goblet cells [31, 152]. NE induces the expression of MUC5AC in an epithelial cell line and this mechanism appears to be dependent on the generation of ROS [153, 154]. NE also induces the expression of some cytokines, including IL-8 in airway epithelial cells [155]. NE cleaves the phosphatidylserine receptor on macrophages, thus impairing their ability to clear apoptotic cells [156].

On the other hand NE also inactivates CD14, a cell surface receptor for lipopolysaccharide, thus reducing the inflammatory response to endotoxin [157]. NE is likely to play a role in host defence and NE$^{(-/-)}$ mice have increased susceptibility to overwhelming gram negative bacterial infections, but do not appear to have any increase in spontaneous infections [158, 159].

The role of NE in COPD will only be established when the effect of NE inhibitors has been studied clinically [160]. In guinea-pigs exposed to cigarette smoke an NE inhibitor markedly reduced emphysema and the neutrophil inflammatory response [161]. Although several NE inhibitors have been tested in humans, there are few results reported. It is not certain whether the drugs failed or the clinical trials were not adequately designed. An NE inhibitor MR889 had no effect on urinary desmosine in unselected COPD patients, but a small reduction was seen in patients with a relatively short history [162]. The macrolide antibiotics erythromycin and flurithromycin have also been shown to inhibit NE activity [163] and this might account for their beneficial effect on mucus hypersecretion [164].

OTHER SERINE PROTEASES

Neutrophils also store two other serine proteases cathepsin G and proteinase 3 in their specific granules. These other serine proteases have similar properties to NE and induce mucus secretion in a similar way [31, 32]. Proteinase 3 is potently expressed on the surface of neutrophils after activation with cytokines [165]. Proteinase 3 is potently inhibited by α_1-AT [166]. The NE inhibitors in development inhibit other serine proteases [160].

CYSTEINE PROTEASES

Lysosomal cysteine proteases (cathepsins) may also be involved in COPD [167, 168]. Cathepsin S expression is induced by interferon-γ in several cell types, including smooth muscle cells. Overexpression of IFN-γ induces emphysema in mice and there is increased expression of cathepsins B, D, H, L and S [169]. Cathepsin inhibitors markedly reduce the emphysema-induced IL-13 in transgenic mice, indicating the elastolytic potential of this cathepsin [170]. Several other cathepsins also have elastolytic activity, including cathepsins B, L and S, which are expressed in alveolar macrophages [35, 171]. The role of cathepsins in COPD is uncertain. Increased concentrations of cathepsin L have been detected in BAL fluid of patients with emphysema [172] and alveolar macrophages from patients with COPD secrete more cysteine protease activity than macrophages from normal smokers or non-smokers [36]. The endogenous inhibitors of cathepsins are cystatins and stefins, but little is known about their role in COPD. Cystatin C concentrations are increased in BAL fluid of patients with COPD [172].

MATRIX METALLOPROTEINASES

There is increasing evidence for a role for MMPs in COPD [173]. In patients with emphysema there is an increase in BAL concentrations and macrophage expression of MMP1 (collagenase) and MMP9 (gelatinase B) [47, 174, 175]. There is an increase in activity of MMP9 in the lung parenchyma of patients with emphysema [176]. MMP1 expression is also increased in the lungs of patients with emphysema, with predominant localisation to type II pneumocytes [177]. Alveolar macrophages from normal smokers express more MMP9 than those from normal subjects [38] and there is an ever greater increase in cells from patients with COPD [37], which have greatly enhanced elastolytic activity [36]. Indeed, using the MMP inhibitor marimastat it was shown that MMPs account for most of the elastolytic activity released from alveolar macrophages from COPD patients over prolonged periods [36].

The interest in MMPs has been heightened by the demonstration that emphysema induced by chronic cigarette exposure is prevented in MMP12$^{-/-}$ (macrophage metalloelastase) mice

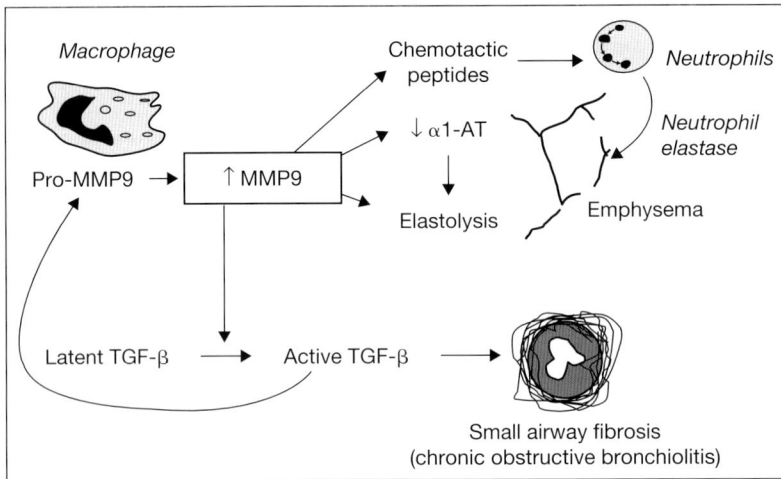

Figure 1.6 Possible interrelationship between small airway fibrosis and emphysema in COPD. Transforming growth factor (TGF)-β is activated by matrix metalloproteinase-9 (MMP9) and is in turn activated by MMP9.

[178]. In MMP12$^{-/-}$ mice emphysema induced by IL-13 and IFN-γ overexpression is reduced [169, 170] and there is a marked reduction in the recruitment of monocytes into the lung. This may be because MMPs generate chemotactic peptides which promote macrophage recruitment to the parenchyma and airways. MMPs may activate the latent form of TGF-β to its active form. In addition, mice in which the integrin αvβ6 is deleted (Itgb6-null mice) fail to activate TGF-β and develop age-related emphysema which is prevented in MMP12$^{-/-}$ mice and by overexpression of TGF-β1 [179]. This suggests that TGF-β1 down-regulates MMP12 under normal conditions and absence TGF-β results in excessive MMP12 and emphysema. MMP9$^{-/-}$ mice are not protected against emphysema induced by cigarette smoke, but are protected from small airway fibrosis [180]. TGF-β1 is activated by MMP9 [181]; this may be mediated *via* MMP9-induced proteolytic cleavage of latent TGF-binding protein-1, resulting in release of TGF-β1 [182]. This mechanism, therefore, could be a link between elastolysis induced by MMP9 and simultaneous production of fibrosis by activation of TGF-β1 (Figure 1.6). Thus, MMP12 is a prominent MMP in the mouse, and while present in humans does not appear to be as important as MMP9.

ANTIPROTEASES

Normally proteases are counteracted by an excess of endogenous antiproteases. The major inhibitors of serine proteases are α$_1$-AT in lung parenchyma and airway epithelium-derived SLPI in the airways. Other serine protease inhibitors include elafin and α$_1$-antichymotrypsin. Serine protease inhibitors inactivate NE and other serine proteases such as proteinase-3 [183]. Multiple genetic variants of α$_1$-AT are now recognised that give rise to reduced circulating active α$_1$-AT concentrations [184, 185]. The best described deficiency that results in early onset emphysema is the ZZ type on which a single amino acid substitution (Gly342→Lys) results in structural alterations in α$_1$-AT resulting in failure of its normal posttranslational modification and secretion by hepatocytes leading to very low plasma concentrations. Whether heterozygotes and other genetic variants that reduce circulating α$_1$-AT concentrations to a lesser extent than the ZZ phenotype also predispose to emphysema is more debatable [186]. ZZ α$_1$-AT deficiency is a rare cause of emphysema accounting for <1% of patients, but it was proposed long ago that cigarette smoking may oxidise α_1-AT resulting in impaired antiprotease function and increased NE activity [187]. The mechanism appears to be due to oxidative stress and oxidation of methionine at positions 351 or 358 impairs anti-NE activity of α_1-AT [137].

SLPI is the other major serine proteinase inhibitor in the airways [188]. Like α_1-AT, SLPI may be inactivated by oxidative stress, and also by cleavage through its active site by cathepsins L and S [189] and in patients with emphysema proteolytic fragments of SLPI are found in BAL fluid which contributes to the reduced anti-NE activity in these patients. This inactivation of SLPI not only impairs its anti-NE activity, but also its anti-microbial and anti-inflammatory roles. SLPI down-regulates LPS-induced TNF-α and MMP secretion from monocytes [190, 191] and this may be mediated by an inhibitory effect on IκBα degradation, resulting in inhibition of NF-κB [192]. The roles of elafin and α_1-antichymotryptase in COPD are less well defined [193, 194].

Four tissue inhibitors of MMPs (TIMP1–4) counteract MMPs [195]. TIMP-1 secretion from alveolar macrophages is increased in response to inflammatory stimuli, but the increase is blunted in cells derived from COPD patients, so favouring increased elastolysis [36, 37]. An increased frequency of loss of function mutations of TIMP-2 has been described in patients with COPD [196].

AMPLIFYING MECHANISMS IN COPD

The inflammatory changes and protease imbalance in COPD are also seen in cigarette smokers without COPD but to a lesser extent [10, 12, 36, 47, 48], suggesting that the accelerated decline in lung function in COPD may be due to amplification of the normal pulmonary inflammatory response to irritants. This may be due to increased production of inflammatory mediators and enzymes, or because of defective endogenous anti-inflammatory or antiprotease mechanisms. These differences might be explained by polymorphisms in the genes encoding cytokines, proteases, anti-inflammatory proteins and antiproteases [197, 198].

Another hypothesis is that these differences are due to latent virus infection [199]. The latent adenovirus sequence E1A is more commonly detected in the lungs of patients with emphysema than in matched smoking control subjects and is correlated with an increased inflammatory response [12]. Adenovirus infection amplifies the inflammatory response to cigarette smoke in the airways of guinea-pigs [34]. Transfection of E1A into a human epithelial cell line results in increased activation of the transcription factor NF-κB with consequent increased release of IL-8 in response to cell activation and increased production of TGF-β1, providing a molecular mechanism for the amplification in inflammatory response [200, 201].

Another molecular mechanism that may underlie the amplification of inflammation in COPD may involve impaired activity of HDAC in alveolar macrophages. In macrophages from cigarette smokers there is impaired activity of HDAC, which is involved in switching off the transcription of inflammatory genes by reversing the acetylation of core histones that is associated with their activation [49, 50]. In COPD there is even more marked reduction in HDAC activity in peripheral lung of COPD patients than smokers without airway obstruction [145]. This may lead to amplification of the expression of inflammatory genes, as is seen in alveolar macrophages from patients with COPD [37, 48]. There is also increased activation of NF-κB in these cells from patients with COPD [39, 40].

Although smoking is the major causal mechanism in COPD, quitting smoking does not appear to result in resolution of the inflammatory response in the airways, particularly in advanced disease [12, 202, 203]. This suggests that there are perpetuating mechanisms that maintain the chronic inflammatory process once it has become established. This may account for presentation of COPD in patients who stopped smoking many years before their first symptoms develop. The mechanisms of disease persistence are currently unknown.

CORTICOSTEROID RESISTANCE

Inhaled corticosteroids are now the mainstay of chronic asthma therapy and the recognition that chronic inflammation is also present in COPD provided a rationale for their use in COPD. Indeed, inhaled corticosteroids are now widely prescribed in the treatment of COPD and are used almost as frequently as in asthma. However, the inflammation in COPD is not suppressed even by high doses of inhaled or oral corticosteroids [46, 47, 204]. This may reflect the fact that neutrophilic inflammation in humans is not suppressible by cortico-steroids as neutrophil survival is prolonged by steroids [205, 206]. Approximately 10% of patients with stable COPD show some symptomatic and objective improvement with oral corticosteroids and it is likely that these patients have concomitant asthma, as both diseases are very common. Indeed, airway hyperresponsiveness, a characteristic of asthma, may predict the rate of decline in COPD [207]. A response to corticosteroids is predicted by increased numbers of eosinophils in sputum and an increase in exhaled NO [71, 72], both characteristic features of asthma.

Four large studies have shown that high doses of inhaled corticosteroids fail to reduce the progression of COPD [208].

It seems likely that there is an *active* resistance to corticosteroids in COPD. High doses of corticosteroids fail to reduce cytokine and chemokines that should be suppressed by corticosteroid treatment [46, 47]. The molecular mechanisms of corticosteroid resistance are not yet known, but may be the same mechanisms that result in amplification of inflammatory responses. Thus reduction in HDAC activity in macrophages [49] may prevent the anti-inflammatory action of corticosteroids, which is dependent on recruitment of HDACs to the inflammatory gene complex [50]. Similarly, latent adenovirus appears to induce corticosteroid resistance in experiments on animals [209]. Oxidative stress through the domain of peroxynitrite may inactivate and degrade HDAC2 which is required for the antiinflammatory action of corticosteroids [210].

FUTURE RESEARCH

Our understanding of the cellular and molecular mechanisms involved in COPD is at an early stage compared with our knowledge of asthma. Although both diseases involve inflammation in the respiratory tract, the pattern of inflammation, the results of the inflammatory process and the therapeutic response are markedly different. This review has focused on some key questions that are now being addressed in COPD, although it is by no means comprehensive.

Although activation of several inflammatory cells has now been identified in COPD, their relative importance and sequential role in producing the typical pathology of COPD are still poorly understood. However, it is likely that cigarette smoke and other irritants activate resident cells, including macrophages, epithelial cells and dendritic cells, which then signal the influx of other inflammatory cells, including neutrophils, monocytes and T-lymphocytes from the circulation. These cells all release multiple mediators of inflammation, although the pattern of mediators differs from those found in asthma. The pathological process is predominantly located in the lung periphery with involvement of small airways and lung parenchyma. However, the relationship between inflammation and fibrosis in small airways and destruction of lung parenchyma and mucus hypersecretion are uncertain and there are differences in the preponderance of these mechanisms between patients and at different stages of the disease. There is a need for better techniques for studying small airway function.

There appears to be an amplification of the inflammatory process between smokers who do not have airflow limitation and the minority of smokers with accelerated decline of lung function who develop COPD. The molecular basis for this amplification needs further investigation, but possible mechanisms relate to genetic differences in inflammatory, proteolytic or protective mechanisms or acquired latent viral infections. The mechanisms of amplification may also be linked to the relative steroid resistance found in COPD and a plausible link is deficiency in HDAC activation that both amplifies inflammatory gene expression and impairs the anti-inflammatory response to corticosteroids.

Much further research is now needed to answer some of these key questions. However, availability of tissues from patients with COPD and patients who have a similar cigarette smoke exposure without COPD and the development of novel molecular and cellular techniques make it likely that rapid progress will be made. This will make it possible to predict which smokers will develop COPD and may identify new targets for the development of novel therapies that suppress this chronic inflammatory process. Many new drugs for COPD are already in development [211] and several are about to enter clinical trials.

SUMMARY

COPD is a leading cause of death and disability, but has only recently been extensively explored from a cellular and molecular perspective. There is a chronic inflammation that leads to fixed narrowing of small airways and alveolar wall destruction (emphysema). This is characterised by increased numbers of alveolar macrophages, neutrophils and cytotoxic T-lymphocytes, and the release of multiple inflammatory mediators (lipids, chemokines, cytokines, growth factors). A high level of oxidative stress may amplify this inflammation. There is also increased elastolysis and evidence for involvement of several elastolytic enzymes, including serine proteases, cathepsins and matrix metalloproteinases. The inflammation and proteolysis in COPD is an amplification of the normal inflammatory response to cigarette smoke. This inflammation, in marked contrast to asthma, appears to be resistant to corticosteroids, prompting a search for novel anti-inflammatory therapies that may prevent the relentless progression of the disease.

REFERENCES

1. Barnes PJ. Chronic obstructive pulmonary disease. *N Engl J Med* 2000; 343:269–280.
2. Barnes PJ, Shapiro SD, Pauwels RA. Chronic obstructive pulmonary disease: molecular and cellular mechanisms. *Eur Respir J* 2003; 22:672–688.
3. Barnes PJ. New concepts in COPD. *Ann Rev Med* 2003; 54:113–129.
4. GOLD. Global Initiative for Chronic Obstructive Lung Disease (GOLD): Global strategy for the diagnosis, management and prevention of chronic obstructive pulmonary disease. *NHLBI/WHO Workshop Report* 2003; www.goldcopd.com/workshop/index.html.
5. Saetta M, Turato G, Maestrelli P, Mapp CE, Fabbri LM. Cellular and structural bases of chronic obstructive pulmonary disease. *Am J Respir Crit Care Med* 2001; 163:1304–1309.
6. Fabbri LM, Romagnoli M, Corbetta L, Casoni G, Busljetic K, Turato G et al. Differences in airway inflammation in patients with fixed airflow obstruction due to asthma or chronic obstructive pulmonary disease. *Am J Respir Crit Care Med* 2003; 167:418–424.
7. Saetta M, Di Stefano A, Turato G, Facchini FM, Corbino L, Mapp CE et al. CD8+ T-lymphocytes in peripheral airways of smokers with chronic obstructive pulmonary disease. *Am J Respir Crit Care Med* 1998; 157:822–826.
8. Di Stefano A, Capelli A, Lusuardi M, Balbo P, Vecchio C, Maestrelli P et al. Severity of airflow limitation is associated with severity of airway inflammation in smokers. *Am J Respir Crit Care Med* 1998; 158:1277–1285.
9. Pesci A, Balbi B, Majori M, Cacciani G, Bertacco S, Alciato P et al. Inflammatory cells and mediators in bronchial lavage of patients with chronic obstructive pulmonary disease. *Eur Respir J* 1998; 12: 380–386.

10. Keatings VM, Collins PD, Scott DM, Barnes PJ. Differences in interleukin-8 and tumor necrosis factor-α in induced sputum from patients with chronic obstructive pulmonary disease or asthma. *Am J Respir Crit Care Med* 1996; 153:530–534.

11. Fabbri L, Beghe B, Caramori G, Papi A, Saetta M. Similarities and discrepancies between exacerbations of asthma and chronic obstructive pulmonary disease. *Thorax* 1998; 53:803–808.

12. Retamales I, Elliott WM, Meshi B, Coxson HO, Pare PD, Sciurba FC *et al.* Amplification of inflammation in emphysema and its association with latent adenoviral infection. *Am J Respir Crit Care Med* 2001; 164:469–473.

13. Lacoste JY, Bousquet J, Chanez P. Eosinophilic and neutrophilic inflammation in asthma, chronic bronchitis and chronic obstructive pulmonary disease. *J Allergy Clin Immunol* 1993; 92:537–548.

14. Finkelstein R, Fraser RS, Ghezzo H, Cosio MG. Alveolar inflammation and its relation to emphysema in smokers. *Am J Respir Crit Care Med* 1995; 152:1666–1672.

15. Di Stefano A, Maestrelli P, Roggeri A, Turato G, Calabro S, Potena A *et al.* Upregulation of adhesion molecules in the bronchial mucosa of subjects with chronic obstructive bronchitis. *Am J Respir Crit Care Med* 1994; 149:803–810.

16. Sparrow D, Glynn RJ, Cohen M, Weiss ST. The relationship of the peripheral leukocyte count and cigarette smoking to pulmonary function among adult men. *Chest* 1984; 86:383–386.

17. Stanescu D, Sanna A, Veriter C, Kostianev S, Callagni PG, Fabbri LM *et al.* Airways obstruction, chronic expectoration and rapid decline in FEV_1 in smokers are associated with increased levels of sputum neutrophils. *Thorax* 1996; 51:267–271.

18. Terashima T, Wiggs B, English D, Hogg JC, van Eeden SF. Phagocytosis of small carbon particles (PM10) by alveolar macrophages stimulates the release of polymorphonuclear leukocytes from bone marrow. *Am J Respir Crit Care Med* 1997; 155:1441–1447.

19. Macnee W, Wiggs B, Belzberg AS, Hogg JC. The effect of cigarette smoking on neutrophil kinetics in human lungs. *N Engl J Med* 1989; 321:924–928.

20. Keatings VM, Barnes PJ. Granulocyte activation markers in induced sputum: comparison between chronic obstructive pulmonary disease, asthma and normal subjects. *Am J Respir Crit Care Med* 1997; 155:449–453.

21. Yamamoto C, Yoneda T, Yoshikawa M, Fu A, Tokuyama T, Tsukaguchi K *et al.* Airway inflammation in COPD assessed by sputum levels of interleukin-8. *Chest* 1997; 112:505–510.

22. Peleman RA, Rytila PH, Kips JC, Joos GF, Pauwels RA. The cellular composition of induced sputum in chronic obstructive pulmonary disease. *Eur Respir J* 1999; 13:839–843.

23. Richards GA, Theron AJ, Van der Merwe CA, Anderson R. Spirometric abnormalities in young smokers correlate with increased chemiluminescence responses of activated blood phagocytes. *Am Rev Respir Dis* 1989; 139:181–187.

24. Condliffe AM, Kitchen E, Chilvers ER. Neutrophil priming: pathophysiological consequences and underlying mechanisms. *Clin Sci (Lond)* 1998; 94:461–471.

25. Noguera A, Batle S, Miralles C, Iglesias J, Busquets X, Macnee W *et al.* Enhanced neutrophil response in chronic obstructive pulmonary disease. *Thorax* 2001; 56:432–437.

26. Traves SL, Culpitt S, Russell REK, Barnes PJ, Donnelly LE. Elevated levels of the chemokines GRO-α and MCP-1 in sputum samples from COPD patients. *Thorax* 2002; 57:590–595.

27. Tanino M, Betsuyaku T, Takeyabu K, Tanino Y, Yamaguchi E, Miyamoto K *et al.* Increased levels of interleukin-8 in BAL fluid from smokers susceptible to pulmonary emphysema. *Thorax* 2002; 57:405–411.

28. Bazzoni F, Cassatella MA, Rossi F, Ceska M, Dewald B, Baggiolini M. Phagocytosing neutrophils produce and release high amounts of the neutrophil-activating peptide 1/interleukin 8. *J Exp Med* 1991; 173:771–774.

29. Hogg JC, Walker BA. Polymorphonuclear leucocyte traffic in lung inflammation. *Thorax* 1995; 50:819–820.

30. Pettersen CA, Adler KB. Airways inflammation and COPD: epithelial–neutrophil interactions. *Chest* 2002; 121:S142–S150.

31. Sommerhoff CP, Nadel JA, Basbaum CB, Caughey GH. Neutrophil elastase and cathepsin G stimulate secretion from cultured bovine airway gland serous cells. *J Clin Invest* 1990; 85:682–689.

32. Witko-Sarsat V, Halbwachs-Mecarelli L, Schuster A, Nusbaum P, Ueki I, Canteloup S *et al.* Proteinase 3, a potent secretagogue in airways, is present in cystic fibrosis sputum. *Am J Respir Cell Mol Biol* 1999; 20:729–736.

33. Barnes PJ. Macrophages as orchestrators of COPD. *J COPD* 2004; 1:59–70.

34. Meshi B, Vitalis TZ, Ionescu D, Elliott WM, Liu C, Wang XD et al. Emphysematous lung destruction by cigarette smoke. The effects of latent adenoviral infection on the lung inflammatory response. Am J Respir Cell Mol Biol 2002; 26:52–57.

35. Punturieri A, Filippov S, Allen E, Caras I, Murray R, Reddy V et al. Regulation of elastinolytic cysteine proteinase activity in normal and cathepsin K-deficient human macrophages. J Exp Med 2000; 192:789–800.

36. Russell RE, Thorley A, Culpitt SV, Dodd S, Donnelly LE, Demattos C et al. Alveolar macrophage-mediated elastolysis: roles of matrix metalloproteinases, cysteine, and serine proteases. Am J Physiol Lung Cell Mol Physiol 2002; 283.L867–L873.

37. Russell RE, Culpitt SV, DeMatos C, Donnelly L, Smith M, Wiggins J et al. Release and activity of matrix metalloproteinase-9 and tissue inhibitor of metalloproteinase-1 by alveolar macrophages from patients with chronic obstructive pulmonary disease. Am J Respir Cell Mol Biol 2002; 26:602–609.

38. Lim S, Roche N, Oliver BG, Mattos W, Barnes PJ, Fan CK. Balance of matrix metalloprotease-9 and tissue inhibitor of metalloprotease-1 from alveolar macrophages in cigarette smokers. Regulation by interleukin-10. Am J Respir Crit Care Med 2000; 162:1355–1360.

39. Di Stefano A, Caramori G, Capelli A, Lusuardi M, Gnemmi I, Ioli F et al. Increased expression of NF-kB in bronchial biopsies from smokers and patients with COPD. Eur Resp J 2002; 20:556–563.

40. Caramori G, Romagnoli M, Casolari P, Bellettato C, Casoni G, Boschetto P et al. Nuclear localisation of p65 in sputum macrophages but not in sputum neutrophils during COPD exacerbations. Thorax 2003; 58:348–351.

41. Capelli A, Di Stefano A, Gnemmi I, Balbo P, Cerutti CG, Balbi B et al. Increased MCP-1 and MIP-1b in bronchoalveolar lavage fluid of chronic bronchitis. Eur Respir J 1999; 14:160–165.

42. de Boer WI, Sont JK, van Schadewijk A, Stolk J, van Krieken JH, Hiemstra PS. Monocyte chemoattractant protein 1, interleukin 8, and chronic airways inflammation in COPD. J Pathol 2000; 190:619–626.

43. Traves SL, Smith SJ, Barnes PJ, Donnelly LE. Specific CXC but not CC chemokines cause elevated monocyte migration in COPD: a role for CXCR2. J Leukoc Biol 2004; 76:441–450.

44. Saetta M, Mariani M, Panina-Bordignon P, Turato G, Buonsanti C, Baraldo S et al. Increased expression of the chemokine receptor CXCR3 and its ligand CXCL10 in peripheral airways of smokers with chronic obstructive pulmonary disease. Am J Respir Crit Care Med 2002; 165:1404–1409.

45. Tomita K, Caramori G, Lim S, Ito K, Hanazawa T, Oates T et al. Increased p21CIP1/WAF1 and B cell lymphoma leukemia-xL expression and reduced apoptosis in alveolar macrophages from smokers. Am J Respir Crit Care Med 2002; 166:724–731.

46. Keatings VM, Jatakanon A, Worsdell YM, Barnes PJ. Effects of inhaled and oral glucocorticoids on inflammatory indices in asthma and COPD. Am J Respir Crit Care Med 1997; 155:542–548.

47. Culpitt SV, Nightingale JA, Barnes PJ. Effect of high dose inhaled steroid on cells, cytokines and proteases in induced sputum in chronic obstructive pulmonary disease. Am J Respir Crit Care Med 1999; 160:1635–1639.

48. Culpitt SV, Rogers DF, Shah P, de Matos C, Russell RE, Donnelly LE et al. Impaired inhibition by dexamethasone of cytokine release by alveolar macrophages from patients with chronic obstructive pulmonary disease. Am J Respir Crit Care Med 2003; 167:24–31.

49. Ito K, Lim S, Caramori G, Chung KF, Barnes PJ, Adcock IM. Cigarette smoking reduces histone deacetylase 2 expression, enhances cytokine expression and inhibits glucocorticoid actions in alveolar macrophages. FASEB J 2001; 15:1100–1102.

50. Ito K, Barnes PJ, Adcock IM. Glucocorticoid receptor recruitment of histone deacetylase 2 inhibits IL-1b-induced histone H4 acetylation on lysines 8 and 12. Mol Cell Biol 2000; 20:6891–6903.

51. Ito K, Tomita T, Barnes PJ, Adcock IM. Oxidative stress reduces histone deacetylase (HDAC)2 activity and enhances IL-8 gene expression: role of tyrosine nitration. Biochem Biophys Res Commun 2004; 315:240–245.

52. Ito K, Lim S, Caramori G, Cosio B, Chung KF, Adcock IM et al. A molecular mechanism of action of theophylline: Induction of histone deacetylase activity to decrease inflammatory gene expression. Proc Natl Acad Sci USA 2002; 99:8921–8926.

53. Donnelly LE, Jones GE, Newton R, Barnes PJ. The anti-inflammatory action of resveratrol on human airway epithelial cells is not mediated via estrogen or glucocorticosteroid receptors. Am J Resp Crit Care Med 2003; 165:A614.

54. Donnelly LE, Newton R, Kennedy GE, Fenwick PS, Leung RH, Ito K et al. Anti-inflammatory effects of resveratrol in lung epithelial cells: molecular mechanisms. Am J Physiol Lung Cell Mol Physiol 2004; 287:L774–L783.

55. Majo J, Ghezzo H, Cosio MG. Lymphocyte population and apoptosis in the lungs of smokers and their relation to emphysema. *Eur Respir J* 2001; 17:946–953.

56. Saetta M, Baraldo S, Corbino L, Turato G, Braccioni F, Rea F *et al*. CD8+ve cells in the lungs of smokers with chronic obstructive pulmonary disease. *Am J Respir Crit Care Med* 1999; 160:711–717.

57. O'Shaughnessy TC, Ansari TW, Barnes NC, Jeffery PK. Inflammation in bronchial biopsies of subjects with chronic bronchitis: inverse relationship of CD8+ T lymphocytes with FEV1. *Am J Respir Crit Care Med* 1997; 155:852–857.

58. Vukmanovic-Stejic M, Vyas B, Gorak-Stolinska P, Noble A, Kemeny DM. Human Tc1 and Tc2/Tc0 CD8 T-cell clones display distinct cell surface and functional phenotypes. *Blood* 2000; 95:231–240.

59. Leckie MJ, Jenkins GR, Khan J, Smith SJ, Walker C, Barnes PJ *et al*. Sputum T-lymphocytes in asthma, COPD and healthy subjects have the phenotype of activated intraepithelial T cells (CD69+ CD103+). *Thorax* 2003; 58:23–29.

60. de Jong JW, Belt-Gritter B, Koeter GH, Postma DS. Peripheral blood lymphocyte cell subsets in subjects with chronic obstructive pulmonary disease: association with smoking, IgE and lung function. *Respir Med* 1997; 91:67–76.

61. Kim WD, Kim WS, Koh Y, Lee SD, Lim CM, Kim DS *et al*. Abnormal peripheral blood T-lymphocyte subsets in a subgroup of patients with COPD. *Chest* 2002; 122:437–444.

62. Majori M, Corradi M, Caminati A, Cacciani G, Bertacco S, Pesci A. Predominant TH1 cytokine pattern in peripheral blood from subjects with chronic obstructive pulmonary disease. *J Allergy Clin Immunol* 1999; 103:458–462.

63. Hill AT, Campbell EJ, Hill SL, Bayley DL, Stockley RA. Association between airway bacterial load and markers of airway inflammation in patients with stable chronic bronchitis. *Am J Med* 2000; 109:288–295.

64. Cosio MG, Majo J, Cosio MG. Inflammation of the airways and lung parenchyma in COPD: role of T cells. *Chest* 2002; 121:S160–S165.

65. Hogg JC, Chu F, Utokaparch S, Yamada Y, Elliott WM, Buzatu L *et al*. The nature of small airway obstruction in chronic pulmonary obstructive disease. *N Engl J Med* 2004; 350:2645–2653.

66. Prieto A, Reyes E, Bernstein ED, Martinez B, Monserrat J, Izquierdo JL *et al*. Defective natural killer and phagocytic activities in chronic obstructive pulmonary disease are restored by glycophosphopeptical (inmunoferon). *Am J Respir Crit Care Med* 2001; 163:1578–1583.

67. Zeidel A, Beilin B, Yardeni I, Mayburd E, Smirnov G, Bessler H. Immune response in asymptomatic smokers. *Acta Anaesthesiol Scand* 2002; 46:959–964.

68. Hashimoto S, Kobayashi A, Kooguchi K, Kitamura Y, Onodera H, Nakajima H. Upregulation of two death pathways of perforin/granzyme and FasL/Fas in septic acute respiratory distress syndrome. *Am J Respir Crit Care Med* 2000; 161:237–243.

69. Takubo Y, Guerassimov A, Ghezzo H, Triantafillopoulos A, Bates JH, Hoidal JR *et al*. Alpha1-antitrypsin determines the pattern of emphysema and function in tobacco smoke-exposed mice: parallels with human disease. *Am J Respir Crit Care Med* 2002; 166:1596–1603.

70. Turato G, Zuin R, Saetta M. Pathogenesis and pathology of copd. *Respiration* 2001; 68:117–128.

71. Brightling CE, Monteiro W, Ward R, Parker D, Morgan MD, Wardlaw AJ *et al*. Sputum eosinophilia and short-term response to prednisolone in chronic obstructive pulmonary disease: a randomised controlled trial. *Lancet* 2000; 356:1480–1485.

72. Papi A, Romagnoli M, Baraldo S, Braccioni F, Guzzinati I, Saetta M *et al*. Partial reversibility of airflow limitation and increased exhaled NO and sputum eosinophilia in chronic obstructive pulmonary disease. *Am J Respir Crit Care Med* 2000; 162:1773–1777.

73. Saetta M, Di Stefano A, Maestrelli P, Graziella T, Rugieri MP, Roggeri A *et al*. Airway eosinophilia in chronic bronchitis during exacerbations. *Am J Resp Crit Care Med* 1994; 150:1646–1652.

74. Saetta M, Di Stefano A, Maestrelli P, Turato G, Mapp CE, Pieno M *et al*. Airway eosinophilia and expression of interleukin-5 protein in asthma and in exacerbations of chronic bronchitis. *Clin Exp Allergy* 1996; 26:766–774.

75. Liu H, Lazarus SC, Caughey GH, Fahy JV. Neutrophil elastase and elastase-rich cystic fibrosis sputum degranulate human eosinophils *in vitro*. *Am J Physiol* 1999; 276:L28-L34.

76. Banchereau J, Briere F, Caux C, Davoust J, Lebecque S, Liu YJ *et al*. Immunobiology of dendritic cells. *Annu Rev Immunol* 2000; 18:767–811.

77. Holt PG, Stumbles PA. Regulation of immunologic homeostasis in peripheral tissues by dendritic cells: the respiratory tract as a paradigm. *J Allergy Clin Immunol* 2000; 105:421–429.

78. Huang Q, Liu D, Majewski P, Schulte LC, Korn JM, Young RA *et al*. The plasticity of dendritic cell responses to pathogens and their components. *Science* 2001; 294:870–875.

79. Francus T, Klein RF, Staiano-Coico L, Becker CG, Siskind GW. Effects of tobacco glycoprotein (TGP) on the immune system. II. TGP stimulates the proliferation of human T cells and the differentiation of human B cells into Ig secreting cells. *J Immunol* 1988; 140:1823–1829.

80. Zeid NA, Muller HK. Tobacco smoke induced lung granulomas and tumors: association with pulmonary Langerhans cells. *Pathology* 1995; 27:247–254.

81. Casolaro MA, Bernaudin JF, Saltini C, Ferrans VJ, Crystal RG. Accumulation of Langerhans' cells on the epithelial surface of the lower respiratory tract in normal subjects in association with cigarette smoking. *Am Rev Respir Dis* 1988; 137:406 411.

82. Soler P, Moreau A, Basset F, Hance AJ. Cigarette smoking-induced changes in the number and differentiated state of pulmonary dendritic cells/Langerhans cells. *Am Rev Respir Dis* 1989; 139: 1112–1117.

83. Tazi A, Soler P, Hance AJ. Adult pulmonary Langerhans' cell histiocytosis. *Thorax* 2000; 55:405–416.

84. Tazi A, Moreau J, Bergeron A, Dominique S, Hance AJ, Soler P. Evidence that Langerhans cells in adult pulmonary Langerhans cell histiocytosis are mature dendritic cells: importance of the cytokine microenvironment. *J Immunol* 1999; 163:3511–3515.

85. D'Hulst A, Vermeulen KY, Pauwels RA. Cigarette smoke exposure causes increase in pulmonary dendritic cells. *Am J Respir Crit Care Med* 2002; 164:A604.

86. Mio T, Romberger DJ, Thompson AB, Robbins RA, Heires A, Rennard SI. Cigarette smoke induces interleukin-8 release from human bronchial epithelial cells. *Am J Respir Crit Care Med* 1997; 155:1770–1776.

87. Hellermann GR, Nagy SB, Kong X, Lockey RF, Mohapatra SS. Mechanism of cigarette smoke condensate-induced acute inflammatory response in human bronchial epithelial cells. *Respir Res* 2002; 3:22.

88. Floreani AA, Wyatt TA, Stoner J, Sanderson SD, Thompson EG, Allen-Gipson D *et al*. Smoke and C5a induce airway epithelial ICAM-1 and cell adhesion. *Am J Respir Cell Mol Biol* 2003; 29:472–482.

89. Takizawa H, Tanaka M, Takami K, Ohtoshi T, Ito K, Satoh M *et al*. Increased expression of transforming growth factor-beta1 in small airway epithelium from tobacco smokers and patients with chronic obstructive pulmonary disease (COPD). *Am J Respir Crit Care Med* 2001; 163:1476–1483.

90. Kasahara Y, Tuder RM, Taraseviciene-Stewart L, Le Cras TD, Abman S, Hirth PK *et al*. Inhibition of VEGF receptors causes lung cell apoptosis and emphysema. *J Clin Invest* 2000; 106:1311–1319.

91. Adler KB, Li Y. Airway epithelium and mucus: intracellular signaling pathways for gene expression and secretion. *Am J Respir Cell Mol Biol* 2001; 25:397–400.

92. Aarbiou J, Rabe KF, Hiemstra PS. Role of defensins in inflammatory lung disease. *Ann Med* 2002; 34: 96–101.

93. Pilette C, Ouadrhiri Y, Godding V, Vaerman JP, Sibille Y. Lung mucosal immunity: immunoglobulin-A revisited. *Eur Respir J* 2001; 18:571–588.

94. Demoly P, Simony-Lafontaine J, Chanez P, Pujol JL, Lequeux N, Michel FB *et al*. Cell proliferation in the bronchial mucosa of asthmatics and chronic bronchitics. *Am J Respir Crit Care Med* 1994; 150: 214–217.

95. Franklin WA, Veve R, Hirsch FR, Helfrich BA, Bunn PA, Jr. Epidermal growth factor receptor family in lung cancer and premalignancy. *Semin Oncol* 2002; 29:3–14.

96. Repine JE, Bast A, Lankhorst I. Oxidative stress in chronic obstructive pulmonary disease. *Am J Respir Crit Care Med* 1997; 156:341–357.

97. Macnee W. Oxidative stress and lung inflammation in airways disease. *Eur J Pharmacol* 2001; 429:195–207.

98. Henricks PA, Nijkamp FP. Reactive oxygen species as mediators in asthma. *Pulm Pharmacol Ther* 2001; 14:409–420.

99. Beckman JS, Koppenol WH. Nitric oxide, superoxide, and peroxynitrite: the good, the bad, and the ugly. *Am J Physiol* 1996; 271:C1432–C1437.

100. Morrow JD. The isoprostanes: their quantification as an index of oxidant stress status *in vivo*. *Drug Metab Rev* 2000; 32:377–385.

101. Kawikova I, Barnes PJ, Takahashi T, Tadjkarimi S, Yacoub MH, Belvisi MG. 8-Epi-PGF2 alpha, a novel non-cyclooxygenase derived prostaglandin, is a potent constrictor of guinea-pig and human airways. *Am J Respir Crit Care Med* 1996; 153:590–596.

102. Okazawa A, Kawikova I, Cui ZH, Skoogh BE, Lotvall J. 8-Epi-PGF2 alpha induces airflow obstruction and airway plasma exudation *in vivo*. *Am J Respir Crit Care Med* 1997; 155:436–441.

103. Janssen LJ. Isoprostanes: an overview and putative roles in pulmonary pathophysiology. *Am J Physiol Lung Cell Mol Physiol* 2001; 280:L1067–L1082.

104. van der Vliet A, Eiserich JP, Shigenaga MK, Cross CE. Reactive nitrogen species and tyrosine nitration in the respiratory tract: epiphenomena or a pathobiologic mechanism of disease? *Am J Respir Crit Care Med* 1999; 160:1–9.

105. Eiserich JP, Hristova M, Cross CE, Jones AD, Freeman BA, Halliwell B *et al.* Formation of nitric oxide-derived inflammatory oxidants by myeloperoxidase in neutrophils. *Nature* 1998; 391:393–397.

106. Gaut JP, Byun J, Tran HD, Lauber WM, Carroll JA, Hotchkiss RS *et al.* Myeloperoxidase produces nitrating oxidants *in vivo. J Clin Invest* 2002; 109:1311–1319.

107. Cantin AM, Fells GA, Hubbard RC, Crystal RG. Antioxidant macromolecules in the epithelial lining fluid of the normal human lower respiratory tract. *J Clin Invest* 1990; 86:962–971.

108. Choi AM, Alam J. Heme oxygenase-1: function, regulation, and implication of a novel stress-inducible protein in oxidant-induced lung injury. *Am J Respir Cell Mol Biol* 1996; 15:9–19.

109. Lim S, Groneberg D, Fischer A, Oates T, Caramori G, Mattos W *et al.* Expression of heme oxygenase isoenzymes 1 and 2 in normal and asthmatic airways. Effect of inhaled corticosteroids. *Am J Respir Crit Care Med* 2000; 162:1912–1918.

110. Montuschi P, Kharitonov SA, Barnes PJ. Exhaled carbon monoxide and nitric oxide in COPD. *Chest* 2001; 120:496–501.

111. Comhair SA, Erzurum SC. Antioxidant responses to oxidant-mediated lung diseases. *Am J Physiol Lung Cell Mol Physiol* 2002; 283:L246–L255.

112. Avissar N, Finkelstein JN, Horowitz S, Willey JC, Coy E, Frampton MW *et al.* Extracellular glutathione peroxidase in human lung epithelial lining fluid and in lung cells. *Am J Physiol* 1996; 270:L173–L182.

113. Bowler RP, Crapo JD. Oxidative stress in airways: is there a role for extracellular superoxide dismutase? *Am J Respir Crit Care Med* 2002; 166:S38–S43.

114. Barnes PJ, Karin M. Nuclear factor-kB: a pivotal transcription factor in chronic inflammatory diseases. *New Engl J Med* 1997; 336:1066–1071.

115. Janssen-Heininger YM, Poynter ME, Baeuerle PA. Recent advances towards understanding redox mechanisms in the activation of nuclear factor kB. *Free Radic Biol Med* 2000; 28:1317–1327.

116. Adcock IM, Brown CR, Kwon OJ, Barnes PJ. Oxidative stress induces NF-kB DNA binding and inducible NOS mRNA in human epithelial cells. *Biochem Biophys Res Commun* 1994; 199:1518–1524.

117. Rusznak C, Devalia JL, Sapsford RJ, Davies RJ. Ozone-induced mediator release from human bronchial epithelial cells *in vitro* and the influence of nedocromil sodium. *Eur Respir J* 1996; 9:2298–2305.

118. Tomita K, Barnes PJ, Adcock IM. The effect of oxidative stress on histone acetylation and IL-8 release. *Biochem Biophys Res Comm* 2003; 301:572–577.

119. Rahman I. Oxidative stress, chromatin remodeling and gene transcription in inflammation and chronic lung diseases. *J Biochem Mol Biol* 2003; 36:95–109.

120. Xanthoudakis S, Curran T. Redox regulation of AP-1: a link between transcription factor signaling and DNA repair. *Adv Exp Med Biol* 1996; 387:69–75.

121. Devalia JL, Bayram H, Rusznak C, Calderon M, Sapsford RJ, Abdelaziz MA *et al.* Mechanisms of pollution-induced airway disease: *in vitro* studies in the upper and lower airways. *Allergy* 1997; 52:45–51; discussion 57–58.

122. Ogura M, Kitamura M. Oxidant stress incites spreading of macrophages *via* extracellular signal-regulated kinases and p38 mitogen-activated protein kinase. *J Immunol* 1998; 161:3569–3574.

123. Forman HJ, Torres M. Reactive oxygen species and cell signaling: respiratory burst in macrophage signaling. *Am J Respir Crit Care Med* 2002; 166:S4–S8.

124. Pryor WA, Stone K. Oxidants in cigarette smoke. Radicals, hydrogen peroxide, peroxynitrate, and peroxynitrite. *Ann N Y Acad Sci* 1993; 686:12–27.

125. Britton JR, Pavord ID, Richards KA, Knox AJ, Wisniewski AF, Lewis SA *et al.* Dietary antioxidant vitamin intake and lung function in the general population. *Am J Respir Crit Care Med* 1995; 151:1383–1387.

126. Schunemann HJ, Freudenheim JL, Grant BJ. Epidemiologic evidence linking antioxidant vitamins to pulmonary function and airway obstruction. *Epidemiol Rev* 2001; 23:248–267.

127. Kharitonov SA, Barnes PJ. Exhaled markers of pulmonary disease. *Am J Respir Crit Care Med* 2001; 163:1693–1772.

128. Montuschi P, Barnes PJ. Analysis of exhaled breath condensate for monitoring airway inflammation. *Trends Pharmacol Sci* 2002; 23:232–237.

129. Paredi P, Kharitonov SA, Barnes PJ. Analysis of expired air for oxidation products. *Am J Respir Crit Care Med* 2002; 166:S31–S37.

130. Dekhuijzen PNR, Aben KHH, Dekker I, Aarts LPHJ, Wielders PLM, van Herwarden CLA *et al.* Increased exhalation of hydrogen peroxide in patients with stable and unstable chronic obstructive pulmonary disease. *Am J Respir Crit Care Med* 1996; 154:813–816.

131. Nowak D, Kasielski M, Antczak A, Pietras T, Bialasiewicz P. Increased content of thiobarbituric acid-reactive substances and hydrogen peroxide in the expired breath condensate of patients with stable chronic obstructive pulmonary disease: no significant effect of cigarette smoking. *Respir Med* 1999; 93:389–396.

132. Montuschi P, Collins JV, Ciabattoni G, Lazzeri N, Corradi M, Kharitonov SA *et al.* Exhaled 8-isoprostane as an *in vivo* biomarker of lung oxidative stress in patients with COPD and healthy smokers. *Am J Respir Crit Care Med* 2000; 162:1175–1177.

133. Biernacki WA, Kharitonov SA, Barnes PJ. Increased leukotriene B4 and 8-isoprostane in exhaled breath condensate of patients with exacerbations of COPD. *Thorax* 2003; 58:294–298.

134. Pratico D, Basili S, Vieri M, Cordova C, Violi F, Fitzgerald GA. Chronic obstructive pulmonary disease is associated with an increase in urinary levels of isoprostane $F_2\alpha$-III, an index of oxidant stress. *Am J Respir Crit Care Med* 1998; 158:1709–1714.

135. Rahman I, Morrison D, Donaldson K, Macnee W. Systemic oxidative stress in asthma, COPD, and smokers. *Am J Respir Crit Care Med* 1996; 154:1055–1060.

136. Rahman I, van Schadewijk AA, Crowther AJ, Hiemstra PS, Stolk J, Macnee W *et al.* 4-Hydroxy-2-nonenal, a specific lipid peroxidation product, is elevated in lungs of patients with chronic obstructive pulmonary disease. *Am J Respir Crit Care Med* 2002; 166:490–495.

137. Taggart C, Cervantes-Laurean D, Kim G, McElvaney NG, Wehr N, Moss J *et al.* Oxidation of either methionine 351 or methionine 358 in alpha1-antitrypsin causes loss of anti-neutrophil elastase activity. *J Biol Chem* 2000; 275:27258–27265.

138. Vestbo J, Sorensen T, Lange P, Brix A, Torre P, Viskum K. Long-term effect of inhaled budesonide in mild and moderate chronic obstructive pulmonary disease: a randomised controlled trial. *Lancet* 1999; 353:1819–1823.

139. Pauwels RA, Lofdahl CG, Laitinen LA, Schouten JP, Postma DS, Pride NB *et al.* Long-term treatment with inhaled budesonide in persons with mild chronic obstructive pulmonary disease who continue smoking. *N Engl J Med* 1999; 340:1948–1953.

140. Burge PS, Calverley PMA, Jones PW, Spencer S, Anderson JA, Maslen T. Randomised, double-blind, placebo-controlled study of fluticasone propionate in patients with moderate to severe chronic obstructive pulmonary disease; the ISOLDE trial. *Br Med J* 2000; 320:1297–1303.

141. Lung Health Study Research Group. Effect of inhaled triamcinolone on the decline in pulmonary function in chronic obstructive pulmonary disease. *N Engl J Med* 2000; 343:1902–1909.

142. Hutchison KA, Matic G, Meshinchi S, Bresnick EH, Pratt WB. Redox manipulation of DNA binding activity and BuGR epitope reactivity of the glucocorticoid receptor. *J Biol Chem* 1991; 266:10505–10509.

143. Okamoto K, Tanaka H, Ogawa H, Makino Y, Eguchi H, Hayashi S *et al.* Redox-dependent regulation of nuclear import of the glucocorticoid receptor. *J Biol Chem* 1999; 274:10363–10371.

144. Barnes PJ, Shapiro SD, Pauwels RA. Chronic obstructive pulmonary disease: molecular and cellular mechanisms. *Eur Respir J* 2003; 22:672–688.

145. Ito K, Watanabe S, Kharitonov S, Hanazawa T, Adcock IM, Barnes PJ. Histone deacetylase activity and gene expression in COPD patients. *Eur Respir J* 2001; 18:316S.

146. Gotoh Y, Cooper JA. Reactive oxygen species- and dimerization-induced activation of apoptosis signal-regulating kinase 1 in tumor necrosis factor-α signal transduction. *J Biol Chem* 1998; 273:17477–17482.

147. Gottlieb DJ, Stone PJ, Sparrow D, Gale ME, Weiss ST, Snider GL *et al.* Urinary desmosine excretion in smokers with and without rapid decline of lung function: the Normative Aging Study. *Am J Respir Crit Care Med* 1996; 154:1290–1295.

148. Stockley RA. Proteases and antiproteases. *Novartis Found Symp* 2001; 234:189–199.

149. Senior RM, Tegner H, Kuhn C, Ohlsson K, Starcher BC, Pierce JA. The induction of pulmonary emphysema with human leukocyte elastase. *Am Rev Respir Dis* 1977; 116:469–475.

150. Damiano VV, Tsang A, Kucich U, Abrams WR, Rosenbloom J, Kimbel P *et al.* Immunolocalization of elastase in human emphysematous lungs. *J Clin Invest* 1986; 78:482–493.

151. Owen CA, Campbell MA, Boukedes SS, Campbell EJ. Cytokines regulate membrane-bound leukocyte elastase on neutrophils: a novel mechanism for effector activity. *Am J Physiol* 1997; 272:L385–L393.

152. Takeyama K, Agusti C, Ueki I, Lausier J, Cardell LO, Nadel JA. Neutrophil-dependent goblet cell degranulation: role of membrane-bound elastase and adhesion molecules. *Am J Physiol* 1998; 275:L294–L302.

153. Voynow JA, Young LR, Wang Y, Horger T, Rose MC, Fischer BM. Neutrophil elastase increases MUC5AC mRNA and protein expression in respiratory epithelial cells. *Am J Physiol* 1999; 276:L835–L843.
154. Fischer BM, Voynow JA. Neutrophil elastase induces MUC5AC gene expression in airway epithelium *via* a pathway involving reactive oxygen species. *Am J Respir Cell Mol Biol* 2002; 26:447–452.
155. Nakamura H, Yoshimura K, McElvaney NG, Crystal RG. Neutrophil elastase in respiratory epithelial lining fluid of individuals with cystic fibrosis induces interleukin-8 gene expression in a human bronchial epithelial cell line. *J Clin Invest* 1992; 89:1478–1484.
156. Vandivier RW, Fadok VA, Hoffmann PR, Bratton DL, Penvari C, Brown KK et al. Elastase-mediated phosphatidylserine receptor cleavage impairs apoptotic cell clearance in cystic fibrosis and bronchiectasis. *J Clin Invest* 2002; 109:661–670.
157. Le Barillec K, Si-Tahar M, Balloy V, Chignard M. Proteolysis of monocyte CD14 by human leukocyte elastase inhibits lipopolysaccharide-mediated cell activation. *J Clin Invest* 1999; 103:1039–1046.
158. Belaaouaj A, McCarthy R, Baumann M, Gao Z, Ley TJ, Abraham SN et al. Mice lacking neutrophil elastase reveal impaired host defense against gram negative bacterial sepsis. *Nat Med* 1998; 4: 615–618.
159. Shapiro SD. Neutrophil elastase: path clearer, pathogen killer, or just pathologic? *Am J Respir Cell Mol Biol* 2002; 26:266–268.
160. Ohbayashi H. Neutrophil elastase inhibitors as treatment for COPD. *Expert Opin Investig Drugs* 2002; 11:965–980.
161. Wright JL, Farmer SG, Churg A. Synthetic serine elastase inhibitor reduces cigarette smoke-induced emphysema in guinea-pigs. *Am J Respir Crit Care Med* 2002; 166:954–960.
162. Luisetti M, Sturani C, Sella D, Madonini E, Galavotti V, Bruno G et al. MR889, a neutrophil elastase inhibitor, in patients with chronic obstructive pulmonary disease: a double-blind, randomized, placebo-controlled clinical trial. *Eur Respir J* 1996; 9:1482–1486.
163. Gorrini M, Lupi A, Viglio S, Pamparana F, Cetta G, Iadarola P et al. Inhibition of human neutrophil elastase by erythromycin and flurythromycin, two macrolide antibiotics. *Am J Respir Cell Mol Biol* 2001; 25:492–499.
164. Goswami SK, Kivity S, Marom Z. Erythromycin inhibits respiratory glycoconjugate secretion from human airways *in vitro*. *Am Rev Respir Dis* 1990; 141:72–78.
165. Campbell EJ, Campbell MA, Owen CA. Bioactive proteinase 3 on the cell surface of human neutrophils: quantification, catalytic activity, and susceptibility to inhibition. *J Immunol* 2000; 165:3366–3374.
166. Duranton J, Bieth JG. Inhibition of proteinase 3 by alpha1-antitrypsin *in vitro* predicts very fast inhibition *in vivo*. *Am J Respir Cell Mol Biol* 2003; 29:57–61.
167. Turk V, Turk B, Turk D. Lysosomal cysteine proteases: facts and opportunities. *EMBO J* 2001; 20: 4629–4633.
168. Chapman HA, Riese RJ, Shi GP. Emerging roles for cysteine proteases in human biology. *Annu Rev Physiol* 1997; 59:63–88.
169. Wang Z, Zheng T, Zhu Z, Homer RJ, Riese RJ, Chapman HA, Jr. et al. Interferon gamma induction of pulmonary emphysema in the adult murine lung. *J Exp Med* 2000; 192:1587–1600.
170. Zheng T, Zhu Z, Wang Z, Homer RJ, Ma B, Riese RJ, Jr. et al. Inducible targeting of IL-13 to the adult lung causes matrix metalloproteinase- and cathepsin-dependent emphysema. *J Clin Invest* 2000; 106:1081–1093.
171. Reddy VY, Zhang QY, Weiss SJ. Pericellular mobilization of the tissue-destructive cysteine proteinases, cathepsins B, L, and S, by human monocyte-derived macrophages. *Proc Natl Acad Sci USA* 1995; 92:3849–3853.
172. Takeyabu K, Betsuyaku T, Nishimura M, Yoshioka A, Tanino M, Miyamoto K et al. Cysteine proteinases and cystatin C in bronchoalveolar lavage fluid from subjects with subclinical emphysema. *Eur Respir J* 1998; 12:1033–1039.
173. Shapiro SD, Senior RM. Matrix metalloproteinases. Matrix degradation and more. *Am J Respir Cell Mol Biol* 1999; 20:1100–1102.
174. Finlay GA, O'Driscoll LR, Russell KJ, D'Arcy EM, Masterson JB, FitzGerald MX et al. Matrix metalloproteinase expression and production by alveolar macrophages in emphysema. *Am J Respir Crit Care Med* 1997; 156:240–247.
175. Betsuyaku T, Nishimura M, Takeyabu K, Tanino M, Venge P, Xu S et al. Neutrophil granule proteins in bronchoalveolar lavage fluid from subjects with subclinical emphysema. *Am J Respir Crit Care Med* 1999; 159:1985–1991.

176. Ohnishi K, Takagi M, Kurokawa Y, Satomi S, Konttinen YT. Matrix metalloproteinase-mediated extracellular matrix protein degradation in human pulmonary emphysema. *Lab Invest* 1998; 78:1077–1087.

177. Imai K, Dalal SS, Chen ES, Downey R, Schulman LL, Ginsburg M *et al.* Human collagenase (matrix metalloproteinase-1) expression in the lungs of patients with emphysema. *Am J Respir Crit Care Med* 2001; 163:786–791.

178. Hautamaki RD, Kobayashi DK, Senior RM, Shapiro SD. Requirement for macrophage metalloelastase for cigarette smoke-induced emphysema in mice. *Science* 1997; 277:2002–2004.

179. Morris DG, Huang X, Kaminski N, Wang Y, Shapiro SD, Dolganov G *et al.* Loss of integrin avb6-mediated TGF-β activation causes MMP12-dependent emphysema. *Nature* 2003; 422:169–173.

180. Lanone S, Zheng T, Zhu Z, Liu W, Lee CG, Ma B *et al.* Overlapping and enzyme-specific contributions of matrix metalloproteinases-9 and -12 in IL-13-induced inflammation and remodeling. *J Clin Invest* 2002; 110:463–474.

181. Yu Q, Stamenkovic I. Cell surface-localized matrix metalloproteinase-9 proteolytically activates TGF-beta and promotes tumor invasion and angiogenesis. *Genes Dev* 2000; 14:163–176.

182. Dallas SL, Rosser JL, Mundy GR, Bonewald LF. Proteolysis of latent transforming growth factor-β (TGF-β)-binding protein-1 by osteoclasts. A cellular mechanism for release of TGF-β from bone matrix. *J Biol Chem* 2002; 277:21352–21360.

183. Rooney CP, Taggart C, Coakley R, McElvaney NG, O'Neill SJ. Anti-proteinase 3 antibody activation of neutrophils can be inhibited by α1-antitrypsin. *Am J Respir Cell Mol Biol* 2001; 24:747–754.

184. Mahadeva R, Lomas DA. Genetics and respiratory disease. 2. Alpha 1-antitrypsin deficiency, cirrhosis and emphysema. *Thorax* 1998; 53:501–505.

185. Carrell RW, Lomas DA. Alpha1-antitrypsin deficiency—a model for conformational diseases. *N Engl J Med* 2002; 346:45–53.

186. Lomas DA, Mahadeva R. Alpha1-antitrypsin polymerization and the serpinopathies: pathobiology and prospects for therapy. *J Clin Invest* 2002; 110:1585–1590.

187. Carp H, Janoff A. Possible mechanisms of emphysema in smokers. *In vitro* suppression of serum elastase-inhibitory capacity by fresh cigarette smoke and its prevention by antioxidants. *Am Rev Respir Dis* 1978; 118:617–621.

188. Vogelmeier C, Hubbard RC, Fells GA, Schnebli HP, Thompson RC, Fritz H *et al.* Anti-neutrophil elastase defense of the normal human respiratory epithelial surface provided by the secretory leukoprotease inhibitor. *J Clin Invest* 1991; 87:482–488.

189. Taggart CC, Lowe GJ, Greene CM, Mulgrew AT, O'Neill SJ, Levine RL *et al.* Cathepsin B, L, and S cleave and inactivate secretory leucoprotease inhibitor. *J Biol Chem* 2001; 276:33345–33352.

190. Jin FY, Nathan C, Radzioch D, Ding A. Secretory leukocyte protease inhibitor: a macrophage product induced by and antagonistic to bacterial lipopolysaccharide. *Cell* 1997; 88:417–426.

191. Zhang Y, DeWitt DL, McNeely TB, Wahl SM, Wahl LM. Secretory leukocyte protease inhibitor suppresses the production of monocyte prostaglandin H synthase-2, prostaglandin E2 and matrix metalloproteinases. *J Clin Invest* 1997; 99:894–900.

192. Taggart CC, Greene CM, McElvaney NG, O'Neill S. Secretory leucoprotease inhibitor prevents lipopolysaccharide-induced IkBa degradation without affecting phosphorylation or ubiquitination. *J Biol Chem* 2002; 277:33648–33653.

193. Sallenave JM. The role of secretory leukocyte proteinase inhibitor and elafin (elastase-specific inhibitor/skin-derived antileukoprotease) as alarm antiproteinases in inflammatory lung disease. *Respir Res* 2000; 1:87–92.

194. Ishii T, Matsuse T, Teramoto S, Matsui H, Hosoi T, Fukuchi Y *et al.* Association between α1-antichymotrypsin polymorphism and susceptibility to chronic obstructive pulmonary disease. *Eur J Clin Invest* 2000; 30:543–548.

195. Cawston T, Carrere S, Catterall J, Duggleby R, Elliott S, Shingleton B *et al.* Matrix metalloproteinases and TIMPs: properties and implications for the treatment of chronic obstructive pulmonary disease. *Novartis Found Symp* 2001; 234:205–218.

196. Hirano K, Sakamoto T, Uchida Y, Morishima Y, Masuyama K, Ishii Y *et al.* Tissue inhibitor of metalloproteinases-2 gene polymorphisms in chronic obstructive pulmonary disease. *Eur Respir J* 2001; 18:748–752.

197. Barnes PJ. Molecular genetics of chronic obstructive pulmonary disease. *Thorax* 1999; 54:245–252.

198. Lomas DA, Silverman EK. The genetics of chronic obstructive pulmonary disease. *Respir Res* 2001; 2:20–26.

199. Hogg JC. Role of latent viral infections in chronic obstructive pulmonary disease and asthma. *Am J Respir Crit Care Med* 2001; 164:S71–S75.
200. Gilmour PS, Rahman I, Hayashi S, Hogg JC, Donaldson K, Macnee W. Adenoviral E1A primes alveolar epithelial cells to PM(10)-induced transcription of interleukin-8. *Am J Physiol Lung Cell Mol Physiol* 2001; 281:L598–L606.
201. Higashimoto Y, Elliott WM, Behzad AR, Sedgwick EG, Takei T, Hogg JC et al. Inflammatory mediator mRNA expression by adenovirus E1A-transfected bronchial epithelial cells. *Am J Respir Crit Care Med* 2002; 166:200–207.
202. Turato G, Di Stefano A, Maestrelli P, Mapp CE, Ruggieri MP, Roggeri A et al. Effect of smoking cessation on airway inflammation in chronic bronchitis. *Am J Respir Crit Care Med* 1995; 152:1262–1267.
203. Rutgers SR, Postma DS, ten Hacken NH, Kauffman HF, Van der Mark TW, Koeter GH et al. Ongoing airway inflammation in patients with COPD who do not currently smoke. *Thorax* 2000; 55:12–18.
204. Loppow D, Schleiss MB, Kanniess F, Taube C, Jorres RA, Magnussen H. In patients with chronic bronchitis a four week trial with inhaled steroids does not attenuate airway inflammation. *Respir Med* 2001; 95:115–121.
205. Meagher LC, Cousin JM, Seckl JR, Haslett C. Opposing effects of glucocorticoids on the rate of apoptosis in neutrophilic and eosinophilic granulocytes. *J Immunol* 1996; 156:4422–4428.
206. Nightingale JA, Rogers DF, Chung KF, Barnes PJ. No effect of inhaled budesonide on the response to inhaled ozone in normal subjects. *Am J Respir Crit Care Med* 2000; 161:479–486.
207. Tashkin DP, Altose MD, Connett JE, Kanner RE, Lee WW, Wise RA. Methacholine reactivity predicts changes in lung function over time in smokers with early chronic obstructive pulmonary disease. The Lung Health Study Research Group. *Am J Respir Crit Care Med* 1996; 153:1802–1811.
208. Highland KB, Strange C, Heffner JE. Long-term effects of inhaled corticosteroids on FEV1 in patients with chronic obstructive pulmonary disease. A meta-analysis. *Ann Intern Med* 2003; 138:969–973.
209. Yamada K, Elliott WM, Brattsand R, Valeur A, Hogg JC, Hayashi S. Molecular mechanisms of decreased steroid responsiveness induced by latent adenoviral infection in allergic lung inflammation. *J Allergy Clin Immunol* 2002; 109:35–42.
210. Barnes PJ, Ito K, Adcock IM. A mechanism of corticosteroid resistance in COPD: inactivation of histone deacetylase. *Lancet* 2004; 363:731–733.
211. Barnes PJ. New treatments for COPD. *Nat Rev Drug Discov* 2002; 1:437–445.

2

Pathophysiology of airflow limitation in COPD

S. Khirani, G. Polese, G. Morlini, A. Rossi

INTRODUCTION

Chronic obstructive pulmonary disease (COPD) is one of the few respiratory disorders including an assertion about lung function in the definition, which indeed contains the statement on the reduction of forced expiratory flows [1]. The pathophysiology of COPD is a complex and attractive subject [2]. It includes abnormalities in lung and chest wall mechanics, in pulmonary gas exchanges, in respiratory and skeletal muscles structure and function and so on [3]. COPD is a heterogeneous disease in terms of clinical, physiological, and pathological presentation [4]. Probably the starting point is the inflammation of the airways [5, 6] and the final events are severe physical disability and premature death. In this complexity, airflow limitation is a central element, and to some extent the bridge, connecting biological defects with clinical phenotypes. Definitely, airflow limitation is a key mechanism determining dyspnoea, progressive disability and ventilatory failure in patients with COPD [7].

Understanding the pathophysiology of airflow limitation is an essential step to alleviate the suffering of those patients with effective interventions such as pharmacological therapy, rehabilitation, changes in lifestyle and so on [1, 8–11]. The literature on airflow limitation in COPD is abundant [12–15]. Hence, it is beyond the scope of this chapter to provide a complete, definitive, state-of-the-art work on such a vast topic. Rather, it will be focused on the important distinction between airway obstruction and airflow limitation and on the tight relationship between the latter and pulmonary hyperinflation. It is our 'prejudice', and surely not only ours, that airway/airflow obstruction and airflow limitation should not be thought of as synonymous, not only in the textbooks but also in clinical practice.

AIRWAY OBSTRUCTION AND AIRFLOW LIMITATION

Although COPD characterises the disease with the expression *'obstructive'*, and the term *'airflow obstruction'* is preserved in the definition in some recent national guidelines [10, 11], other recent international guidelines [1, 8, 9] have a preference for the term *'airflow limitation'* in their definition. The former emphasises that, whatever the underlying pathophysiological mechanism, the final result is a reduced expiratory flow due to smaller bronchial calibre (airway obstruction); the latter points out that obstruction of the airways – due to pathological

Sonia Khirani*, PhD, Doctor in Biomedical Engineering, Ospedale Riuniti di Bergamo, Bergamo, Italy.
Guido Polese, MD, Pulmonary Division, Ospedale Riuniti di Bergamo, Bergamo, Italy.
Giacomo Morlini, RRT, Respiratory Therapist, Ospedale Riuniti di Bergamo, Bergamo, Italy.
Andrea Rossi, MD, Director, Pulmonary Division, Ospedale Riuniti di Bergamo, Bergamo, Italy.
*Recipient of a European Respiratory Society Fellowship (No. 174).

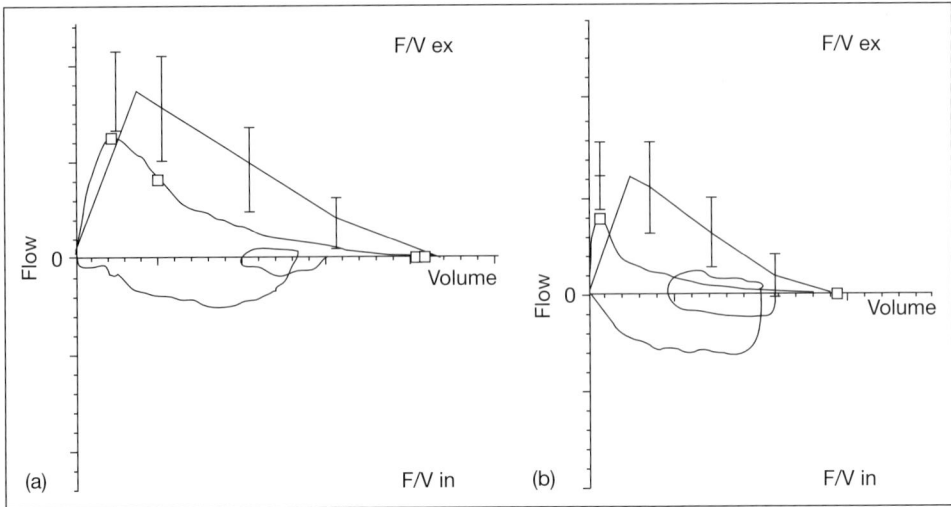

Figure 2.1 Flow-volume curves in COPD with small airway obstruction (a) and with airflow limitation (b). Flow-volume curve at rest (small circle) followed by a forced expiratory manoeuvre. (a) The curve at rest is not reaching the maximum expiratory flow-volume curve obtained during the forced expiratory manoeuvre, indicating that the subject is not flow limited at rest. The particular shape of the flow-volume curve during the forced expiratory manoeuvre is characteristic of the presence of small airway obstruction (FEV_1% predicted pre-bronchodilator = 73.7%; FEV_1/FVC post-bronchodilator = 60.7%). (b) The curve at rest is reaching the maximum expiratory flow-volume curve obtained during the forced expiratory manoeuvre, indicating that the subject is flow limited at rest. (FEV_1% predicted pre-bronchodilator = 60.7%; FEV_1/FVC post-bronchodilator = 44.2%). Black line (triangle shape): expected FV curve. 100-75-50-25% of expired volume. F/V ex, F/V in: expiratory and inspiratory part of FV curve, respectively. FEV_1: forced expiratory volume in 1 second.

(mainly inflammatory) changes in the bronchial wall, and altered mucus secretion and transport – is one of the mechanisms leading to reduced expiration, the other being the loss of lung elastic recoil and alveolar attachments sustaining the small airways. These are the consequence of destructive events occurring in the peripheral lung [16]. Both airway obstruction and loss of lung elastic recoil contribute to the presence and degree of airflow limitation.

Airflow limitation might be considered a more complex pathophysiological phenomenon than airway obstruction (Figure 2.1a). The latter may be determined by a simple straightforward event such as, for a example, bronchoconstriction due to bronchial smooth muscle contraction in asthma, whereas the former implies more complicated physiological mechanisms, such as dynamic compression of the small airways, upward movement of the equal pressure point (EPP), 'choke point' theory, etc. [17, 18].

The clinical implications of this distinction are that:

■ The destruction of the lung parenchyma is essentially an irreversible phenomenon whereas bronchial inflammation and obstruction can be treated with anti-inflammatory drugs and bronchodilators;
■ The presence of airflow limitation is more relevant in the pathophysiology and clinical diagnosis (exercise tolerance, respiratory failure, etc.) of COPD than simple airway obstruction.

A potential opposition to the widespread use of the term 'expiratory airflow limitation' is that it would imply a condition of 'unlimited expiratory airflow' which does not exist even in a 'pure' physiological condition. Normal subjects are not flow-limited at rest, but they may exhibit expiratory flow limitation with increasing levels of ventilation up to the maximum exercise capacity. Many physiologists prefer to restrict the definition of expiratory flow limitation to the condition in which 'expiratory flow cannot augment at a given volume, for example by active contraction of the expiratory muscles, as the expiratory flows lie on the maximum expiratory flow-volume curve generated by the forced expiratory manoeuvre' (Figure 2.1b) [18].

DIAGNOSIS AND STAGING OF COPD

The preliminary diagnosis of suspected COPD is based clearly on [1, 8–11, 19–23]:

■ risk exposure (e.g., cigarette smoking, occupational, urban and indoor pollution);
■ symptoms such as chronic cough and phlegm, and exercise dyspnoea; and
■ signs such as modifications in the thorax configuration, changes in lung sounds etc.

The diagnosis of COPD needs to be confirmed by spirometry. Independently, whether the term obstruction or limitation is used, all of the national and international guidelines on 'assessment and management of COPD' indicate the measurement of FEV_1 (forced expiratory volume in one second) as the landmark parameter of respiratory function

■ to make the diagnosis of COPD;
■ to stage the severity of the disease; and
■ to assess its progression.

The FEV_1 is measured on the volume/time or flow/volume tracing of a forced expiratory manoeuvre. This manoeuvre is recorded from the point of maximal inspiration to complete expiration at the maximum possible speed for at least 6–9 s to measure also the FVC (forced vital capacity).

A value of the FEV_1/FVC ratio <0.7 after bronchodilator indicates existing COPD, independent of age, gender, ethnicity, height, weight and so on [1, 8–11]. The obvious limitations of such an absolute index are well known [24]. However, there is general agreement that a simple tool for the diagnosis of COPD is urgently needed to disclose the large underdiagnosis of a disease whose impact on public health has been clearly documented [25].

Some years ago, the European Respiratory Society (ERS) guidelines on COPD [26] were indicating a predicted FEV_1/VC (vital capacity) ratio <88 and 89% for males and females respectively, as the parameter for the diagnosis of COPD. However, this ratio (Tiffeneau's index) [27] required both a forced and a slow complete expiration, i.e., two different manoeuvres. In addition, there was the necessity to select the appropriate predicted values [1]. The GOLD committee and ATS/ERS joint committee on COPD guidelines concluded that, despite all of the known limitations, a single FVC manoeuvre was more likely to meet the requirements of a simple tool to liberate the diagnosis of COPD from its severe underestimation.

The value of the percent of the predicted FEV_1 (FEV_1% predicted) was then suggested to stage the severity of COPD (Table 2.1, Figure 2.2). The interesting relationship recently found by Hogg et al. [28] between some inflammatory changes in the small airways and the reported staging of COPD is also shown in Table 2.1.

Table 2.1 Staging of severity of COPD

With a post-bronchodilator FEV_1/FVC <0.7:	
■ FEV_1% predicted >80%	mild
■ 50%< FEV_1% predicted <80%	moderate
■ 30%< FEV_1% predicted <50%	severe
■ FEV_1% predicted <30%	very severe

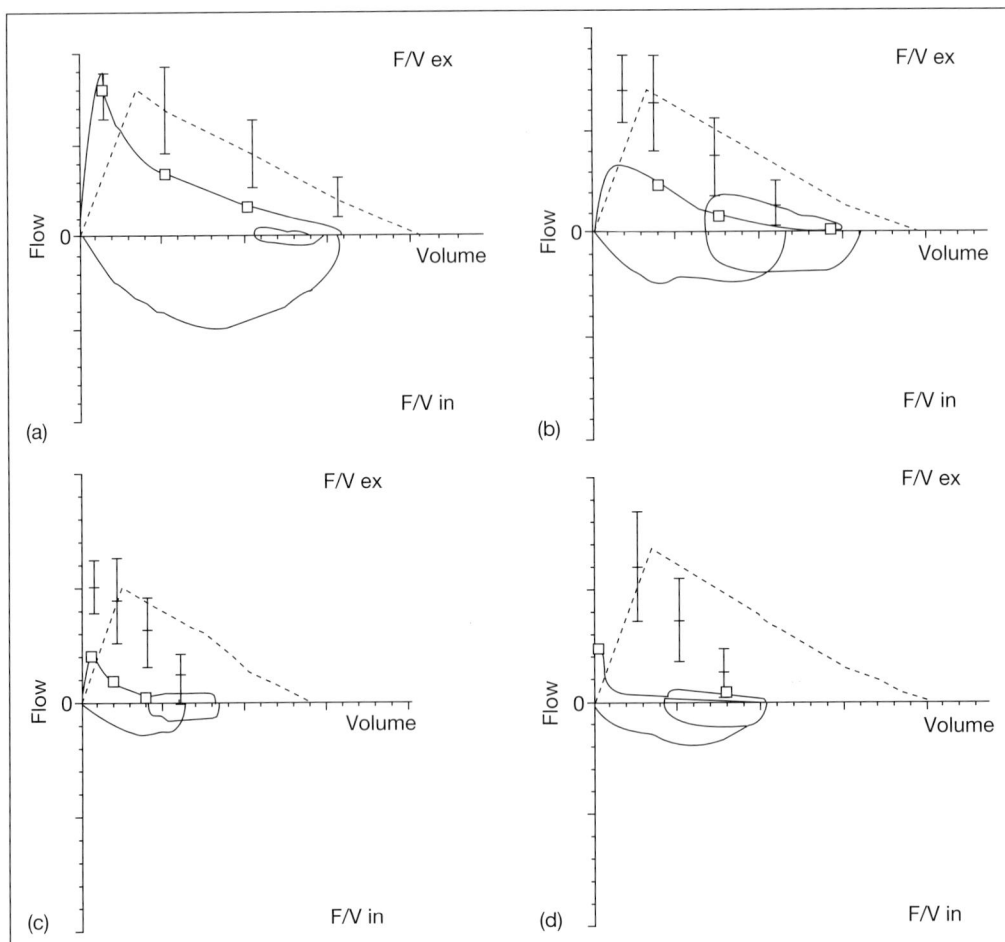

Figure 2.2 Flow-volume (FV) curves of patients with diverse degrees of COPD. (a) mild (FEV$_1$% predicted
>80%); (b) moderate (FEV$_1$% predicted = 56%); (c) severe (FEV$_1$% predicted = 37%); (d) very severe (FEV$_1$%
predicted = 21%). Dotted line: Triangle shape expected FV curve. ⌐ 100-75-50-25% of expired volume. F/V ex,
F/V in: expiratory and inspiratory part of FV curve, respectively.

After the landmark publications by Fletcher and colleagues [19, 20], the progression of the
disease has been commonly assessed by measuring the annual decline in the FEV$_1$. This is
accelerated in smokers and in COPD patients compared to normal subjects (50–100 vs. 30 ml/
year, respectively). The accelerated FEV$_1$ decline leads to disability and premature death.
Smoking cessation slows down the rate of the FEV$_1$ decline at any age [8, 9, 15, 19, 20].

It should be recalled here that the value of both FVC and FEV$_1$ could be affected by the
speed of the inspiration preceding the forced expiration and by the presence and duration
of the end-inspiratory pause. If the forced expiratory manoeuvre is preceded by a slow
inspiration with a long (about 4–5 s) inspiratory pause, expiratory flows are smaller than
those obtained by a forced expiration preceded by a fast inspiration and without any end-
inspiratory pause [29–31]. Therefore, the forced expiratory manoeuvre for spirometry needs
to be standardised. To obtain maximal flows, the inspiration should be at maximum speed,
followed immediately by the forced expiration, without any pause [31].

COPD AND ASTHMA

COPD when coexists with other anomalies of airways and lungs, among them chronic bronchitis and emphysema, [32, 33], and in some patients, perhaps, features of asthma [4]. In fact, COPD may also be the consequence of advanced asthma when some important reversibility of airway obstruction exists, for example an increase of FEV_1 >20–25% from pre-bronchodilator value, but without reaching any more the normal spirometric values (Figure 2.3). This has been known for many years as the 'Dutch Hypothesis' [34]. The different phenotypes of COPD are frequently concomitant in such a way that at an evolved stage of disease, it becomes difficult to distinguish the contribution of each. However, a recent paper by Lapperre et al. [4], addressing the heterogeneity of COPD, concluded that airflow limitation, airway inflammation and features commonly associated with asthma are separate and largely independent factors in the pathophysiology of COPD. Another recent elegant paper by Fabbri et al. [35] showed that the characteristics of inflammation in asthma are different from whose in COPD, even at the same level of airflow obstruction, suggesting that asthma and COPD remain two different diseases even at advanced stages, and that different therapeutic strategies are thus warranted. In this connection, it should be noted that COPD is no longer considered a disease with irreversible or poorly reversible airflow obstruction [1, and ERS old guidelines]. Some degrees of reversibility exist in COPD [36–38], but the value of FEV_1/FVC always remains <0.7.

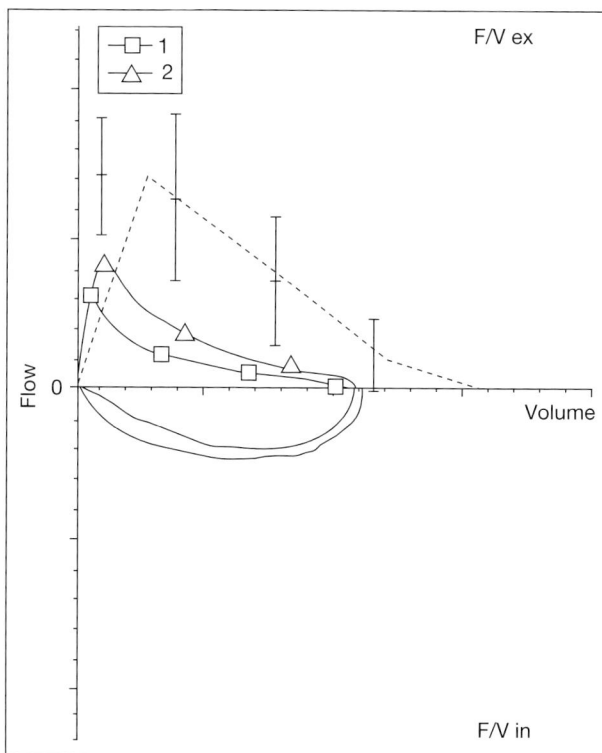

Figure 2.3 Flow-volume curve showing reversibility airway obstruction. Increase of FEV_1 of 29% from pre-bronchodilator value, but without reaching normal spirometric values. 1-line with square symbols: FV curve pre-bronchodilator (FEV_1% predicted = 52%); 2-line with triangle symbols: FV curve post-bronchodilator (FEV_1% predicted = 67%); dotted line: expected FV curve. 100-75-50-25% of expired volume. F/V ex, F/V in: expiratory and inspiratory part of FV curve, respectively.

SMALL AIRWAYS IN COPD

COPD is the consequence of an abnormal inflammatory response to inhalation of noxious agents such as cigarette smoking (the main etiological agent), occupational exposure, and environmental pollution [5, 6]. However, individual factors also play an important role (e.g. enzymatic deficiencies, immunological troubles). In fact, only a portion (estimated at between 15 and 40%) of heavy smokers develop a clinically detectable disease [5, 15, 33]. At present, the factors determining individual susceptibility are still largely obscure. By contrast, both the pathogenesis and pathophysiology of COPD have been extensively investigated, with impressive progress in our scientific knowledge of some of the key mechanisms underlying the disease [5, 6, 15].

In their pioneering work almost 40 years ago, Hogg et al. [39] addressed the structure-function correlation in COPD. They concluded that the main site of airway obstruction was in the small airways, i.e., the bronchioles with an internal diameter <2 mm, and they found that the nature of that obstruction was mucus plugging, fibrosis, distortion, narrowing and obliteration of small airways. Measurements of pulmonary resistance and partitioning between central and peripheral airway resistance were performed on excised human lungs by means of the peripheral catheter technique [40]. Hogg [15] showed that widespread pathological changes in small airways occur in COPD without detectable abnormalities of routine pulmonary function tests such as spirometry and/or, at that time, measurement of total pulmonary resistance [41]. This is due to the negligible contribution of peripheral airway resistance to total resistance. In his classic editorial, Mead defined the small airways 'the lungs' silent zone' [42]. However, parenchyma beyond the obstructed small airways should be ventilated via collateral channels such that the distribution of ventilation should be markedly abnormal, and presumably gas exchange would be impaired. As a matter of fact, this prediction was confirmed, almost 30 years later, by the experimental data from Barbera et al. [43]. They used the multiple inert gas expiratory technique (MIGET) and showed that both the distribution of perfusion and the distribution of ventilation were determined by small airway abnormalities and parenchymal destruction, with a poor correlation with FEV_1 [43].

Ten years after Hogg's paper [39], Cosio et al. [44], from the same group of investigators, published a momentous study on the relationship between structural changes in small airways and pulmonary function tests. By examining samples from open lung biopsies of localised pulmonary lesions in smokers, they found that the primary lesion was a progressive inflammatory reaction leading to fibrosis with connective tissue deposition in the small airways. These lesions could be detected by the so-called 'tests for small airways function' [45] such as measurements of closing capacity [46, 47], volume of isoflow [48], and slope of the phase III of the single breath washout curve [44, 47]. These tests showed abnormalities in smokers at a time when the pathological changes were still potentially reversible and when other tests were not appreciably changed. Some years later, a group of researchers made some measurements in vivo, and confirmed that in some patients with asthma and in all patients with COPD there was a significant increase in total airway resistance [49]. This was due to an increase in both central and peripheral resistance. However, whilst central resistance increased by 50% on average, the resistance of the small airways exhibited a five-fold increase.

Recently, Hogg et al. [28] reported extensive information on the nature of small airway obstruction in COPD. In a large investigation, the small airways were assessed in surgically resected lung tissue from 159 patients. They found that 'progression of COPD was associated with the accumulation of inflammatory mucus exudates in the lumen and infiltration of the bronchial wall by innate and adaptive inflammatory and immune cells'. They also showed a significant correlation between pathological changes in the small airways, mainly wall thickness changes, and the FEV_1% predicted GOLD classification of severity [28]. They also confirmed previous reports that showed a persistence of bronchial inflammation years after stopping smoking, suggesting that inflammation becomes independent of the causal mechanism in severe disease. The reason for this persistence is still unclear.

The final conclusion of this long-standing and elegant series of publications is that pathological abnormalities of the small airways play a pivotal role in the pathogenesis of COPD [15, 22]. In particular, these studies highlighted the importance of inflammation in small airways as a determinant of airway obstruction as well as the progression and severity of the disease [5, 15].

EXPIRATORY AIRFLOW LIMITATION

It has been know for many years that the loss of lung elastic recoil was the major determinant of reduction of expiratory airflow in emphysema [50, 51]. In fact, inspiration is an active event driven by the contraction of the inspiratory muscles, whereas expiration is passively driven by the elastic recoil stored in the preceding inspiration. Although the mechanics of impaired expiration is to some extent self-explanatory in the presence of reduced driving pressure [51], the biological mechanism underlying the relationship between that loss of lung recoil and the reduction of expiratory flow rate was not clear. Saetta et al. [52] addressed that issue and found that the loss of alveolar attachments sustaining the small intrathoracic airways was correlated to the reduction in forced expiratory flow, and that this loss was related to inflammation in the periphery of the lungs. Subsequently, Kim et al. [53] reported that the inflammation and remodelling of the airways and parenchyma could be different in lungs with centrilobular and panlobular emphysema. Finkelstein et al. [54] showed that in centrilobular emphysema the airways were narrower and thicker than in panlobular emphysema, the former being more characteristic in smokers whereas the latter was more related to α_1-antitrypsin deficiency.

The inflammatory response in the periphery of the lungs in patients with COPD, representing an amplification of the inflammatory response to irritants that is seen in normal smokers, plays a paramount role in the pathogenesis of COPD for both the airway obstruction and the loss of lung elastic recoil [15, 16, 21]. The consequence of these pathological changes is a retarded rate of lung emptying during a forced expiration and eventually during the tidal expiration.

The expiratory collapse of airways during passive expiration, mainly induced by the loss of elasticity and destruction of parenchyma, is associated with a dynamic compression, which is the mechanism responsible for the occurrence of expiratory airflow limitation in COPD patients (Figure 2.4) [55]. Airflow limitation means that expiratory flows cannot augment at a given lung volume by increasing the intrathoracic pressure (and so alveolar pressure) through, for example, activation of expiratory muscles. The expiratory flow is already maximal and hence independent of muscle activity [17, 18]. The magnitude of the expiratory flow thus depends upon the elastic recoil pulmonary pressure, stored during the preceding inspiration. In contrast to the conventional belief that the first portion of the forced expiration is effort dependent, Tantucci et al. [56] have recently shown that the peak-expiratory flow may also be in the range of expiratory flow limitation events.

Small airways dynamic compression can, in the case of severe airways wall alterations, also lead to airway closure, which can generate mechanical lesions of small airways due to the repetitive mechanical constraints [57]. These mechanical lesions tend to accelerate the decline of respiratory function.

At this point it has to be mentioned that expiratory flow limitation occurs in all subjects when the level of the maximum flow has been reached. In normal subjects and in patients with mild-to-moderate airway obstruction, airflow limitation occurs during different grades of exercise due to the increased ventilation. By contrast, in severe COPD, airflow limitation occurs during resting breathing (Figure 2.1b). During a normal expiration, there is a pressure difference between the inside (lumen) and the outside (intrathoracic space) of the

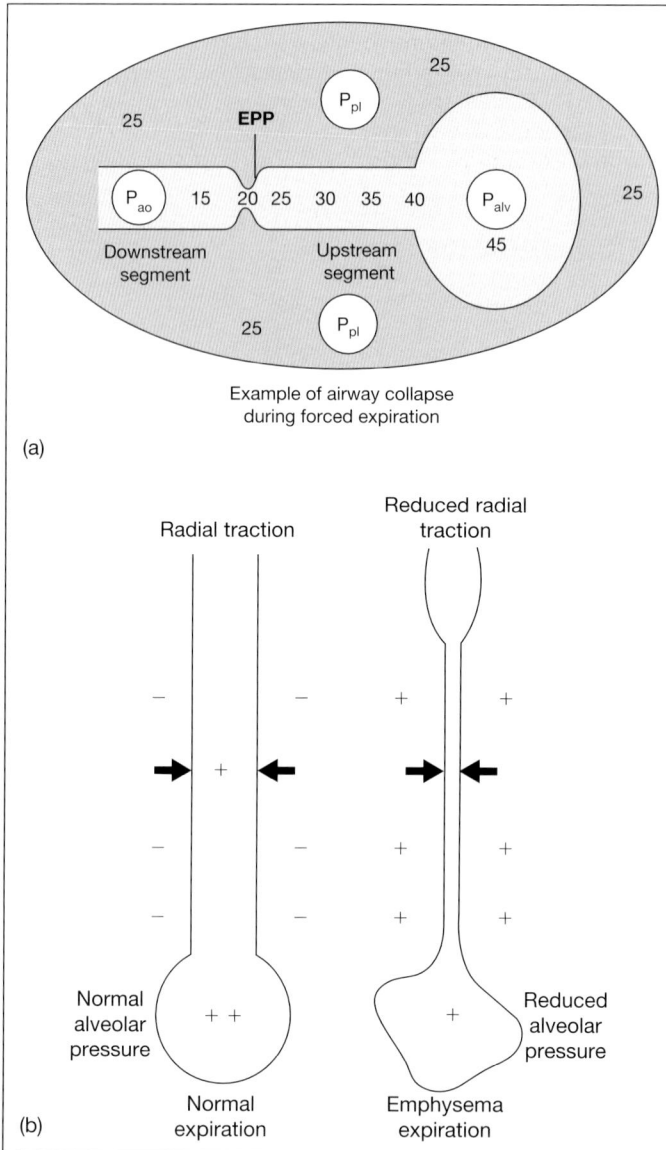

Figure 2.4 Dynamic airway compression. (a) Mechanism of dynamic airway compression. When the pressure outside the airway becomes higher than the pressure inside the airway, dynamic compression takes place. The flow becomes dependent of the difference between pleural pressure (P_{pl}) and airway pressure (P_{ao}) and upstream resistance. EPP: equal pressure point. (b) Dynamic compression at rest in COPD patient. For further explanation, see text. http://oac.med.jhmi.edu/LectureLinks/LectureNotes/Physiology/Mechanics2.Hoh.html

airways to hold them open, but during a forced expiration or in COPD patients, this pressure difference is reversed. When the pressure inside the airways is less than the pleural pressure, airways tend to narrow and/or compress. Expiratory airflows are therefore determined by the elastic recoil force of the lungs and the resistance of the airways upstream of the collapse point [18].

A simple approach would be to consider airflow limitation as a kind of severe airway obstruction. However, airflow limitation, defined as the impinging of tidal expiratory flow on the maximum flow-volume envelope (Figure 2.1b), is not correlated with the degree of airway obstruction assessed and staged by measurement of the FEV_1. This interesting observation was reported by Eltayara *et al.* [58] by comparing the value of $FEV_1\%$ predicted with the results from the negative expiratory pressure (NEP) technique in a population of patients at different stages of COPD. The NEP technique is described extensively elsewhere [7]. Briefly, it is based on the concept that in the presence of expiratory flow limitation, changes in pressure at the airway opening, i.e., downstream of the 'choke point' [18], do not affect expiratory flows. Hence a negative pressure amounting to $-5/-10\,cm\ H_2O$ is applied at the airway opening, i.e., the mouth or the proximal tip of an endotracheal tube, while recording the tidal expiratory flows. As illustrated in Figure 2.5, the expiratory flow is increased by the NEP technique in non-flow limited patients, whereas it remains unaltered if the patient is flow-limited.

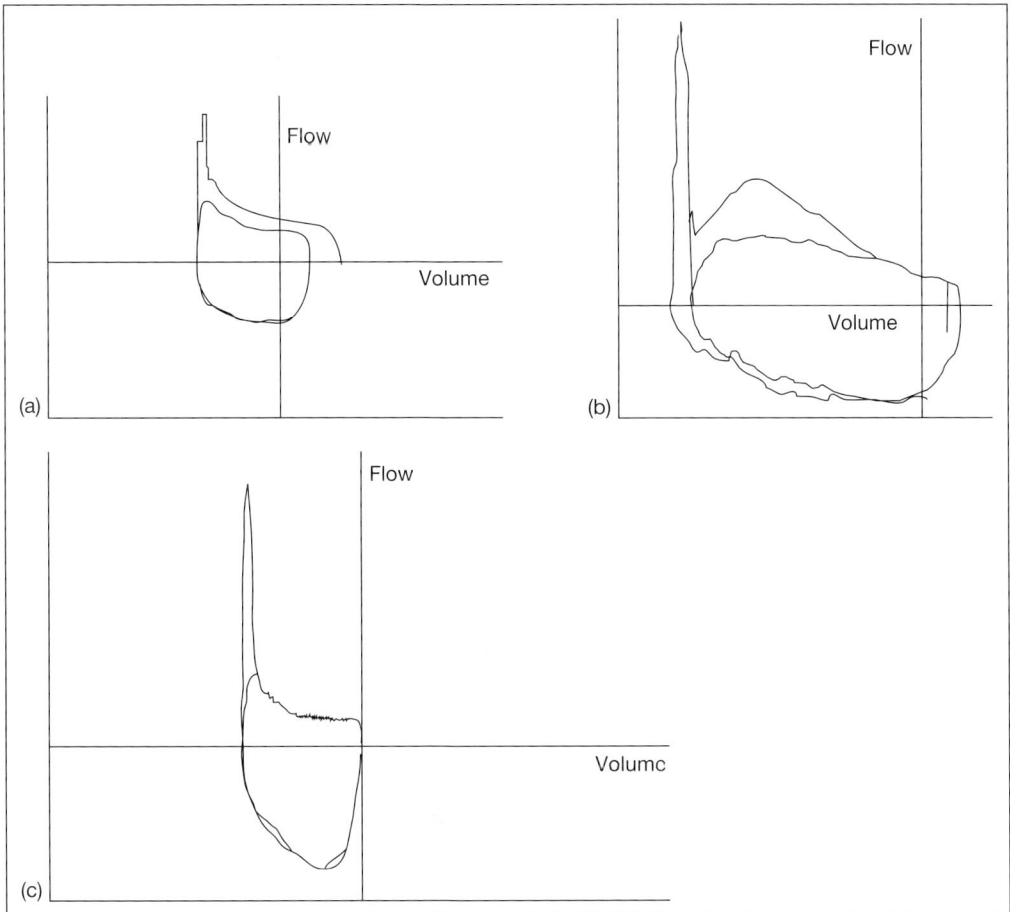

Figure 2.5 Flow-volume loops during tidal breathing of three different patients undergoing the NEP manoeuvre. The degree of expiratory flow limitation is assessed by plotting the breath cycle with NEP application and the preceding control breath cycle. The expiratory part is on the top. No flow limitation (FL) (a), FL under 50% of control expired tidal volume (VT) (b), FL over 50% of control expired VT (c). Zero volume corresponds to the end-expiratory lung volume of the control breaths.

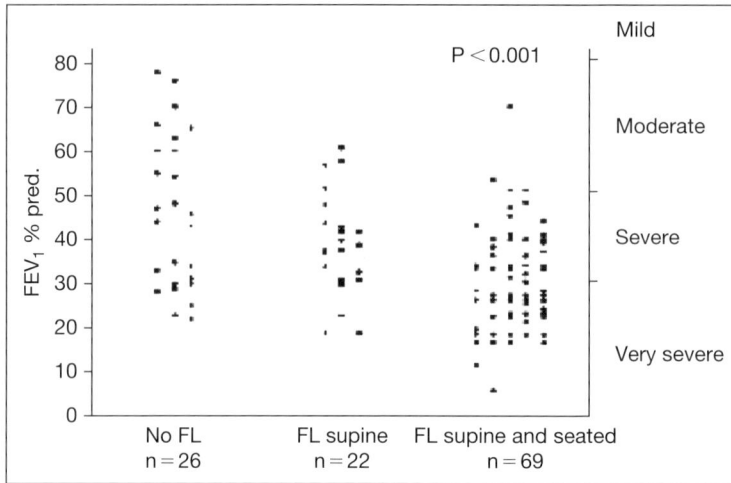

Figure 2.6   Values of FEV_1 (% predicted) in some COPD patients. Patients were classified according to the three-point flow limitation (FL) score. The right ordinate represents the classification of the degree of ventilatory disability according to FEV_1. n = Number of patients; p value refers to significant difference between no FL and FL supine and seated. Modified from Eltayara et al., 1996 [58].

As predicted from the known changes in lung volume [59], flow limitation may be present in the supine posture even when not yet evident in the standing and sitting position [60]. Figure 2.6 shows that the presence of expiratory flow limitation at rest, detected by means of the NEP technique, cannot be predicted from the value of FEV_1. The reason for the poor association between FEV_1 and flow limitation at rest is not completely clear. Presumably, it depends on the variable association between 'bronchitic' lesions of the small airways and 'emphysematous' destruction of the parenchyma in the individual patient. The predominant parenchymal destruction can determine a greater loss of alveolar attachments supporting the small intrapulmonary airways as well as a greater reduction of lung elastic recoil, i.e., the driving force for expiration. In these circumstances, flow limitation would occur earlier than in the patients in whom destruction is less widespread compared to the lesions of the bronchial wall.

PULMONARY HYPERINFLATION

The major consequence of airway obstruction is the increased work of breathing (so-called 'resistive work') while the major straightforward consequence of airflow limitation is pulmonary hyperinflation. This further increases the work of breathing because ventilation occurs toward the upper flat portion of the pressure-volume curve [61] where compliance is lower (so-called 'elastic work'). Although it was known for many years that retarded expiratory flow lead to an increase in the functional residual capacity, the real elucidation of the key role of pulmonary hyperinflation in the pathogenesis of COPD came from a series of studies in the intensive care setting [62, 63].

Pulmonary hyperinflation is defined by an increase in the functional residual capacity (FRC) above the predicted values [57]. FRC is defined by the amount of gas remaining in the lungs and the airways at the end of a tidal expiration [64]. In normal subjects, FRC corresponds to the elastic equilibrium volume of the respiratory system, i.e., the volume at which the inward elastic recoil of the lungs is counterbalanced by the outward elastic recoil of the chest wall. In these circumstances, FRC is approximately 40% of the total lung capacity (TLC) [64]. The act of breathing inflates the lungs through the contraction of the inspiratory muscles. Expiration is passively driven back to the relaxed FRC by the elastic recoil stored during the preceding inspiration.

■ Static Hyperinflation
   In patients with COPD, the static equilibrium volume of the respiratory system is set at a higher lung volume than in normal subjects because of the loss of lung elastic recoil such that the outward elastic recoil of the chest wall raises the relaxed FRC to the volume of the relaxed chest wall, i.e., about 55–60% of TLC.
■ Dynamic Hyperinflation
   This is the main mechanism leading to the remarkable increase of FRC in patients with severe COPD. Due to airway obstruction and expiratory flow limitation, the rate of lung emptying is unduly retarded, first during different levels of exercise and progressively even during resting breathing, preventing a complete expiration to the relaxed FRC in the time available between two consecutive inspiratory efforts. In these circumstances, the inspiratory effort ensues before the complete expiration while the alveolar pressure is still positive to drive the end-expiratory flows (Figure 2.7) [65]. Clearly, the end-expiratory positive alveolar pressure must be counterbalanced by the contracting inspiratory muscles in order to create a subatmospheric pressure in the central airways and generate inspiratory flow [66]. The positive end-expiratory alveolar pressure has been termed intrinsic positive end-expiratory pressure (PEEPi) [67–69] (Figure 2.8).

Breathing at higher lung volume increases the work of ventilation. PEEPi poses an additional burden on the inspiratory muscles [70, 71] whose pressure generating capacity is impaired by hyperinflation because of:

■ changes in the geometric arrangement (decreased area of apposition of diaphragm); and
■ length-tension characteristics of the fibres.

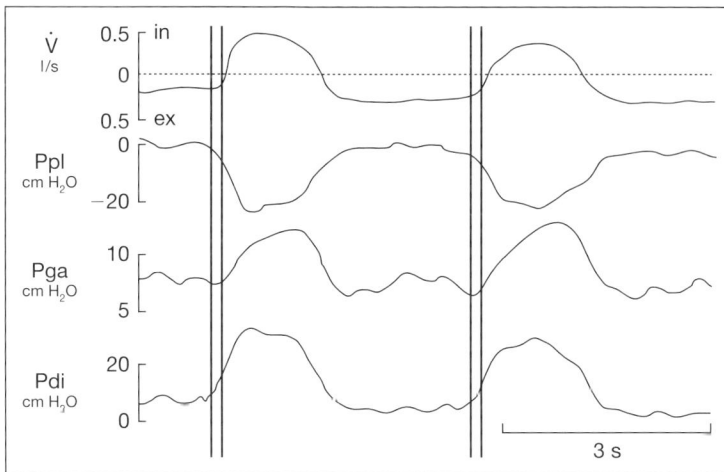

Figure 2.7   Method to determine the level of dynamic intrinsic PEEP (PEEPi$_{dyn}$) during spontaneous un-occluded breathing efforts in a COPD patient. From top to bottom: records of flow, pleural pressure (Ppl), gastric pressure (Pga) and transdiaphragmatic pressure (Pdi). The first vertical line indicates the point corresponding to the onset of the inspiratory effort (Pdi swing). The second vertical line indicates the point corresponding to the start of the inspiratory flow. The dotted horizontal line represents zero flow. in = inspiratory flow; ex = expiratory flow. Note that expiratory flow ends abruptly before inspiration, whereas the Pdi and Ppl swings have already begun and Pga has remained constant during the interval. In this case, PEEPi$_{dyn}$ is measured as the negative deflection in Ppl between the point corresponding to the onset of the Pdi swing and the point of zero flow. From Appendini et al., 1994 [65].

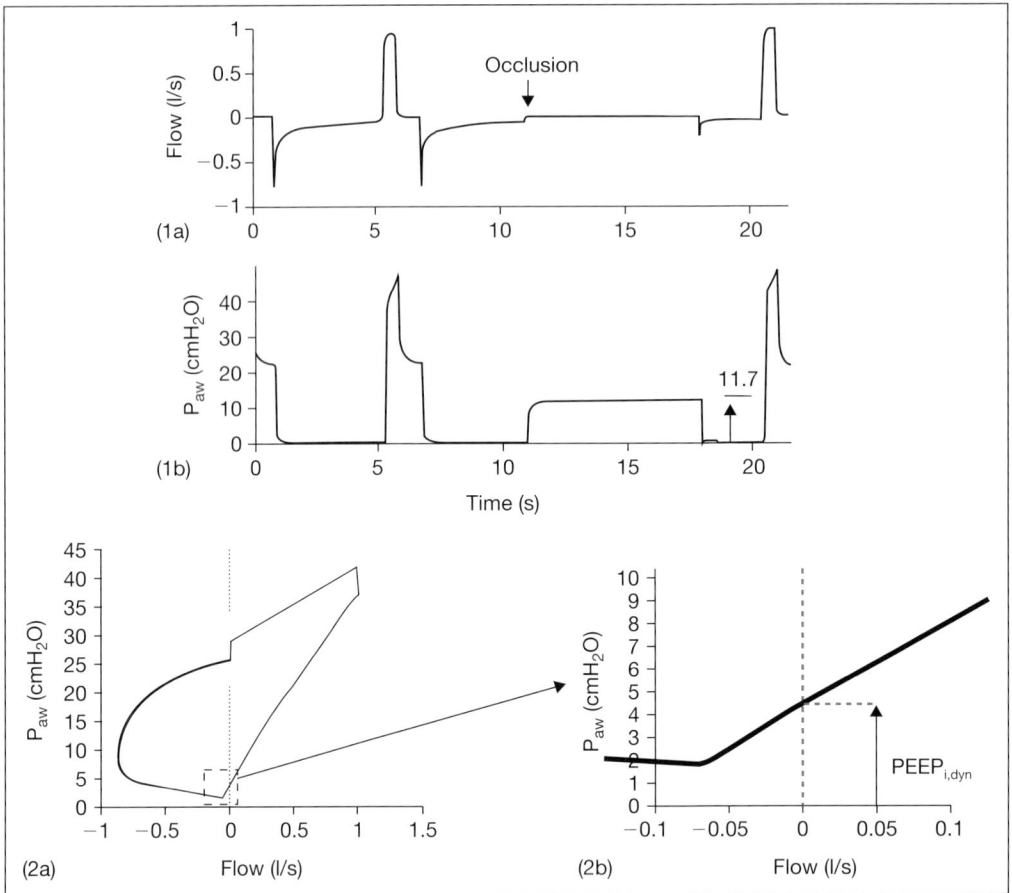

Figure 2.8 (1) Measurement of static intrinsic positive end-expiratory pressure (PEEPi,st) by the end-expiratory occlusion manoeuvre. The arrow in (b) indicates the value of PEEPi,st., (2) (a): airway pressure (P_{aw}) vs. flow diagram. Twenty-two consecutive ventilatory cycles are superimposed. Inspiration is rightward. Note that the start of inspiration precedes the zero flow (dotted line). The target portion (dashed box) is magnified in (b). Dynamic PEEPi (PEEPi,dyn) is measured as the difference between the value of P_{aw} at zero flow and end-expiratory pressure. The small end-expiratory pressure reflects the resistive pressure due to the end-expiratory flow and is included in the value of PEEPi,dyn. From Nucci et al., 2000 [68].

Although it has been shown that some compensatory mechanisms, both in experimental animals [72] and in humans [73], occur (i.e., drop of sarcomeres to match the new configuration of the diaphragmatic dome), the pressure generating capacity of the diaphragm is reduced overall [74].

The tight link between airway obstruction and airflow limitation and pulmonary hyperinflation has an important implication for the assessment of COPD. In fact, spirometry, i.e., measurement of FEV_1 and FVC from a forced expiratory manoeuvre, is necessary for the diagnosis of COPD; FEV_1 is useful for staging the severity of COPD. However, measurement of lung volume is fundamental to understand the pathophysiology of patients with COPD. For example, extreme narrowing or even closure of small airways during the forced expiration can cause an increase in the residual volume and a decrease in FVC. In these circumstances, the FEV_1/FVC ratio may exceed 0.7 and therefore hide a real condition of COPD.

Only measurement of lung volumes can show that the decrease in FVC is associated with an increase in residual volume and hence with closure of the small airways, without a decrease in TLC.

An FEV_1/FVC of <0.7 post-bronchodilator is the first step in the diagnosis of COPD; measurement of lung volumes, i.e., FRC, TLC, and RV (residual volume), is then needed to confirm the diagnosis, to understand apparent spirometric abnormalities misclassified as 'restrictive disorders' by simple spirometry, and to assess the degree of pulmonary hyperinflation. It has been suggested that measurement of the lung diffusion capacity of carbon monoxide (DLCO) may help to reveal the presence and magnitude of emphysema [75]. Therefore, an adequate use of pulmonary function tests is fundamental to understanding the respiratory pathophysiology of patients with COPD at any level. In fact, neither lung volumes nor the DLCO can be predicted by the values coming from simple spirometry. An extensive use of CT scanning for clinical purposes clearly cannot be proposed [75–77].

RESPIRATORY FAILURE

The role of pulmonary hyperinflation in the pathophysiology of respiratory failure in COPD has extensively been reported in other publications, including an official document of the most relevant international scientific societies in the area [78]. Briefly, the increase in airway resistance during a severe exacerbation of COPD determines an increase in both the work of breathing and air trapping. The latter worsens pulmonary hyperinflation which challenges the capacity of the inspiratory muscles to bear the greater ventilatory workload. A compensatory increase in the central drive would be even more deleterious because it would require an additional effort to the inspiratory muscles, which are already overloaded by both the increased work of breathing and the threshold load (PEEPi). In this condition, a decrease in tidal volume associated with an increase in the breathing frequency seems to remain the only means to defend pulmonary ventilation. However, the rapid and shallow breathing pattern is a very poor way to clear CO_2: not surprisingly, in those circumstances an increase in $PaCO_2$ ensues. In addition, a high frequency of breathing generates a short expiratory duration which in turn further worsens pulmonary hyperinflation and its deleterious consequences on the mechanics of breathing in a 'vicious circle' eventually leading to the failure of the ventilatory pump if assisted ventilation is not promptly instituted [78].

In a paper addressing the pathophysiology of chronic ventilator-dependent patients with very extreme COPD, Purro et al. [79] contributed to the elucidation of the general mechanism. They showed that the main characteristics of patients were:

- shallow breathing pattern, i.e., low tidal volume;
- high P 0.1 (an index of the total neuromuscular drive [80]), and high effective inspiratory impedance, i.e., the P 0.1/VT/TI ratio (VT and TI are the tidal volume and the inspiratory duration such that their ratio is the mean inspiratory flow) [81]; and
- high P/Pmax for both transdiaphragmatic (Pdi) and total pleural (Ppl) pressures, indicating that a large amount ($>40\%$) of the total pressure able to be generated by the respiratory muscles was needed for that pattern of breathing [82].

These findings taken together indicate that even in extreme conditions of very severe COPD, the drive to breathe was not only preserved, but was even greater than in stable conditions. However, the mechanical ventilatory load was so large that a big effort was required by the patient's respiratory muscles in order to breathe. As shown by Purro et al. [79], a P 0.1/VT/TI $> 10\,cm\,H_2O/l/s$ and a Pdi/Pdi,max $>40\%$ were associated with the inability to sustain spontaneous breathing for more than a few minutes and patients were chronically ventilator-dependent. In other words, those patients wanted to breathe (high P 0.1), but could not breathe because of the large mechanical load. The ineffective compensatory mechanism with the low tidal volume was resulting in chronic CO_2 retention.

DYSPNOEA

Dyspnoea, an unpleasant sensation of difficult breathing, is one of the most disabling symptoms of COPD, although chronic cough and phlegm can also severely impair the social activity of patients and can be associated with an accelerated decline of FEV_1 [83]. It is generally believed that dyspnoea appears first during exercise and then becomes progressively more evident during physical action of lesser and lesser intensity, until it becomes so severe as to impair daily activities. The Medical Research Council scale for chronic dyspnoea is widely used (Table 2.2).

It is generally accepted that there is some association between the severity of dyspnoea and the degree of airway obstruction. However, it is also well known that the individual correlation between the severity of dyspnoea and the degree of obstruction measured by means of the $FEV_1\%$ predicted is rather poor (Figure 2.9). This depends on several issues such as the condition of respiratory/skeletal muscles and comorbidity, in particular cardiovascular disorders, nutritional status and so on [3]. However, it depends also on the lifestyle of the patient. An additional factor which may delay the adequate consideration of exercise dyspnoea could be the self limitation of those activities that cause the 'unpleasant sensation', for example a more frequent use of the elevators, replacing some distressing activities such as playing tennis with the more relaxing fishing. In terms of lung mechanics, exercise dyspnoea is more related to airflow limitation than to airway obstruction

Table 2.2 Grades of dyspnoea (Medical Research Council scale)

Grade 0:	no dyspnoea
Grade 1:	get breathless with strenuous exercise
Grade 2:	shortness of breath when hurrying on the level or up a slight hill
Grade 3:	walks slower when walking with people of the same age on the level or when walking at my own pace on the level because of shortness of breath
Grade 4:	shortness of breath after walking 100 yards or after a few minutes on the level
Grade 5:	too breathless to leave the house

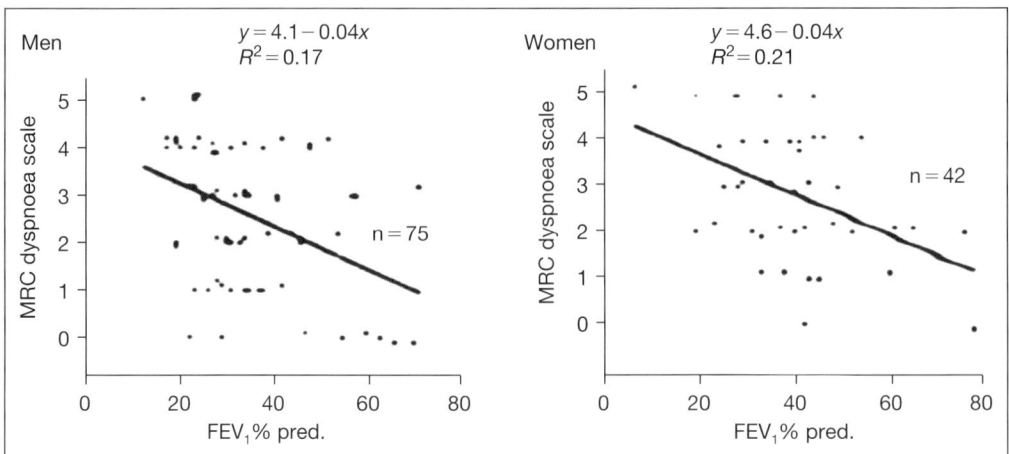

Figure 2.9 Relationship between the degree of dyspnoea (MRC dyspnoea scale) and $FEV_1\%$ predicted in men and women. Significant linear regression equations and variance (R^2) are provided. Modified from Eltayara et al., 1996 [58].

itself. In fact, when expiratory flow limitation occurs during tidal breathing, the increased ventilatory demand generated by exercise can be afforded only through pulmonary hyper-inflation, to find some room for the greater flows and volumes in the flow-volume enve-lope as illustrated in Figure 2.1b. As mentioned previously, pulmonary hyperinflation is a poor compensatory mechanism that can lead to a 'vicious circle' of increasing mechanical load and decreasing pressure generating capacity of the inspiratory muscles. Under those circumstances, the exercise capacity is clearly reduced.

In fact, by comparing COPD patients both with and without flow limitation, in its strict physiological meaning, Boni et al. [84] and Diaz et al. [85] showed that flow limited COPD patients had a much smaller exercise tolerance than COPD patients with significant airway obstruction but without flow limitation [86].

INSPIRATORY CAPACITY

The re-evaluation of measurements of lung volumes to complete the functional assessment of those patients, following simple spirometry, for a better understanding of the patho-physiology of COPD led not only to a much better definition of what are 'obstructive' dis-orders and 'restrictive' disorders, but also to the reconsideration of a spirometric variable known for many years but rather neglected in the clinical setting: the inspiratory capacity (IC), i.e., the sum of the tidal volume and the inspiratory reserve volume [7, 87]. IC is the mirroring value of FRC: any change in the FRC will determine an opposite change in IC, providing that TLC remains largely constant. Since TLC is mainly determined by the elastic properties of the lungs and the chest wall, its changes in general occur over a rather long period of time. An elegant series of studies by Milic-Emili [57] and Casanova et al. [87] showed that IC is significantly correlated with both dyspnoea and the exercise capacity such that IC is a much better predictor of the individual capacity of physical activity than the FEV_1 (Figure 2.10). It is also a good predictor of maximal tidal volume during exercise,

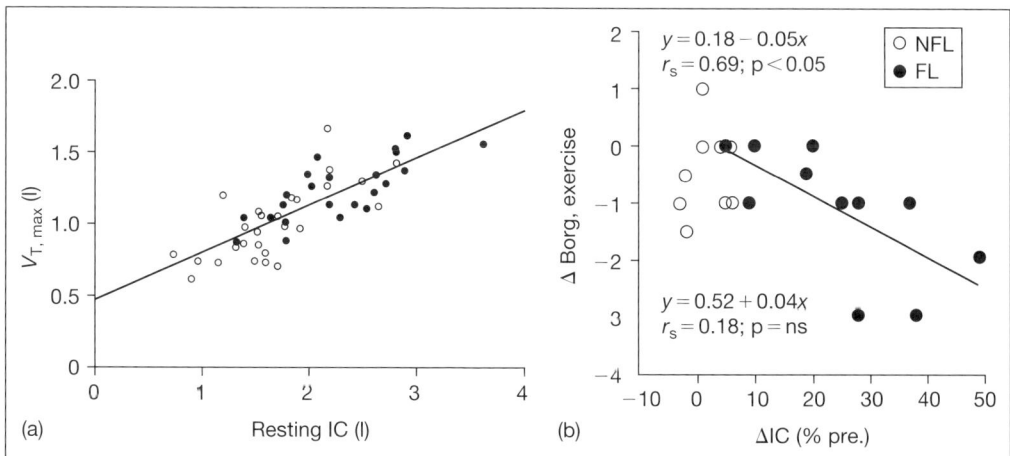

Figure 2.10 Relationship between IC, dyspnoea and exercise capacity. (a) Relationship between peak exercise tidal volume ($V_{T,max}$) and resting inspiratory capacity (IC) for COPD patients. • : Without tidal expiratory flow limitation at rest and o : with flow limitation. Regression line : $V_{T,max} = 0.49 + IC \pm 0.17$ (SEM); r = 0.77, p < 0.0001. From Diaz et al., 2001 [89]. (b) Relationship between reduction in resting IC (ΔIC %pre) and decrease in exertional breathlessness during light exercise (ΔBorg, exercise) after bronchodilatation in COPD patients. A significant correlation is found only with patients with tidal expiratory flow limitation at rest. FL = Flow limitation; NFL = Non flow limitation. From Boni et al., 2002 [84].

and so, of maximal exercise ventilation. IC reflects the real inspiratory reserve, particularly in patients who cannot use the expiratory reserve because of expiratory flow limitation which renders the activation of the expiratory muscles useless.

Significant correlations between IC and the maximal oxygen uptake during exercise have been reported [88, 89], but the major explanation of the variance of maximal oxygen uptake is provided by the assessment of both IC and FEV_1/FVC. However, in COPD patients with expiratory airflow limitation at rest, in the sitting position, maximal oxygen uptake correlates significantly only with IC, while in COPD patients without expiratory airflow limitation the significant correlation is seen between maximal oxygen uptake and FEV_1/FVC. Some studies have also shown that in most COPD patients with expiratory airflow limitation at rest, the IC is lower than normal while in non-airflow limited COPD patients at rest, IC is within normal values [57, 85]. As expiratory airflow limitation limits maximal tidal volume during exercise and maximal exercise ventilation and exercise tolerance, it well explains why IC is a good predictor of these factors.

A significant correlation between arterial PCO_2 and IC was also reported in stable COPD patients, and particularly in patients with expiratory airflow limitation at rest, as their arterial PCO_2 is significantly higher (with a decreased arterial PO_2) than in patients without expiratory airflow limitation. Thus hypercapnic COPD patients with expiratory airflow limitation at rest are characterised by a reduced IC [90]. O'Donnell et al. [91] studied the effects of surgical treatment in COPD by assessing the change in IC and found that measurement of IC provided useful information.

Furthermore, it should be considered that IC is a much easier variable to measure than FRC, and provides the same information. For example, IC can reflect acute changes in hyperinflation due to either a bronchodilator or an increase in ventilation. The former reduces pulmonary hyperinflation and this is well represented by a significant increase in IC; the latter is associated with an increase in FRC to match the greater ventilatory demand and is reflected by a progressive reduction in IC [84].

As the degree of COPD can be evaluated in terms of impairment of exercise capacity and dyspnoea [84, 90], it seems that IC could represent an effective tool to evaluate the status and progress of COPD in patients and to assess the efficacy of therapies [88]. Measurements of both FEV_1 and IC should be analysed to provide complementary information on lung function in COPD.

Further studies are still needed in order to better understand the pathogenesis of COPD and the different mechanisms involved in the process of airflow limitation, as many points remain unclear, due mainly to the complex heterogeneity of the disease. Moreover, strong quantitative methods are required to diagnose the specific targets responsible for airflow limitation, but also to assess the effects of treatments on small airways. The main objective is to find potential therapies that able to slow the progression of COPD. According to Barnes [5], 'new therapies must target the inflammation in small airways as well as emphysema in the lung parenchyma'.

CONCLUSIONS

- Although airflow limitation and airflow obstruction are often used as synonymous, they can have different meanings in the pathophysiology of COPD. That difference may have important clinical implications to predict, for example, the degree of exercise tolerance and the risk of ventilatory failure.
- Small airways are the major site of airflow limitation in COPD and inflammation is root cause of changes in the small airways, associated with parenchymal destruction determining loss of lung elastic recoil and of alveolar attachments supporting the small intrathoracic airways.

- Pulmonary hyperinflation is a major consequence of airflow limitation and has devastating consequences on the mechanics of breathing.
- Measurement of lung volume in addition to simple spirometry is necessary to understand the pathophysiology of patients with COPD.
- Inspiratory capacity is a simple measurement which may help significantly to explain dyspnoea and to predict the degree of exercise tolerance in COPD patients.

REFERENCES

1. Celli BR, MacNee W. ATS/ERS Task Force. Standards for the diagnosis and treatment of patients with COPD: a summary of the ATS/ERS position paper. *Eur Respir J* 2004; 23:932–946.
2. Pride NB, Milic-Emili J. Lung mechanics. In: Calverley P, Pride NB (eds) Chronic Obstructive Lung Disease. Chapman & Hall, London, UK, 1995; pp 135–160.
3. Celli BR, Cote CG, Marin JM, Casanova C, Montes de Oca M, Mendez RA *et al.* The body-mass index, airflow obstruction, dyspnea, and exercise capacity index in chronic obstructive pulmonary disease. *N Engl J Med* 2004; 350:1005–1012.
4. Lapperre TS, Snoeck-Stroband JB, Gosman MME, Stolk J, Sont JK, Jansen DF, Kerstjens HAM, Postma DS, Sterk PJ, and the Groningen and Leiden Universities Corticosteroids in Obstructive Lung Disease (GLUCOLD) Study Group. Dissociation of lung function and airway inflammation in chronic obstructive pulmonary disease. *Am J Respir Crit Care Med* 2004; 170:499–504.
5. Barnes PJ. Small airways in COPD. *N Engl J Med* 2004; 350:2635–2637.
6. Barnes PJ, Kleinert S. COPD – a neglected disease. *Lancet* 2004; 364:564–565.
7. Milic-Emili J. Expiratory flow limitation. *Chest* 2004; 117:219S–223S.
8. Pauwels RA, Buist AS, Calverley PM, Jenkins CR, Hurd SS. The GOLD Scientific Committee. NHLBI/WHO Global Initiative for Chronic Obstructive Lung Disease (GOLD) Workshop Summary. *Am J Respir Crit Care Med* 2001; 163:1256–1276.
9. Global Initiative for Chronic Obstructive Lung Disease (GOLD). Global Strategy for the Diagnosis, Management, and Prevention of Chronic Obstructive Pulmonary Disease NHLBI/WHO Workshop report. NIH Publication update 2004.
10. NICE (National Institute for Clinical Excellence) Guideline on COPD. National clinical guideline on management of chronic obstructive pulmonary disease in adults in primary and secondary care. *Thorax* 2004; 59 (suppl 1).
11. O'Donnell DE, Aaron S, Bourbeau J, Hernandez P, Marciniuk D, Balter M *et al.* State of the art compendium: Canadian Thoracic Society recommendations for the management of chronic obstructive pulmonary disease. *Can Respir J* 2004; 11 (suppl B):7B–59B.
12. Mead J, Turner JM, Macklem PT, Little JB. Significance of the relationship between lung recoil and maximum expiratory flow. *J Appl Physiol* 1967; 22:95–108.
13. Pride NB, Permutt S, Riley RL, Bromberger-Barnea B. Determinants of maximal expiratory flow from the lungs. *J Appl Physiol* 1967; 23:646–662.
14. Hyatt RE. Expiratory flow limitation. *J Appl Physiol* 1983; 55:1–7.
15. Hogg JC. Pathophysiology of airflow limitation in chronic obstructive pulmonary disease. *Lancet* 2004; 364:709–721.
16. Cosio MG, Guerassimov A. Chronic obstructive pulmonary disease. Inflammation of small airways and lung parenchyma. *Am J Respir Crit Care Med* 1999; 160:S21–S25.
17. Fry DL, Hyatt RF. Pulmonary mechanics. A unified analysis of the relationship between pressure, volume and gasflow in the lungs of normal and diseased human subjects. *Am J Med* 1960; 29:672–689.
18. Hyatt RE. Forced expiration. In: Macklem PT, Mead J (eds) Handbook of Physiology, Section 3: The Respiratory System. Mechanics of Breathing, Part 1, vol. III. American Physiological Society, Bethesda, Maryland, 1986, chap. 19, pp 295–314.
19. Fletcher C, Peto R, Tinker C, Speizer FE. The natural history of chronic bronchitis and emphysema. Oxford: Oxford University Press, 1976.
20. Fletcher C, Peto R. The natural history of chronic airflow obstruction. *Br Med J* 1977; 1:1645–1648.
21. Barnes PJ. New concepts in chronic obstructive pulmonary disease. *Annu Rev Med* 2003; 54:113–129.
22. Calverley PMA, Walker P. Chronic obstructive pulmonary disease. *Lancet* 2003; 362:1053–1061.
23. Sutherland ER, Cherniack RM. Management of chronic obstructive pulmonary disease. *N Engl J Med* 2004; 350:2689–2697.

24. Viegi G, Pedreschi M, Pistelli F, Di Pede F, Baldacci S, Carozzi L, Giuntini C. Prevalence of airways obstruction in a general population: European Respiratory Society vs American Thoracic Society definition. *Chest* 2000; 117(5 suppl 2):339S–345S.

25. European Lung White Book. The first comprehensive survey on respiratory health in Europe. European Respiratory Society Journals, The Charlesworth Group, Huddersfield, UK, 2003.

26. Siafakas NM, Vermeire P, Pride NB, Paoletti P, Gibson J, Howard P *et al.* Optimal assessment and management of chronic obstructive pulmonary disease (COPD). The European Respiratory Society Task Force. *Eur Respir J* 1995; 8:1398–1420.

27. Tiffeneau R, Pinelli A. Air circulant et air captif dans l'exploration de la fonction ventilatrice pulmonaire. *Paris Méd* 1947; 37:624–628.

28. Hogg JC, Chu F, Utokaparch S, Woods R, Elliott WM, Buzatu L *et al.* The nature of small airway obstruction in chronic obstructive pulmonary disease. *N Engl J Med* 2004; 350:2645–2653.

29. D'Angelo E, Prandi E, Milic-Emili J. Dependence of maximal flow-volume curves on time-course of preceding inspiration. *J Appl Physiol* 1993; 75:1155–1159.

30. D'Angelo E, Prandi E, Marazzini L, Milic-Emili J. Dependence of maximal flow-volume curves on time-course of preceding inspiration in patients with chronic obstructive lung disease. *Am J Respir Crit Care Med* 1994; 150:1581–1586.

31. Milic-Emili J. Recent advances in spirometry and flow-volume loop. *Sem Respir Crit Care Med* 1998; 19:309–316.

32. Snider GL. 1. Changes in COPD occurrence. Chronic obstructive pulmonary disease: a definition and implications of structural determinants of airflow obstruction for epidemiology. *Am Rev Respir Dis* 1989; 140:S3–S8.

33. Cosio Piqueras MG, Cosio MG. Disease of the airways in chronic obstructive pulmonary disease. *Eur Respir J* 2001; 18(suppl 34):41S–49S.

34. Postma DS, Boezen HM. Rationale for the Dutch hypothesis. Allergy and airway hyperresponsiveness as genetic factors and their interaction with environment in the development of asthma and COPD. *Chest* 2004; 126(2 suppl):96S–104S.

35. Fabbri LM, Romagnoli M, Corbetta L, Casoni G, Busljetic K, Turato G *et al.* Differences in airway inflammation in patients with fixed airflow obstruction due to asthma or chronic obstructive pulmonary disease. *Am J Respir Crit Care Med* 2003; 167:418–424.

36. Dahl R, Greefhorst LAPM, Nowak D, Nonikov V, Byrne AM, Thomson MH, Till D, Della Cioppa G, on behalf of the Formoterol in Chronic Obstructive Pulmonary Disease I (FICOPD I) Study Group. Inhaled formoterol dry powder versus ipratropium bromide in chronic obstructive pulmonary disease. *Am J Respir Crit Care Med* 2001; 164:778–784.

37. Rennard SI, Anderson W, ZuWallack R, Broughton J, Bailey W, Friedman M *et al.* Use of a long-acting inhaled β_2-adrenergic agonist, salmeterol xinafoate, in patients with chronic obstructive pulmonary disease. *Am J Respir Crit Care Med* 2001; 163:1087–1092.

38. Rossi A, Kristufek P, Levine BE, Thomson MH, Till D, Kottakis J, Della Cioppa G, for the Formoterol in Chronic Obstructive Pulmonary Disease (FICOPD) II Study Group. Comparison of the efficacy, tolerability, and safety of formoterol dry powder and oral, slow-release theophylline in the treatment of COPD. *Chest* 2002; 121:1058–1069.

39. Hogg JC, Macklem PT, Thurlbeck WM. Site and nature of airway obstruction in chronic obstructive lung disease. *New Engl J Med* 1968; 278:1355–1360.

40. Macklem PT, Mead J. Resistance of central and peripheral airways measured by a retrograde catheter. *J Appl Physiol* 1967; 22:395–401.

41. Mead J, Whittenberger JL. Physical properties of human lungs measured during spontaneous respiration. *J Appl Physiol* 1953; 5:770–796.

42. Mead J. The lung's 'quiet zone'. *N Engl J Med* 1970; 282:1318–1319.

43. Barbera JA, Roca J, Ferrer A, Felez MA, Diaz O, Roger N, Rodriguez-Roisin R. Mechanisms of worsening gas exchange during acute exacerbations of chronic obstructive pulmonary disease. *Eur Respir J* 1997; 10:1285–1291.

44. Cosio M, Ghezzo H, Hogg JC, Corbin R, Loveland M, Dosman J, Macklem PT. The relations between structural change in small airways and pulmonary function tests. *N Engl J Med* 1978; 298:1277–1281.

45. Sadoul P, Milic-Emili J, Simonsson BG, Clark TJH (eds) Small Airways in Health and Disease. Proceedings of a symposium. Copenhagen, 29th–30th March 1979. Excerpta Medica, Amsterdam, 1979.

46. Dollfuss RE, Milic-Emili J, Bates DV. Regional ventilation of the lung studied with boluses of [133]xenon. *Respir Physiol* 1967; 2:234–246.

47. McCarthy DS, Spencer R, Greene R, Milic-Emili J. Measurement of 'closing volume' as a simple and sensitive test for early detection of small airway disease. *Am J Med* 1972; 52:747–753.

48. Despas PJM, Leroux M, Macklem PT. Site of airway obstruction in asthma as determined by measuring maximal expiratory flow breathing air and a helium-oxygen mixture. *J Clin Invest* 1972; 51:3235–3243.

49. Yanai M, Sekizawa K, Ohrui T, Sasaki H, Takishima T. Site of airway obstruction in pulmonary disease: direct measurement of intrabronchial pressure. *J Appl Physiol* 1992; 72:1016–1023.

50. Mead J, Lindgren I, Gaensler EA. The mechanical properties of the lungs in emphysema. *J Clin Invest* 1955; 34:1005–1016.

51. Gibson GJ, Pride NB, Davis J, Schroter RC. Exponential description of the static pressure-volume curve of normal and diseased lung. *Am Rev Respir Dis* 1979; 120:799–811.

52. Saetta M, Ghezzo H, Kim WD, King M, Angus GE, Wang NS, Cosio MG. Loss of alveolar attachments in smokers. A morphometric correlate of lung function impairment. *Am Rev Respir Dis* 1985; 132:894–900.

53. Kim WD, Eidelman DH, Izquierdo JL, Ghezzo H, Saetta MP, Cosio MG. Centrilobular and panlobular emphysema in smokers. *Am Rev Respir Dis* 1991; 144:1385–1390.

54. Finkelstein R, Ma H-D, Ghezzo H, Whittaker K, Fraser RS, Cosio MG. Morphometric of small airway in smokers and its relationship to emphysema type and hyperresponsiveness. *Am J Respir Crit Care Med* 1995, 152:267–276.

55. Pride NB, Macklem PT. Lung mechanics in disease. In: Macklem PT, Mead J (eds) Handbook of Physiology, Section 3: The Respiratory System. Mechanics of Breathing. Part 2, vol. III. American Physiological Society, Bethesda, Maryland, 1986, chap. 37, pp 659–692.

56. Tantucci C, Duguet A, Giampiccolo P, Similowski T, Zelter M, Derenne JP. The best peak expiratory flow is flow-limited and effort-independent in normal subjects. *Am J Respir Crit Care Med* 2002; 165:1304–1308.

57. Milic-Emili J. Lésions mécaniques des voies aériennes périphériques. Un rôle dans la pathogenèse de la BPCO chez les fumeurs? *Rev Mal Respir* 2003; 20:833–840.

58. Eltayara L, Becklake MR, Volta CA, Milic-Emili J. Relationship between chronic dyspnea and expiratory flow limitation in patients with chronic obstructive pulmonary disease. *Am J Respir Crit Care Med* 1996; 154:1726–1734.

59. Agostoni E. Statics. In: Campbell EJM, Agostoni E, Newsom Davis J (eds) The Respiratory Muscles. Mechanics and Neural Control. Second Edition. Lloyd-Luke (Medical Books) Ltd., London, 1970, chap. III, pp 48–79.

60. Tantucci C, Grassi V. Flow limitation: an overview. *Monaldi Arch Chest Dis* 1999; 54:353–357.

61. Rahn H, Otis AB, Chadwick LE, Fenn WO. The pressure-volume diagram of the thorax and lung. *Am J Physiol* 1946; 140:161–178.

62. Rossi A, Polese G, Brandi G. Dynamic Hyperinflation. In: Marini JJ, Roussos C (eds) Ventilatory Failure. *Update in Intensive Care and Emergency Medicine*, 15. Springer-Verlag, Berlin, Heidelberg, 1991, pp 199–218.

63. Calverley PM, Koulouris NG. Flow limitation and dynamic hyperinflation: key concepts in modern respiratory physiology. *Eur Respir J* 2005; 25:186–199.

64. Agostoni E, Mead J. Statics of the respiratory system. In: Macklem PT, Mead J (eds) Handbook of Physiology. Section 3. vol. I. The Respiratory System: Mechanics of Breathing. American Physiology Society, Bethesda, Maryland, 1964, pp 387–409.

65. Appendini L, Patessio A, Zanaboni S, Carone M, Gukov B, Donner CF, Rossi A. Physiologic effects of positive end expiratory pressure and mask pressure support during exacerbations of chronic obstructive pulmonary disease. *Am J Respir Crit Care Med* 1994; 149:1069–1076.

66. Dal Vecchio L, Polese G, Poggi R, Rossi A. 'Intrinsic' positive end-expiratory pressure in stable patients with chronic obstructive pulmonary disease. *Eur Respir J* 1990; 3:74–80.

67. Rossi A, Polese G, Brandi G, Conti G. Intrinsic positive end-expiratory pressure (PEEPi). *Intensive Care Med* 1995; 21:522–536.

68. Nucci G, Mergoni M, Briccchi C, Polese G, Cobelli C, Rossi A. On-line monitoring of intrinsic PEEP in ventilator-dependent patients. *J Appl Physiol* 2000; 89:985–995.

69. Tobin MJ, Brochard L, Rossi A. Assessment of Respiratory Muscle Function in the Intensive Care Unit, chap. 10, pp 610–619. In ATS/ERS Statement on Respiratory Muscle Testing. *Am J Respir Crit Care Med* 2002; 166:518–624.

70. Laghi F, Tobin MJ. Disorders of the respiratory muscles. *Am J Respir Crit Care Med* 2003; 168:10–48.

71. Sahebjami H, Sathianpitayakul E. Influence of body weight on the severity of dyspnea in chronic obstructive pulmonary disease. *Am J Respir Crit Care Med* 2000; 161:886–890.

72. Farkas GA, Roussos C. Adaptability of the hamster diaphragm to exercise and/or emphysema. *J Appl Physiol* 1982; 53:1263–1272.

73. Similowski T, Yan S, Gauthier AP, Macklem PT, Bellemare F. Contractile properties of the human diaphragm during chronic hyperinflation. *N Engl J Med* 1991; 325:917–923.

74. Rochester DF. The diaphragm in COPD. Better than expected, but not good enough. *N Engl J Med* 1991; 325:961–962.

75. Cerveri I, Dore R, Corsico A, Zoia MC, Pellegrino R, Brusasco V, Pozzi E. Assessment of emphysema in COPD: a functional and radiologic study. *Chest* 2004; 125:1714–1718.

76. Baldi S, Miniati M, Bellina CR, Battolla L, Catapano G, Begliomini E *et al*. Relationship between extent of pulmonary emphysema by high-resolution computed tomography and lung elastic recoil in patients with chronic obstructive pulmonary disease. *Am J Respir Crit Care Med* 2001; 164:585–589.

77. Newell JD, Jr, Hogg JC, Snider GL. Report of a workshop: quantitative computed tomography scanning in longitudinal studies of emphysema. *Eur Respir J* 2004; 23:769–775.

78. International Consensus Conferences in Intensive Care Medicine: Noninvasive Positive Pressure Ventilation in Acute Respiratory Failure. Organized jointly by the American Thoracic Society, the European Respiratory Society, the European Society of Intensive Care Medicine, and the Société de Réanimation de Langue Française, and approved by the ATS Board of Directors, December 2000. *Am J Respir Crit Care Med* 2001; 163:283–291.

79. Purro A, Appendini L, De Gaetano A, Gudjonsdottir M, Donner CF, Rossi A. Physiologic determinants of ventilator dependence in long-term mechanically ventilated patients. *Am J Respir Crit Care Med* 2000; 161(4 Pt 1):1115–1123.

80. Whitelaw WA, Derenne JP, Milic-Emili J. Occlusion pressure as a measure of respiratory center output in conscious man. *Respir Physiol* 1975; 23:181–199.

81. Milic-Emili J. Recent advances in clinical assessment of control of breathing. *Lung* 1982; 160:1–17.

82. Roussos CS, Macklem PT. Diaphragmatic fatigue in man. *J Appl Physiol* 1977; 43:189–197.

83. Vestbo J, Prescott E, Lange P. Association of chronic mucus hypersecretion with FEV1 decline and chronic obstructive pulmonary disease morbidity. Copenhagen City Heart Study Group. *Am J Respir Crit Care Med* 1996; 153:1530–1535.

84. Boni E, Corda L, Franchini D, Chiroli P, Damiani GP, Pini L *et al*. Volume effect and exertional dyspnoea after bronchodilator in patients with COPD with and without expiratory flow limitation at rest. *Thorax* 2002; 57:528–532.

85. Diaz O, Villafranca C, Ghezzo H, Borzone G, Leiva A, Milic-Emili J, Lisboa C. Role of inspiratory capacity on exercise tolerance in COPD patients with and without tidal expiratory flow limitation at rest. *Eur Respir J* 2000; 16:269–275.

86. Carlson DJ, Ries AL, Kaplan RM. Predicting maximal exercise tolerance in patients with COPD. *Chest* 1991; 100:307–311.

87. Casanova C, Cote C, de Torres JP, Aguirre-Jaime A, Marin JM, Pinto-Plata V, Celli BR. The inspiratory to total lung capacity ratio predicts mortality in patients with COPD. *Am J Respir Crit Care Med* 2004.

88. Murariu C, Ghezzo H, Milic-Emili J, Gautier H. Exercise limitation in obstructive lung disease. *Chest* 1998; 114:965–968.

89. Diaz O, Villafranca C, Ghezzo H, Borzone G, Leiva A, Milic-Emili J, Lisboa C. Breathing pattern and gas exchange at peak exercise in COPD patients with and without tidal flow limitation at rest. *Eur Respir J* 2001; 17:1120–1127.

90. O'Donnell DE, D'Arsigny C, Fitzpatrick M, Webb KA. Exercise hypercapnia in advanced chronic obstructive pulmonary disease. The role of lung hyperinflation. *Am J Respir Crit Care Med* 2002; 166:663–668.

91. O'Donnell DE, Lam M, Webb KA. Spirometric correlates of improvement in exercise performance after anti-cholinergic therapy in chronic obstructive pulmonary disease. *Am J Respir Crit Care Med* 1999; 160:542–549.

3

Beta-adrenoceptor agonists: basic pharmacology

L. B. Fernandes, P. J. Henry, R. G. Goldie

INTRODUCTION

β_2-Adrenoceptor agonist bronchodilators are widely used in the treatment of both chronic obstructive pulmonary disease (COPD) and asthma and provide rapid and effective bronchodilation. The primary role of this class of bronchodilators is to reverse airway smooth muscle contraction caused by a variety of excitatory airway mediators in these diseases.

COPD is a disease state characterised by airflow limitation that is not fully reversible. The limitation of airflow develops progressively and is usually associated with an abnormal inflammatory response of the lungs to noxious particles or gases. COPD is characterised by inflammation throughout the respiratory system, including bronchial and bronchiolar airways, parenchyma and pulmonary vasculature. Increased numbers of inflammatory cells [macrophages, T-lymphocytes (predominantly CD8$^+$) and neutrophils] in the airways is also a feature of this disease [1, 2]. Activation of inflammatory cells releases a variety of mediators, including leukotriene B$_4$ (LTB$_4$), interleukin-8 (IL-8) and tumour necrosis factor-α (TNF-α), that in turn contribute to widespread degenerative changes to the structure of the respiratory tract and promote neutrophilic inflammation [2–6]. An imbalance between proteases that digest elastin and other structural proteins and antiproteases that protect against this damage is thought to contribute to the progression of this disease [7]. Oxidative stress may also be involved in the pathogenesis of COPD. It is likely that cigarette smoke and other factors associated with COPD can initiate an inflammatory reaction in the airways that leads to this disease. The airflow obstruction seen in COPD patients is usually accompanied by airway hyperresponsiveness. This chronic airflow obstruction especially affects small airways, with lung elasticity also lost due to enzymatic destruction of the lung parenchyma, resulting in progressively worsening emphysema. COPD is characterised by shortness of breath, cough, sputum production and exercise limitation, with acute exacerbations resulting in worsening of symptoms. Inhaled bronchodilators, including β_2-adrenoceptor agonists, have been shown to ameliorate respiratory symptoms and improve the quality of life for COPD patients and are recommended in the management of acute exacerbations of this disease. Unfortunately, β_2-adrenoceptor agonists fail to provide lasting improvements in the deteriorating lung function seen in COPD.

Lynette B. Fernandes, BSc, PhD, Lecturer in Pharmacology, Western Australian Institute for Medical Research, Pharmacology Unit, School of Medicine & Pharmacology, The University of Western Australia, Australia.

Peter J. Henry, BSc, PhD, Senior Lecturer in Pharmacology, Western Australian Institute for Medical Research, Pharmacology Unit, School of Medicine & Pharmacology, The University of Western Australia, Australia.

Roy G. Goldie, BSc, PhD, Executive Dean, Faculty of Health Sciences, Western Australian Institute for Medical Research, Pharmacology Unit, School of Medicine & Pharmacology, The University of Western Australia, Australia.

Much of what is known of the basic and clinical pharmacology of β_2-adrenoceptor agonist bronchodilators was established in studies from the 1970s and 1980s. The actions of β_2-adrenoceptor agonists in the respiratory tract have been extensively reviewed by us [8]. However, significant advances in β_2-adrenoceptor agonist development and therapy in COPD and asthma have been made in recent years [9]. This review will focus on the basic pharmacology of β_2-adrenoceptor agonists, with a particular emphasis on COPD therapy.

THE β-ADRENOCEPTOR AND ITS ASSOCIATED SIGNAL TRANSDUCTION PROCESSES

β-ADRENOCEPTOR SUBTYPES

The β-adrenoceptor is a single polypeptide glycoprotein moiety [10], embedded in the plasma membrane of the cell [11]. Three functionally distinct subtypes of β-adrenoceptor (β_1, β_2, and β_3) are known to exist and have been cloned. β-Adrenoceptors are found throughout the human lung and are predominantly of the β_2-subtype. While small populations of β_1-adrenoceptors exist in airway smooth muscle, their functional significance is unclear [12, 13]. β_3-Adrenoceptors are unlikey to exist in the respiratory tract given that β_3-adrenoceptor mRNA has not been detected in human lung [14] and β_3-adrenoceptor agonists failed to induce airway smooth muscle relaxation in human isolated bronchi [15].

ADENYLYL CYCLASE

Agonist binding to all β-adrenoceptor subtypes activates membrane-bound adenylyl cyclase *via* a guanine nucleotide regulatory protein (G_s) to convert adenosine 5′-triphosphate (ATP) to cyclic adenosine 3′, 5′-monophosphate (cAMP) [16] (Figure 3.1). cAMP is produced continuously following β-adrenoceptor activation and is inactivated by hydrolysis to 5′-AMP, *via* the action of phosphodiesterases. cAMP acts as an intracellular messenger to regulate many aspects of cellular function including those of smooth muscle contractile proteins. Thus, cAMP activates cAMP-dependent protein kinases to modify cellular enzyme function *via* protein phosphorylation. For example, phosphorylation, and thus inactivation, of myosin light chain kinase reduces its kinase activity which precludes its interaction with contractile protein

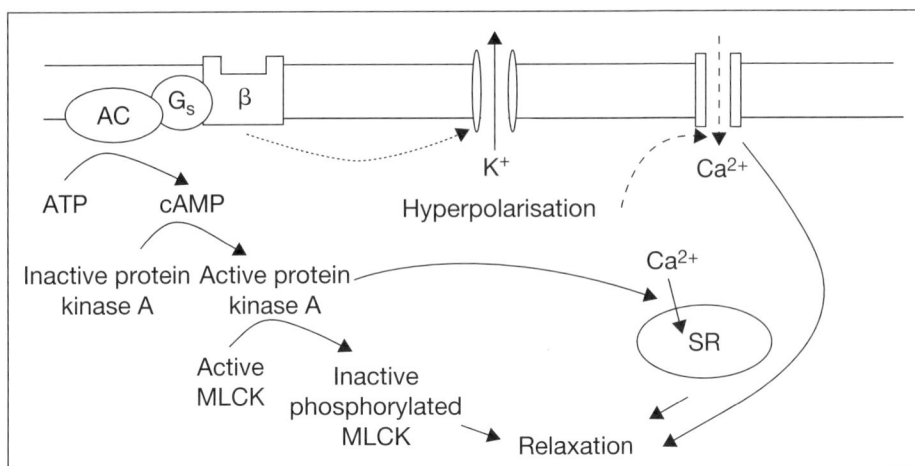

Figure 3.1   Main pathways promoting airway smooth muscle relaxation associated with the β-adrenoceptor-effector system. The dashed lines indicate inhibition of Ca^{2+} entry into the cell *via* voltage-gated Ca^{2+} channels. The dotted line indicates that the exact mechanism is yet to be defined [adapted from 17].

myosin and promotes relaxation of airway smooth muscle [17]. In addition, β-adrenoceptor agonists may also decrease airway smooth muscle tone *via* an interaction with plasma membrane potassium channels (Figure 3.1). This results in hyperpolarisation of the cell membrane and inhibition of calcium influx *via* voltage-dependent calcium channels [18].

DISTRIBUTION AND DENSITY OF β-ADRENOCEPTORS IN THE PERIPHERAL LUNG

Radioligand binding and autoradiographic studies have been critical to evaluations of the distribution of β-adrenoceptors in both animal and human lung tissue. Over 25 years ago, the presence of high densities of β-adrenoceptors was demonstrated in rabbit and rat lung membranes [19] and in human lung membrane preparations [20]. Subsequent studies in guinea-pig [21, 22] and hamster lung [23] confirmed that the lung was densely populated with β-adrenoceptors. Furthermore, lung parenchyma contained heterogeneous populations of both β$_1$- and β$_2$-adrenoceptors [22, 24, 25]. However, the most important information, i.e., the location of these receptors within the normal structure of the lung, was not revealed in detail until autoradiographic assessments were completed. Light-microscopic autoradiography [26] enabled the detection and localisation of β-adrenoceptor subtypes in airways and lung parenchyma from many animal species including ferret [27], guinea-pig [28], rabbit [29], rat [30], mouse [31] and pig [28] as well as from the human [32, 33].

In human lung, the greatest density of β-adrenoceptors was found in alveolar septae [34]. Approximately 78% of the total human lung tissue volume consists of alveolar tissue, with only 8% being vascular smooth muscle, 3% is airway smooth muscle and the remaining 11% is connective tissue and cartilage [35]. Furthermore, β-adrenoceptor numbers were 3 times higher in the alveolar wall than over bronchial smooth muscle and 1.4 times higher than over bronchiolar smooth muscle. Thus, approximately 96% of the β-adrenoceptor population was located in alveolar tissue. However, as might be expected, significant numbers of β-adrenoceptors were found in bronchial and bronchiolar airway smooth muscle, as well as in airway epithelium and in vascular endothelium and smooth muscle.

β-ADRENOCEPTOR AGONISTS

ADRENALINE

The β$_2$-adrenoceptor agonists used in the therapy of both COPD and asthma are all derivatives of the endogenous catecholamine adrenaline (Figure 3.2). Although adrenaline activates α- and β$_1$-adrenoceptors, it is the powerful β$_2$-adrenoceptor-mediated effects of adrenaline that are most important. Adrenaline is not effective when taken orally since it is rapidly metabolised by gastrointestinal and hepatic monoamine oxidase (MAO). Accordingly, adrenaline is administered by parenteral (subcutaneous) injection if required in emergency conditions.

ISOPRENALINE

This N-isopropyl derivative of adrenaline has no significant agonist effect at α-adrenoceptors and was the first β-adrenoceptor-selective agonist introduced into asthma therapy. Isoprenaline, like adrenaline, is also a catecholamine and so is not useful orally since it is metabolised rapidly by catechol-O-methyltransferase (COMT). However, significant cardiac stimulation induced *via* activation of β$_1$-adrenoceptors, even after inhalational administration, reduces its acceptability as a bronchodilator.

SELECTIVE β$_2$-ADRENOCEPTOR AGONISTS

The development and introduction of β$_2$-adrenoceptor-selective agonists that could be given orally or by inhalation and had extended durations of action compared with adrenaline or

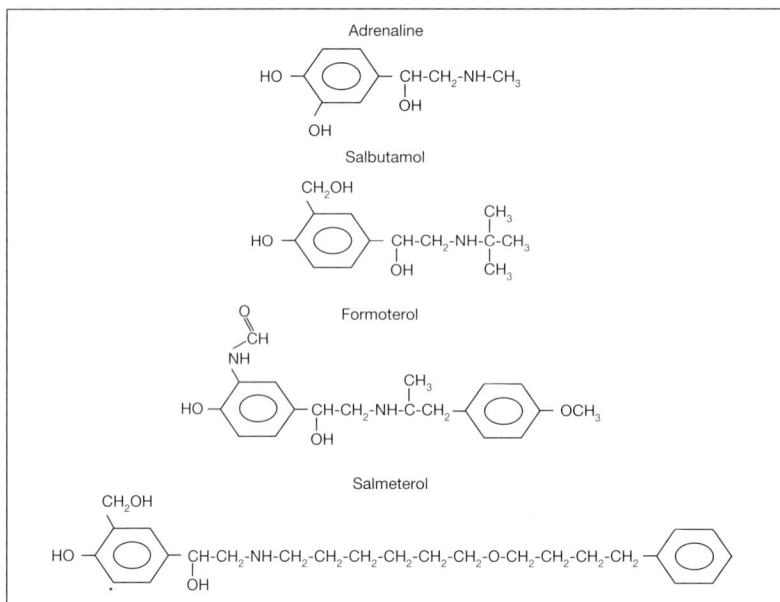

Figure 3.2 β-Adrenoceptor agonists.

isoprenaline was a major therapeutic advance. Orciprenaline, the first of this new generation of bronchodilator amines, is a resorcinol derivative rather than a catecholamine and
thus is not inactivated by extraneuronal COMT. Furthermore, this tertiary amine is not
metabolised by MAO. Although orciprenaline is metabolised by sulpho-conjugation,
enough free drug is absorbed to make it an effective oral bronchodilator. However, selectivity for the β_2-adrenoceptor is only slightly improved over that of isoprenaline [36] and thus
activation of cardiovascular β-adrenoceptors remains an issue in terms of the production of
unwanted side-effects.

Salbutamol [37], terbutaline [38] and fenoterol [39] possess much greater selectivity for
β_2-adrenoceptors than orciprenaline. These compounds are active orally, as well as by
inhalation and intravenous injection. All of the newer orally active β_2-adrenoceptor agonists
are used in various inhalation formulations. The great virtue of being able to administer
these new β_2-adrenoceptor agonists by inhalation is that small but highly effective doses can
be delivered to the lung giving the desired therapeutic effect rapidly (onset 5–10 min) and
with an extended duration of action (up to 6 h). Administration of these therapies by inhalation also results in negligible plasma concentrations of the active drug. Concerns over the
negative impact of the chronic use of fenoterol in asthmatics resulted in its restricted therapeutic use [40].

LONG-ACTING β_2-ADRENOCEPTOR AGONISTS

Members of the first generation of β_2-adrenoceptor-selective agonist bronchodilators, such
as salbutamol, are considered to be short-acting since they have a duration of action of
4–6 h. These agents are effective and provide rapid symptom relief in a large proportion of
patients. However, in some patients, these short-acting drugs need to be administered several times a day for adequate symptom relief. In addition, treatment of nocturnal symptoms
in susceptible patients may be problematic given the relatively short duration of action of
these drugs. In order to provide effective treatment in individuals whose symptoms were

not adequately managed with short-acting agents, β_2-adrenoceptor agonist bronchodilators were developed that had durations of action of up to 12 h.

Salmeterol [41] (Figure 3.2) was specifically designed to prolong the duration of action of the short-acting β_2-adrenoceptor agonist salbutamol. While formoterol (Figure 3.2) was not deliberately designed to have this property, it was found to have a 12-h duration of action when administered by inhalation [42]. The agonist activity profiles of formoterol and salmeterol are distinct, suggesting that the extended duration of action of these agents is achieved *via* different mechanisms. Furthermore, salmeterol is a partial β_2-adrenoceptor agonist, whereas formoterol has higher intrinsic activity and is a full agonist [43, 44]. Unlike salbutamol, which is hydrophilic, both salmeterol and formoterol possess lipophilic properties which allow them to remain in airway tissues in close proximity to β_2-adrenoceptors. This partly explains why the duration of action of these long-acting β_2-adrenoceptor agonist bronchodilators is at least 12 h. In addition to being lipophilic, formoterol is also water soluble, ensuring rapid access to the β_2-adrenoceptor and thus rapid bronchodilator activity. The exact mechanism by which formoterol exerts its prolonged effects is unclear but may result from its lipophilicity, allowing formoterol to enter the plasma membrane where it is held for a prolonged period. From this site, formoterol diffuses over time to activate the β_2-adrenoceptor. Inhaled formoterol has also been shown to have a longer duration of action than orally administered formoterol, probably as a result of high concentrations building in the bronchial periciliary fluid [45]. In contrast, salmeterol, being highly lipophilic, probably diffuses more slowly to the β_2-adrenoceptor laterally through the cell membrane and has a slower onset of action [46, 47]. Salmeterol contains the saligenin head of salbutamol that binds to the active site of the β_2-adrenoceptor. This saligenin head is coupled to a long aliphatic side chain that significantly increases the lipophilicity of salmeterol. The side chain then binds to a discrete 'exosite' that anchors it to the receptor and enables repetitive receptor activation [48].

DELIVERY OF β_2-ADRENOCEPTOR AGONISTS

The metered dose inhaler (MDI) is the most commonly prescribed patient-operated device for the delivery of COPD and asthma therapies that include β_2-adrenoceptor agonists. The popularity of the MDI is by virtue of its effectiveness and ability to deliver a wide range of drugs [49]. Indeed, salbutamol, when administered *via* MDI and spacer, is as effective and more cost effective when compared with delivery *via* a nebuliser [50]. MDIs were formulated with a combination of the chlorofluorocarbon (CFC) propellants 11 and 12. However, due to the ozone-depleting potential of CFCs, the ozone-friendly propellant hydrofluoroalkane 134a (HFA 134a) has now replaced CFCs. Studies have demonstrated that the effectiveness and safety of salbutamol/HFA 134a is comparable to that of salbutamol/CFC [51, 52].

SITES OF THERAPEUTIC ACTION

AIRWAY SMOOTH MUSCLE

Both contraction studies *in vitro* [53] and autoradiographic studies have confirmed that β_2-adrenoceptors are expressed and mediate relaxation to β-adrenoceptor agonists in human airway smooth muscle [33]. Agonist stimulation of β_2-adrenoceptors reverses airway obstruction primarily by causing relaxation of central and peripheral airway smooth muscle. However, given that β_2-adrenoceptors are widely distributed throughout the lung, the beneficial actions of β_2-adrenoceptor agonists may in part be the result of actions at other sites. For example, reversal or blunting of the actions of inflammatory mediators causing airway wall oedema would be expected to relieve that component of bronchial obstruction.

INFLAMMATORY CELLS

It has long been known that β_2-adrenoceptors are expressed on inflammatory cells including mast cells [54, 55], peripheral blood lymphocytes [56–58], polymorphonuclear leukocytes [59–61], peritoneal macrophages [62], alveolar macrophages, [63], platelets [64] and eosinophils [57, 65]. The established effects of β_2-adrenoceptor stimulation in some of these cells may be relevant to the therapeutic benefits of these agents in COPD and asthma.

The relatively short-acting β_2-adrenoceptor agonist bronchodilators such as salbutamol and terbutaline have been shown to suppress pro-inflammatory mediator release from inflammatory cells in vitro. For example, in the case of lymphocytes, inhibition of lymphokine secretion (and of proliferation) is well established [66, 67]. In polymorphonuclear leukocytes, inhibition of superoxide radical generation and leukotriene release has been reported [68, 69]. In the case of human lung mast cells, salbutamol is a potent inhibitor of antigen-induced release of histamine and leukotrienes [70, 71]. Indeed, salbutamol is 10–100 times more potent than disodium cromoglycate in this regard [72]. However, while the early response to allergen is inhibited by β_2-adrenoceptor agonists, their impact on the late response is much less impressive [73]. Thus, the anti-inflammatory effect of monotherapy with inhaled, short-acting β_2-adrenoceptor agonist bronchodilators is minimal [74–76]. Accordingly, it is generally accepted that it is the airway smooth muscle relaxant activity of β_2-adrenoceptor agonists that is the action of primary importance in COPD and asthma.

The advent of long acting β_2-adrenoceptor agonist bronchodilators such as formoterol and salmeterol has re-ignited the question of whether or not a real therapeutic benefit is obtained in terms of the suppression of mediator release from inflammatory cells, even though these agents are also delivered by inhalation. It could be argued that the longer duration of action of these agents increases the likelihood of such an effect. Predictably, long-acting β_2-adrenoceptor agonists have been shown in animal studies both in vivo and in vitro to effectively suppress pro-inflammatory mediator release and cytokine production and/or release from inflammatory cells. These actions have been demonstrated in human and/or animal T-lymphocytes [77], macrophages [78], mast cells [79–81], eosinophils [82, 83] and neutrophils [84]. Furthermore, these agonists are also known to inhibit chemotaxis and recruitment of eosinophils [82, 85, 86] and to delay apoptosis in these cells [87]. However, it is now clear that monotherapy with long-acting agents such as salmeterol does not provide any significant anti-inflammatory effect [88, 89].

EPITHELIUM AND SECRETORY CELLS

The deleterious impact of mucous hypersecretion and impaired mucociliary clearance on the effective bronchial lumen diameter and thus on bronchial airflow, can be life-threatening in severe COPD and asthma. Submucosal glands in human airways contain β_2-adrenoceptors [32], the stimulation of which increases mucus secretion. Furthermore, the systemic administration of β-adrenoceptor agonists in rats has been shown to increase secretory cell numbers in the airway [90], an effect that would be detrimental to effective mucociliary clearance. Furthermore, the transport of water and ions across the airway epithelium is critical to the maintenance of a sufficient liquid layer on the surface of the airways as well as effective mucociliary clearance. β_2-Adrenoceptor agonists have been shown to stimulate chloride ion and hence water secretion towards the lumen [91]. Importantly, β_2-adrenoceptor agonists also stimulate increases in ciliary beat frequency in vitro [92, 93] and in vivo [94]. β_2-Adrenoceptor-mediated increases in water on the surface of the airways and cilia beat frequency both enhance mucociliary clearance. However, in patients with significantly damaged bronchial epithelium it seems likely that cilia function will be impaired, raising the possibility that in some patients β_2-adrenoceptor agonist-stimulated mucous secretion could be detrimental. It is important to note, however, that airway smooth muscle is the primary site of therapeutic action, with lower doses of β_2-adrenoceptor agonist required to produce bronchodilatation compared with enhanced mucociliary clearance [95].

Pathogens such as *Pseudomonas aeruginosa* and *Haemophilus influenzae* colonise the respiratory tract, causing damage to and loss of airway epithelium. Indeed, *Pseudomonas aeruginosa*, which frequently colonises the respiratory tract, contains pyocyanin and elastase that disrupt airway epithelium as well as slow cilia beat frequency in human nasal respiratory epithelium *in vitro* [96]. Importantly, salmeterol reduced epithelial damage caused by *Pseudomonas aeruginosa* and *Haemophilus influenzae* [97, 98] and attenuated pyocyanin-induced slowing of cilia beat frequency [99, 100]. These data suggest that β_2-adrenoceptor agonists may protect epithelial function in the presence of respiratory pathogens.

Damage to airway epithelium, in a similar manner to other tissue systems, initiates repair processes that require migration of bronchial epithelial cells from the edge of the wound in order to restore the epithelial layer. That isoprenaline has been found to increase bronchial epithelial cell migration *in vitro* [101], suggests that β_2-adrenoceptor agonists may hasten airway epithelial repair following insults due to, for example, respiratory tract viral infections.

COMBINATION THERAPY

LONG-ACTING β_2-ADRENOCEPTOR AGONISTS AND GLUCOCORTICOIDS

The scientific rationale for the use of long-acting β_2-adrenoceptor agonists in combination with a corticosteroid has recently been summarised [102]. The use of long-acting β_2-adrenoceptor agonists has been examined in asthmatic patients whose symptoms persisted despite treatment with low-dose glucocorticoids [103–105]. Patients suffering from moderate-to-severe COPD may benefit from regular inhaled glucocorticoid treatment [106, 107]. These studies demonstrate that interactions between β_2-adrenoceptor agonists and glucocorticoids are predominantly positive, with combinations of the two drugs improving airway limitation and exacerbation rates in COPD and asthma patients. While this is particularly true for long-acting β_2-adrenoceptor agonists, the exact mechanism remains unclear. For example, the effects of long-acting β_2-adrenoceptor agonists and glucocorticoids may be merely additive; with the former causing prolonged bronchodilation and the latter reducing or reversing airway inflammation. Alternately, there may be true synergy between these agents with long-acting β_2-adrenoceptor agonists enhancing the effects of glucocorticoids [102, 108]. It has been suggested that long-acting β_2-adrenoceptor agonists may have 'steroid-enhancing' or 'steroid-sparing' effects. However, it is important to note that monotherapy with long-acting β_2-adrenoceptor agonists is less effective than inhaled glucocorticoids alone, suggesting that these terms need to be used cautiously [109].

Based on the complementary roles of β_2-adrenoceptor agonists and glucocorticoids, the long-acting β_2-adrenoceptor agonist salmeterol and the glucocorticoid fluticasone have been combined in a single inhaler with the potential to treat both the airway smooth muscle dysfunction and inflammatory components of COPD and asthma. Such combination products have the potential to limit overuse of β_2-adrenoceptor agonist bronchodilators in the absence of anti-inflammatory therapy, thus ensuring that β_2-adrenoceptor agonists are not used as monotherapy in moderate-to-severe COPD patients. However, the use of 'fixed' combination inhalers may be associated with the overuse of both drugs in disease management as control over individual drug dosages is lost.

DUAL D_2-RECEPTOR AND β_2-ADRENOCEPTOR AGONISTS

A different approach to combination therapy is to incorporate multiple pharmacological actions within the one drug molecule. Airway hyperreactivity, a feature of both COPD and asthma, is associated with neural reflex pathways that include sensory afferent nerves.

While the receptors that modulate the activity of these airway nerves have yet to be characterised, reflex nerve activity may be controlled by modulating the activity of afferent nerves. For example, dopamine, *via* stimulation of D_2-receptors, may play a role in the control of lung function by reducing the ability of sensory nerves to produce harmful reflex activity. Indeed, D_2-receptor mRNA has been detected in rat vagal afferent neurones [110] and dorsal root ganglia [111], nerves associated with reflex pathways. Thus, D_2-receptor agonists should reduce reflex bronchoconstriction, dyspnoea, cough and mucus production, without any direct bronchodilator activity. A dual dopamine D_2-receptor and β_2-adrenoceptor agonist was hoped to combine the modulating effects of a dopamine D_2-receptor agonist on sensory afferent nerves with the bronchodilator action of a β_2-adrenoceptor agonist in the one molecule. The dual dopamine D_2-receptor and β_2-adrenoceptor agonist sibenadet (Viozan) has now been investigated for its efficacy in relieving COPD symptoms [112, 113]. However, while sibenadet was well tolerated, there was a lack of sustained benefit in clinical studies resulting in development of this drug being discontinued [112].

CONCLUSIONS

The airway smooth muscle relaxant effect of β_2-adrenoceptor agonists is their primary beneficial action in COPD and asthma, although positive therapeutic influences on mucus production and clearance and bronchial oedema may also occur. β_2-Adrenoceptor agonists appear to be largely ineffective in suppressing or controlling airway inflammation in asthmatics and are likely to be equally ineffective in COPD patients. Unfortunately, in COPD, bronchodilator therapies do not alter the long-term decline in lung function. However, β_2-adrenoceptor agonist bronchodilators and anticholinergics and theophylline, given alone or in combination, can relieve symptoms and help to reverse exacerbations. The introduction of long-acting β_2-adrenoceptor agonists has produced significant improvements in symptoms in COPD patients and thus has had a positive impact on quality of life in these patients. The use of combination bronchodilator/corticosteroid regimes further assists in the management of this disease.

REFERENCES

1.   Jeffery PK. Structural and inflammatory changes in COPD: a comparison with asthma. *Thorax* 1998; 53:129–136.
2.   Pesci A, Balbi B, Majori M, Cacciani G, Bertacco S, Alciato P, Donner CF. Inflammatory cells and mediators in bronchial lavage of patients with chronic obstructive pulmonary disease. *Eur Respir J* 1998; 12:380–386.
3.   Keatings VM, Collins PD, Scott DM, Barnes PJ. Differences in interleukin-8 and tumor necrosis factor-alpha in induced sputum from patients with chronic obstructive pulmonary disease or asthma. *Am J Respir Crit Care Med* 1996; 153:530–534.
4.   Mueller R, Chanez P, Campbell AM, Bousquet J, Heusser C, Bullock GR. Different cytokine patterns in bronchial biopsies in asthma and chronic bronchitis. *Respir Med* 1996; 90:79–85.
5.   Yamamoto C, Yoneda T, Yoshikawa M, Fu A, Tokuyama T, Tsukaguchi K, Narita N. Airway inflammation in COPD assessed by sputum levels of interleukin-8. *Chest* 1997; 112:505–510.
6.   Hill AT, Bayley D, Stockley RA. The interrelationship of sputum inflammatory markers in patients with chronic bronchitis. *Am J Respir Crit Care Med* 1999; 160:893–898.
7.   Chapman HA, Jr., Shi GP. Protease injury in the development of COPD: Thomas A. Neff Lecture. *Chest* 2000; 117:S295–S299.
8.   Goldie RG, Paterson JW, Lulich KM. Pharmacology and therapeutics of beta-adrenoceptor agonists. In: Page CP, Barnes PJ (eds) Handbook of Experimental Pharmacology. Vol 98. Springer-Verlag, Berlin, 1991; pp 167–205.
9.   Fernandes LB, Henry PJ, Goldie RG. β-Adrenoceptor agonists. In: Page CP, Barnes PJ (eds) Handbook of Experimental Pharmacology. Vol 161. Pharmacology and Therapeutics of Asthma and COPD. Springer, Berlin, 2004; pp 3–35.

10. Gilman AG. G proteins: transducers of receptor-generated signals. *Annu Rev Biochem* 1987; 56:615–649.

11. Stiles GL, Caron MG, Lefkowitz RJ. Beta-adrenergic receptors: biochemical mechanisms of physiological regulation. *Physiol Rev* 1984; 64:661–743.

12. Harms HH. Isoproterenol antagonism of cardioselective beta adrenergic receptor blocking agents: a comparative study of human and guinea-pig cardiac and bronchial beta adrenergic receptors. *J Pharmacol Exp Ther* 1976; 199:329–335.

13. Goldie RG, Spina D, Henry PJ, Lulich KM, Paterson JW. *In vitro* responsiveness of human asthmatic bronchus to carbachol, histamine, beta-adrenoceptor agonists and theophylline. *Br J Clin Pharmacol* 1986b; 22:669–676.

14. Mak JC, Nishikawa M, Haddad EB, Kwon OJ, Hirst SJ, Twort CH, Barnes PJ. Localisation and expression of beta-adrenoceptor subtype mRNAs in human lung. *Eur J Pharmacol* 1996; 302: 215–221.

15. Martin CA, Naline E, Bakdach H, Advenier C. Beta3-adrenoceptor agonists, BRL 37344 and SR 58611A, do not induce relaxation of human, sheep and guinea-pig airway smooth muscle *in vitro*. *Eur Respir J* 1994; 7:1610–1615.

16. Benovic JL, Pike LJ, Cerione RA, Staniszewski C, Yoshimasa T, Codina J *et al*. Phosphorylation of the mammalian beta-adrenergic receptor by cyclic AMP-dependent protein kinase. Regulation of the rate of receptor phosphorylation and dephosphorylation by agonist occupancy and effects on coupling of the receptor to the stimulatory guanine nucleotide regulatory protein. *J Biol Chem* 1985; 260:7094–7101.

17. Thirstrup S. Control of airway smooth muscle tone: II-pharmacology of relaxation. *Respir Med* 2000; 94:519–528.

18. Kume H, Hall IP, Washabau RJ, Takagi K, Kotlikoff MI. Beta-adrenergic agonists regulate Kca channels in airway smooth muscle by cAMP-dependent and -independent mechanisms. *J Clin Invest* 1994; 93:371–379.

19. Rugg EL, Barnett DB, Nahorski SR. Coexistence of beta1 and beta2 adrenoceptors in mammalian lung: evidence from direct binding studies. *Mol Pharmacol* 1978; 14:996–1005.

20. Szentivanyi A. The conformational flexibility of adrenoceptors and the constitutional basis of atopy. *Triangle* 1979; 18:109–115.

21. Barnes PJ, Karliner JS, Dollery CT. Human lung adrenoreceptors studied by radioligand binding. *Clin Sci* 1980; 58:457–461.

22. Engel G, Hoyer D, Berthold R, Wagner H. (+/−)[^{125}Iodo]-cyanopindolol, a new ligand for β-adrenoceptors. Identification and quantitation of subclasses of β adrenoceptors in guinea-pig. *Naunyn Schmiedebergs Arch Pharmacol* 1981; 317:277–285.

23. Benovic JL, Stiles GL, Lefkowitz RJ, Caron MG. Photoaffinity labelling of mammalian beta-adrenergic receptors: metal-dependent proteolysis explains apparent heterogeneity. *Biochem Biophys Res Commun* 1983; 110:504–511.

24. Dickinson K, Richardson A, Nahorski SR. Homogeneity of beta2-adrenoceptors on rat erythrocytes and reticulocytes. A comparison with heterogeneous rat lung beta-adrenoceptors. *Mol Pharmacol* 1981; 19:194–204.

25. Carswell H, Nahorski SR. Beta-adrenoceptor heterogeneity in guinea-pig airways: comparison of functional and receptor labelling studies. *Br J Pharmacol* 1983; 79:965–971.

26. Young WS, 3rd, Kuhar MJ. A new method for receptor autoradiography. *Brain Res* 1979; 179:255–270.

27. Barnes PJ, Basbaum CB, Nadel JA, Roberts JM. Localization of beta-adrenoreceptors in mammalian lung by light microscopic autoradiography. *Nature* 1982; 299:444–447.

28. Goldie RG, Papadimitriou JM, Paterson JW, Rigby PJ, Spina D. Autoradiographic localization of beta-adrenoceptors in pig lung using [^{125}I]-iodocyanopindolol. *Br J Pharmacol* 1986a; 88:621–628.

29. Barnes P, Jacobs M, Roberts JM. Glucocorticoids preferentially increase fetal alveolar beta-adrenoreceptors: autoradiographic evidence. *Pediatr Res* 1984; 18:1191–1194.

30. Finkel MS, Quirion R, Pert C, Patterson RE. Characterization and autoradiographic distribution of the beta-adrenergic receptor in the rat lung. *Pharmacology* 1984; 29:247–254.

31. Henry PJ, Rigby PJ, Goldie RG. Distribution of beta1- and beta2-adrenoceptors in mouse trachea and lung: a quantitative autoradiographic study. *Br J Pharmacol* 1990; 99:136–144.

32. Carstairs JR, Nimmo AJ, Barnes PJ. Autoradiographic visualization of beta-adrenoceptor subtypes in human lung. *Am Rev Respir Dis* 1985; 132:541–547.

33. Spina D, Rigby PJ, Paterson JW, Goldie RG. Autoradiographic localization of beta-adrenoceptors in asthmatic human lung. *Am Rev Respir Dis* 1989; 140:1410–1415.

34. Carstairs JR, Nimmo AJ, Barnes PJ. Autoradiographic localisation of beta-adrenoceptors in human lung. *Eur J Pharmacol* 1984; 103:189–190.

35. Bertram JF, Goldie RG, Papadimitriou JM, Paterson JW. Correlations between pharmacological responses and structure of human lung parenchyma strips. *Br J Pharmacol* 1983; 80:107–114.

36. McEvoy JD, Vall-Spinosa A, Paterson JW. Assessment of orciprenaline and isoproterenol infusions in asthmatic patients. *Am Rev Respir Dis* 1973; 108:490–500.

37. Brittain RT, Farmer JB, Jack D, Martin LE, Simpson WT. α-[-(*t*-butylamino)methyl]-4-hydroxy-*m*-xylene-α^1,α^3-diol (AH.3365) a selective β-adrenergic stimulant. *Nature* 1968; 219:862–863.

38. Bergman J, Persson H, Wetterlin K. 2 new groups of selective stimulants of adrenergic beta-receptors. *Experientia* 1969; 25:899–901.

39. Sasaki T, Takishima T, Sugiura R. Comparison of fenoterol and orciprenaline with regard to broncho-dilating action and beta2-selectivity. *J Int Med Res* 1980; 8:205–216.

40. Beasley R, Pearce N, Crane J, Burgess C. Withdrawal of fenoterol and the end of the New Zealand asthma mortality epidemic. *Int Arch Allergy Immunol* 1995; 107:325–327.

41. Ullman A, Svedmyr N. Salmeterol, a new long acting inhaled beta2 adrenoceptor agonist: comparison with salbutamol in adult asthmatic patients. *Thorax* 1988; 43:674–678.

42. Hekking PR, Maesen F, Greefhorst A, Prins J, Tan Y, Zweers P. Long-term efficacy of formoterol compared to salbutamol. *Lung* 1990; 168:76–82.

43. Linden A, Bergendal A, Ullman A, Skoogh BE, Lofdahl CG. Salmeterol, formoterol, and salbutamol in the isolated guinea-pig trachea: differences in maximum relaxant effect and potency but not in functional antagonism. *Thorax* 1993; 48:547–553.

44. Naline E, Zhang Y, Qian Y, Mairon N, Anderson GP, Grandordy B, Advenier C. Relaxant effects and durations of action of formoterol and salmeterol on the isolated human bronchus. *Eur Respir J* 1994; 7:914–920.

45. Anderson GP, Linden A, Rabe KF. Why are long-acting beta-adrenoceptor agonists long-acting? *Eur Respir J* 1994; 7:569–578.

46. Lotvall J. Pharmacological similarities and differences between beta2-agonists. *Respir Med* 2001; 95:S7–S11.

47. Kottakis J, Cioppa GD, Creemers J, Greefhorst L, Lecler V, Pistelli R *et al.* Faster onset of bronchodilation with formoterol than with salmeterol in patients with stable, moderate to severe COPD: results of a randomized, double-blind clinical study. *Can Respir J* 2002; 9:107–115.

48. Green SA, Spasoff AP, Coleman RA, Johnson M, Liggett SB. Sustained activation of a G protein-coupled receptor *via* "anchored" agonist binding. Molecular localization of the salmeterol exosite within the β2-adrenergic receptor. *J Biol Chem* 1996; 271:24029–24035.

49. Woodcock A. Continuing patient care with metered-dose inhalers. *J Aerosol Med* 1995;8:S5–S10.

50. Newman KB, Milne S, Hamilton C, Hall K. A comparison of albuterol administered by metered-dose inhaler and spacer with albuterol by nebulizer in adults presenting to an urban emergency department with acute asthma. *Chest* 2002; 121:1036–1041.

51. Hawksworth RJ, Sykes AP, Faris M, Mant T, Lee TH. Albuterol HFA is as effective as albuterol CFC in preventing exercise-induced bronchoconstriction. *Ann Allergy Asthma Immunol* 2002; 88:473–477.

52. Langley SJ, Sykes AP, Batty EP, Masterson CM, Woodcock A. A comparison of the efficacy and tolerability of single doses of HFA 134a albuterol and CFC albuterol in mild-to-moderate asthmatic patients. *Ann Allergy Asthma Immunol* 2002; 88:488–493.

53. Goldie RG, Paterson JW, Wale JL. Pharmacological responses of human and porcine lung parenchyma, bronchus and pulmonary artery. *Br J Pharmacol* 1982; 76:515–521.

54. Butchers PR, Skidmore IF, Vardey CJ, Wheeldon A. Characterization of the receptor mediating the antianaphylactic effects of beta-adrenoceptor agonists in human lung tissue *in vitro*. *Br J Pharmacol* 1980; 71:663–667.

55. Hughes JM, Seale JP, Temple DM. Effect of fenoterol on immunological release of leukotrienes and histamine from human lung *in vitro*: selective antagonism by beta-adrenoceptor antagonists. *Eur J Pharmacol* 1983; 95:239–245.

56. Williams LT, Snyderman R, Lefkowitz RJ. Identification of beta-adrenergic receptors in human lymphocytes by (–) (3H) alprenolol binding. *J Clin Invest* 1976; 57:149–155.

57. Koeter GH, Meurs H, Kauffman HF, de Vries K. The role of the adrenergic system in allergy and bronchial hyperreactivity. *Eur J Respir Dis Suppl* 1982; 121:72–78.

58. Sano Y, Watt G, Townley RG. Decreased mononuclear cell beta-adrenergic receptors in bronchial asthma: parallel studies of lymphocyte and granulocyte desensitization. *J Allergy Clin Immunol* 1983; 72:495–503.

59. Galant SP, Duriseti L, Underwood S, Allred S, Insel PA. Beta adrenergic receptors of polymorphonuclear particulates in bronchial asthma. *J Clin Invest* 1980; 65:577–585.

60. Davis PB, Simpson DM, Paget GL, Turi V. Beta-adrenergic responses in drug-free subjects with asthma. *J Allergy Clin Immunol* 1986; 77:871–879.

61. Nielson CP. Beta-adrenergic modulation of the polymorphonuclear leukocyte respiratory burst is dependent upon the mechanism of cell activation. *J Immunol* 1987; 139:2392–2397.

62. Schenkelaars EJ, Bonta IL. Beta2-adrenoceptor agonists reverse the leukotriene C4-induced release response of macrophages. *Eur J Pharmacol* 1984; 107:65–70.

63. Fuller RW, O'Malley G, Baker AJ, MacDermot J. Human alveolar macrophage activation: inhibition by forskolin but not beta-adrenoceptor stimulation or phosphodiesterase inhibition. *Pulm Pharmacol* 1988; 1:101–106.

64. Cook N, Nahorski SR, Barnett DB. Human platelet beta2-adrenoceptors: agonist-induced internalisation and down-regulation in intact cells. *Br J Pharmacol* 1987; 92:587–596.

65. Kraan J, Koeter GH, vd Mark TW, Sluiter HJ, de Vries K. Changes in bronchial hyperreactivity induced by 4 weeks of treatment with antiasthmatic drugs in patients with allergic asthma: a comparison between budesonide and terbutaline. *J Allergy Clin Immunol* 1985; 76:628–636.

66. Bourne HR, Lichtenstein LM, Melmon KL, Henney CS, Weinstein Y, Shearer GM. Modulation of inflammation and immunity by cyclic AMP. *Science* 1974; 184:19–28.

67. Reed CE. Adrenergic bronchodilators: pharmacology and toxicology. *J Allergy Clin Immunol* 1985; 76:335–341.

68. Busse WW, Sosman JM. Isoproterenol inhibition of isolated human neutrophil function. *J Allergy Clin Immunol* 1984; 73:404–410.

69. Mack JA, Nielson CP, Stevens DL, Vestal RE. Beta-adrenoceptor-mediated modulation of calcium ionophore activated polymorphonuclear leucocytes. *Br J Pharmacol* 1986; 88:417–423.

70. Peters SP, Schulman ES, Schleimer RP, MacGlashan DW, Jr., Newball HH, Lichtenstein LM. Dispersed human lung mast cells. Pharmacologic aspects and comparison with human lung tissue fragments. *Am Rev Respir Dis* 1982; 126:1034–1039.

71. Church MK, Young KD. The characteristics of inhibition of histamine release from human lung fragments by sodium cromoglycate, salbutamol and chlorpromazine. *Br J Pharmacol* 1983; 78:671–679.

72. Church MK, Hiroi J. Inhibition of IgE-dependent histamine release from human dispersed lung mast cells by anti-allergic drugs and salbutamol. *Br J Pharmacol* 1987; 90:421–429.

73. Cockcroft DW, Murdock KY. Comparative effects of inhaled salbutamol, sodium cromoglycate, and beclomethasone dipropionate on allergen-induced early asthmatic responses, late asthmatic responses, and increased bronchial responsiveness to histamine. *J Allergy Clin Immunol* 1987; 79:734–740.

74. Juniper EF, Kline PA, Vanzieleghem MA, Ramsdale EH, O'Byrne PM, Hargreave FE. Effect of long-term treatment with an inhaled corticosteroid (budesonide) on airway hyperresponsiveness and clinical asthma in nonsteroid-dependent asthmatics. *Am Rev Respir Dis* 1990; 142:832–836.

75. Haahtela T, Jarvinen M, Kava T, Kiviranta K, Koskinen S, Lehtonen K *et al*. Comparison of a beta2-agonist, terbutaline, with an inhaled corticosteroid, budesonide, in newly detected asthma. *N Engl J Med* 1991; 325:388–392.

76. van Essen-Zandvliet EE, Hughes MD, Waalkens HJ, Duiverman EJ, Pocock SJ, Kerrebijn KF. Effects of 22 months of treatment with inhaled corticosteroids and/or beta-2-agonists on lung function, airway responsiveness, and symptoms in children with asthma. The Dutch Chronic Non-specific Lung Disease Study Group. *Am Rev Respir Dis* 1992; 146:547–554.

77. Holen E, Elsayed S. Effects of beta2 adrenoceptor agonists on T-cell subpopulations. *APMIS* 1998; 106:849–857.

78. Baker AJ, Palmer J, Johnson M, Fuller RW. Inhibitory actions of salmeterol on human airway macrophages and blood monocytes. *Eur J Pharmacol* 1994; 264:301–306.

79. Lau HY, Wong PL, Lai CK. Effects of beta2-adrenergic agonists on isolated guinea-pig lung mast cells. *Agents Actions* 1994; 42:92–94.

80. Bissonnette EY, Befus AD. Anti-inflammatory effect of beta2-agonists: inhibition of TNF-alpha release from human mast cells. *J Allergy Clin Immunol* 1997; 100:825–831.

81. Chong LK, Cooper E, Vardey CJ, Peachell PT. Salmeterol inhibition of mediator release from human lung mast cells by beta-adrenoceptor-dependent and independent mechanisms. *Br J Pharmacol* 1998; 123:1009–1015.

82. Eda R, Sugiyama H, Hopp RJ, Okada C, Bewtra AK, Townley RG. Inhibitory effects of formoterol on platelet-activating factor induced eosinophil chemotaxis and degranulation. *Int Arch Allergy Immunol* 1993; 102:391–398.

83. Rabe KF, Giembycz MA, Dent G, Perkins RS, Evans P, Barnes PJ. Salmeterol is a competitive antagonist at beta-adrenoceptors mediating inhibition of respiratory burst in guinea-pig eosinophils. *Eur J Pharmacol* 1993; 231:305–308.

84. Anderson R, Feldman C, Theron AJ, Ramafi G, Cole PJ, Wilson R. Anti-inflammatory, membrane-stabilizing interactions of salmeterol with human neutrophils *in vitro*. *Br J Pharmacol* 1996; 117:1387–1394.

85. Whelan CJ, Johnson M, Vardey CJ. Comparison of the anti-inflammatory properties of formoterol, salbutamol and salmeterol in guinea-pig skin and lung. *Br J Pharmacol* 1993; 110:613–618.

86. Teixeira MM, Hellewell PG. Evidence that the eosinophil is a cellular target for the inhibitory action of salmeterol on eosinophil recruitment *in vivo*. *Eur J Pharmacol* 1997; 323:255–260.

87. Kankaanranta H, Lindsay MA, Giembycz MA, Zhang X, Moilanen E, Barnes PJ. Delayed eosinophil apoptosis in asthma. *J Allergy Clin Immunol* 2000; 106:77–83.

88. Simons FE. A comparison of beclomethasone, salmeterol, and placebo in children with asthma. Canadian Beclomethasone Dipropionate-Salmeterol Xinafoate Study Group. *N Engl J Med* 1997; 337:1659–1665.

89. Verberne AA, Frost C, Roorda RJ, van der Laag H, Kerrebijn KF. One year treatment with salmeterol compared with beclomethasone in children with asthma. The Dutch Paediatric Asthma Study Group. *Am J Respir Crit Care Med* 1997; 156:688–695.

90. Jones R, Reid L. Beta-agonists and secretory cell number and intracellular glycoproteins in airway epithelium. The effect of isoproterenol and salbutamol. *Am J Pathol* 1979; 95:407–421.

91. Davis B, Marin MG, Yee JW, Nadel JA. Effect of terbutaline on movement of Cl− and Na+ across the trachea of the dog *in vitro*. *Am Rev Respir Dis* 1979; 120:547–552.

92. Verdugo P, Johnson NT, Tam PY. beta-Adrenergic stimulation of respiratory ciliary activity. *J Appl Physiol: Respir, Environ Exercise Physiol* 1980; 48:868–871.

93. Lopez-Vidriero MT, Jacobs M, Clarke SW. The effect of isoprenaline on the ciliary activity of an *in vitro* preparation of rat trachea. *Eur J Pharmacol* 1985; 112:429–432.

94. Wong LB, Miller IF, Yeates DB. Stimulation of ciliary beat frequency by autonomic agonists: *in vivo*. *J Appl Physiol* 1988; 65:971–981.

95. Bennett WD, Chapman WF, Lay JC, Gerrity TR. Pulmonary clearance of inhaled particles 24 to 48 hours post deposition: effect of beta-adrenergic stimulation. *J Aerosol Med* 1993; 6:53–62.

96. Amitani R, Wilson R, Rutman A, Read R, Ward C, Burnett D et al. Effects of human neutrophil elastase and Pseudomonas aeruginosa proteinases on human respiratory epithelium. *Am J Respir Cell Mol Biol* 1991; 4:26–32.

97. Dowling RB, Rayner CF, Rutman A, Jackson AD, Kanthakumar K, Dewar A et al. Effect of salmeterol on Pseudomonas aeruginosa infection of respiratory mucosa. *Am J Respir Crit Care Med* 1997; 155:327–336.

98. Dowling RB, Johnson M, Cole PJ, Wilson R. Effect of salmeterol on Haemophilus influenzae infection of respiratory mucosa *in vitro*. *Eur Respir J* 1998; 11:86–90.

99. Kanthakumar K, Cundell DR, Johnson M, Wills PJ, Taylor GW, Cole PJ, Wilson R. Effect of salmeterol on human nasal epithelial cell ciliary beating: inhibition of the ciliotoxin, pyocyanin. *Br J Pharmacol* 1994; 112:493–498.

100. Kanthakumar K, Taylor GW, Cundell DR, Dowling RB, Johnson M, Cole PJ, Wilson R. The effect of bacterial toxins on levels of intracellular adenosine nucleotides and human ciliary beat frequency. *Pulm Pharmacol* 1996; 9:223–230.

101. Spurzem JR, Gupta J, Veys T, Kneifl KR, Rennard SI, Wyatt TA. Activation of protein kinase A accelerates bovine bronchial epithelial cell migration. *Am J Physiol* 2002; 282:1108–1116.

102. Barnes PJ. Scientific rationale for inhaled combination therapy with long-acting beta2-agonists and corticosteroids. *Eur Respir J* 2002; 19:182–191.

103. Greening AP, Ind PW, Northfield M, Shaw G. Added salmeterol versus higher-dose corticosteroid in asthma patients with symptoms on existing inhaled corticosteroid. Allen & Hanburys Limited UK Study Group. *Lancet* 1994; 344:219–224.

104. Woolcock A, Lundback B, Ringdal N, Jacques LA: Comparison of addition of salmeterol to inhaled steroids with doubling of the dose of inhaled steroids. *Am J Respir Crit Care Med* 1996; 153:1481–1488.

105. Shrewsbury S, Pyke S, Britton M. Meta-analysis of increased dose of inhaled steroid or addition of salmeterol in symptomatic asthma (MIASMA). *Br Med J* 2000; 320:1368–1373.
106. Cazzola M, Santus P, Di Marco F, Boveri B, Castagna F, Carlucci P *et al.* Bronchodilator effect of an inhaled combination therapy with salmeterol + fluticasone + budesonide in patients with COPD. *Respir Med* 2003; 97:453–457.
107. Sin DD, McAlister FA, Man SF, Anthonisen NR. Contemporary management of chronic obstructive pulmonary disease: scientific review. *JAMA* 2003; 290:2301–2312.
108. Kips JC, Pauwels RA. Long-acting inhaled beta(2)-agonist therapy in asthma. *Am J Respir Crit Care Med* 2001; 164:923–932.
109. Lazarus SC, Boushey HA, Fahy JV, Chinchilli VM, Lemanske RF, Jr., Sorkness CA *et al.* Asthma Clinical Research Network for the National Heart, Lung and Blood Institute. Long-acting beta2-agonist monotherapy vs continued therapy with inhaled corticosteroids in patients with persistent asthma: a randomized controlled trial. *JAMA* 2001; 285:2583–2593.
110. Lawrence AJ, Krstew E, Jarrott B. Functional dopamine D2 receptors on rat vagal afferent neurones. *Br J Pharmacol* 1995; 114:1329–1334.
111. Xie GX, Jones K, Peroutka SJ, Palmer PP. Detection of mRNAs and alternatively spliced transcripts of dopamine receptors in rat peripheral sensory and sympathetic ganglia. *Brain Res* 1998; 785:129–135.
112. Hiller FC, Alderfer V, Goldman M. Long-term use of Viozan (sibenadet HCl) in patients with chronic obstructive pulmonary disease: results of a 1-year study. *Respir Med* 2003; 97:S45–S52
113. Laursen LC, Lindqvist A, Hepburn T, Lloyd J, Perrett J, Sanders N, Rocchiccioli K. The role of the novel D2/beta2-agonist, Viozan (sibenadet HCl), in the treatment of symptoms of chronic obstructive pulmonary disease: results of a large scale clinical investigation. *Respir Med* 2003; 97:S23–S33.

4

Beta-adrenoceptor agonists: clinical use

M. Cazzola, M. G. Matera

INTRODUCTION

β_2-Agonists are agents that induce bronchodilation by causing prolonged relaxation of airway smooth muscle. Smooth muscle relaxation is due to β_2-adrenoceptor(β_2-AR)-mediated activation of adenylate cyclase in airway smooth muscle, which in turn increases the concentration of intracellular cyclic adenosine monophosphate (cAMP) [1]. As a consequence of their broncholytic activity, these agents improve lung function, reduce symptoms, and protect against exercise-induced dyspnoea in patients with chronic obstructive pulmonary disease (COPD). Some non-bronchodilator effects have also been observed but their significance is uncertain [2].

Numerous agents of differing pharmacological properties are available for clinical use [3, 4]. β-Agonists are classified by their selectivity, duration of action, affinity, potency and efficacy [4]. Two major classes of β-agonists are currently available, which differ in their duration of action.

SHORT-ACTING β_2-ADRENOCEPTOR AGONISTS

Short-acting β_2-agonists, such as salbutamol and terbutaline, produce >80% of maximal bronchodilator effect within 15 min of administration and last roughly 4–6 h [5, 6]. Generally, the maximum bronchodilator response to inhaled β_2-agonists in COPD occurs significantly later to that observed in asthmatics [7], and, unfortunately, the magnitude of the bronchodilator response to these agonists often falls within the natural variability observed in patients with COPD [8–15]. However, the conventional doses of some agents could be too low in some cases and, for this reason, bronchodilation is not evident.

Barclay *et al.* [16] have demonstrated that several COPD patients, who were not responsive to 200 µg of inhaled salbutamol, presented with some degree of bronchodilation when the dose of this agent was gradually increased. Other studies have reported similar findings [17, 18]. However, the dose–response relationship for salbutamol in patients with largely or completely irreversible COPD is almost flat [19]. Nevertheless, as doses increase, the frequency of adverse effects (i.e., tremor, reflex tachycardia) increases as well [20].

Mario Cazzola, MD, Consultant in Respiratory Medicine, Chief of Respiratory Medicine, Unit of Pneumology and Allergology, Department of Respiratory Medicine, A. Cardarelli Hospital, Naples, Italy.

Maria Gabriella Matera, MD, PhD, Researcher in Pharmacology and Consultant in Clinical Pharmacology, Unit of Pharmacology, Department of Experimental Medicine, School of Medicine, Second University, Naples, Italy.

The increases in vital capacity (VC) are usually higher than those observed for forced expiratory volume in 1 second (FEV_1) [11], and often they are associated with a symptomatic improvement [9], although there is relatively limited information available on the benefits of these agents on clinical aspects.

A recent Cochrane review [21] has documented that the use of short-acting β_2-agonists on a regular basis for at least 7 days in stable COPD is associated with improvements in post-bronchodilator lung function and also a decrease in breathlessness. Patients are far more likely to prefer treatment with β_2-agonists than placebo, and less likely to drop out from such treatment. None of the studies included in this review reported sufficient data or were of sufficient length or size in order to provide reliable information on adverse effects. One randomised clinical trial (RCT) in 985 people with severe disease found a significant increase in lung function in up to half of the patients [22]. Nonetheless, the general opinion is that, despite the accumulation of positive data available for short-acting β_2-agonists, approximately one in three patients have no measurable response in lung function tests after using these agents [23].

Nevertheless, spirometric changes in FEV_1 are not necessarily indicative of the functional benefits of bronchodilators [24]. Patients who do not show 'significant' spirometric improvement can still benefit from β-agonist treatment [25]. Correlation between bronchodilator responsiveness and self-paced walking distance, periods of rest, and end-exercise breathlessness is poor [26]. Even patients who show 'no bronchodilator response' can still have significantly improved exercise performance after supranormal doses of β_2-agonists [27]. Thus, although Berger and Smith [27] found no change in lung function after inhalation of metaproterenol, subjects increased both their treadmill and hall-walking distances significantly with the short-acting β_2-agonist compared with placebo. It is conceivable that the enhanced exercise capacity was the result of reduced lung hyperinflation. It has been noted that symptoms can appear to improve without significant measurable increase in lung function or exercise performance [27, 28]. The short-acting β_2-agonists lessen breathlessness by allowing for more complete lung emptying and by decreasing cough intensity [29, 30]. In particular, it has been documented that these agents reduce breathlessness during exercise mainly through their effect on reducing dynamic hyperinflation and are not reflected by the FEV_1 or forced vital capacity (FVC) [31].

Concerning the utility of long-term treatment of COPD with short-acting β_2-agonists, it is worth considering the findings of Anthonisen et al. [22] who demonstrated that the bronchodilator response to β_2-adrenoceptor agonists (metaproterenol, isoetherine, fenoterol or salbutamol) did not decrease over a 3-year period. However, another study showed that FEV_1 declined faster in subjects treated regularly compared with subjects' treatment on demand [32], but the criteria used in the selection of patients could have an impact on the findings of this study. Indeed, patients who were taking β_2-adrenoceptor agonists regularly presented with a lower FEV_1 at the beginning of the study. This indicates that their disease severity was greater, resulting in a greater decline in FEV_1. In any case, some of these patients may also have had asthmatic features, such as allergy and high reversibility of obstruction, which may have been partly responsible for the annual decline of FEV_1 [33]. van Schaych et al. [34] reported that a fall in FEV_1 did not occur when patients with mild COPD were regularly treated with bronchodilators for 4 years. In this study none of the patients were dependent on steroid and the baseline FEV_1 did not differ between the patients treated continuously and those treated on demand. It is interesting to highlight that bronchodilator dose-response effects were not attenuated after treatment with high-dose inhaled terbutaline (2,000 µg four times a day for 4 weeks), in comparison with the effects of conventional low-dose therapy (500 µg four times a day for 4 weeks) in patients with COPD [35].

Because of their relatively rapid onset of bronchodilation, inhaled short-acting β_2-agonists may be used as required for symptom relief. In effect, their use 'on demand' is often the first treatment choice in patients presenting with mild COPD.

LONG-ACTING β_2-ADRENOCEPTOR AGONISTS

Long-acting versions of β_2-agonists with duration of action that is around 12 h have also been developed. At present, long-acting β_2-agonist (LABA) bronchodilators (formoterol, salmeterol) are an interesting therapeutic option for patients with COPD [36, 37]. These drugs have quite different molecular structures and there are thought to be different mechanisms responsible for the longer duration of action of these two molecules.

ACUTE BRONCHOLYTIC EFFECTS

The onset of action of formoterol is as rapid as that of salbutamol and terbutaline [38, 39], and a significant effect occurs within minutes of inhalation of a therapeutic dose [40, 41]. In particular, it has been demonstrated that inhaled formoterol 12 and 24 µg and inhaled salbutamol 400 and 800 µg are equi-effective doses in inducing a rapid onset of action in patients with stable COPD [42]. The pharmacodynamic properties of salmeterol differ from those of formoterol. In fact, formoterol, but not salmeterol, has as fast an onset of action as salbutamol [43]. It has been documented that in patients with stable COPD, 200 µg salbutamol induced an increase in FEV_1 from baseline of at least 15% in 3.56 min (95% CI: 3.03–4.49), whereas the same increase was observed in 10.08 min (95% CI: 6.16–13.58) after inhalation of 50 µg salmeterol [44].

In a small group of patients with severe-to-very severe COPD, both formoterol and salmeterol induced a functional improvement lasting 12 h [45]. Formoterol 12–36 µg caused a dose-dependent increase in FVC, FEV_1 and flow at 50% expired volume (FEF_{50}), whereas salmeterol 75 µg did not elicit any further increase in bronchodilation than salmeterol 50 µg. Moreover, at the recommended dose, salmeterol 50 µg was more active than formoterol 12 and 24 µg. Nevertheless, Çelik et al. [46] showed that a single dose of formoterol 12 µg and salmeterol 50 µg provided comparable bronchodilation within 12 h. The disparity between results of these two studies could be attributed to the methodological differences in patient selection criteria. In fact, the population enrolled by Çelik et al. [46] was dispersed between mild-to-severe airway obstruction and the baseline characteristics of patients should explain why their data were different from those of Cazzola et al. [45] who recruited only patients with severe COPD. Consequently, it has been argued that formoterol 12 µg is more active in patients with mild-to-moderate COPD and salmeterol 50 µg in patients with severe COPD [37]. In any case, it must be highlighted that a low dose of formoterol 6 µg via Turbuhaler has been demonstrated to cause significant, immediate and long-lasting reductions in airway resistance and effort in breathing in patients with moderate-to-severe 'non-reversible' COPD [47]. Increasing the dose above 6 µg did not enhance these effects [47].

NON-BRONCHOLYTIC EFFECTS

In addition to prolonged bronchodilatation, LABAs exert other additive effects that may be of clinical relevance in COPD (Table 4.1). For example, part of the symptomatic benefit of these agents might be mediated through the reduction of dynamic hyperinflation, as this makes breathing more comfortable and dyspnoea is lessened. Di Marco *et al.* [48] documented that at standard recommended dosage, formoterol elicited a greater acute increase in inspiratory capacity (IC) than salbutamol, salmeterol, and oxitropium bromide, an anticholinergic agent. This increase in IC correlated closely with the improvement of dyspnoea sensation at rest. Ramirez-Venegas *et al.* [49] investigated the short-term (4 h) effects of inhaled salmeterol on the perception of dyspnoea and lung function in patients with COPD. There were significantly higher values for FEV_1 and FVC (at all time periods) and lower values for functional residual capacity (FRC) (at all time periods) and residual volume (RV) (at 4 h) with salmeterol than with placebo. There were significantly lower dyspnoea ratings and for the mean dyspnoea scores during resistive breathing with salmeterol compared with placebo.

LABAs can increase the level of cAMP in neutrophils, thereby inhibiting neutrophil adhesion, accumulation, and activation, and inducing apoptosis [50]. In particular, salmeterol inhibits neutrophil adhesion to bronchial epithelial cells [51]. Formoterol inhibits chemotaxis to platelet-activating factor [52] over the concentration range 10^{-7}–10^{-4} mol/l. Neutrophil activation also is attenuated, as evidenced by reductions in the release of superoxide [53], interleukin (IL)-8 [54], and bacterial permeability-increasing protein [55], which are not associated with the short-acting β_2-agonist salbutamol. However, in general, these effects are only significant at relatively high concentrations (i.e., $>10^{-6}$ mol/l) and are not reversed by propranolol, suggesting that they are not mediated by β_2-adrenoceptors. The end result is a possible reduction in the number and activation status of neutrophils in airway tissue and in the airway lumen [56]. LABAs may also decrease the number of neutrophils that adhere to the vascular endothelium at sites of inflammation and reduce the amount of plasma leakage [57], but the relevance of these findings to COPD patients is unclear.

REGULAR TREATMENT OF COPD WITH LONG-ACTING β_2-AGONISTS

A volume of published evidence sustains the role of LABAs in the treatment of stable COPD [58]. These agents not only induce prolonged bronchodilation, but also translate this action into other health-outcome measures that relate to quality of life, such as the severity of dyspnoea, exercise capacity, and exacerbations.

Table 4.1   Non-broncholytic effects of long-acting β_2-agonists

Reduced lung hyperinflation
Increased diaphragm and intercostal muscle function
Increased mucociliary transport
Mucosae cytoprotection
Antineutrophil activity
Inhibition of airway smooth muscle
Cell proliferation
Inhibition of inflammatory mediator release

IMPACT ON LUNG FUNCTION

Several clinical studies have documented that the protracted treatment of COPD with formoterol or salmeterol can induce a sustained improvement in the respiratory function when compared to placebo, but these agents do not modify the rate of decline in FEV_1 [59–62].

Salmeterol 50 µg twice daily has also been compared with ipratropium bromide 40 µg four times daily in a double-blind, placebo-controlled, 12-week period crossover study involving 411 patients with COPD with FEV_1 values <65% predicted and no clinically significant concurrent disease [60]. During salmeterol treatment, patients did statistically better in terms of all the measured functional parameters. In another study involving 405 patients [61], salmeterol provided similar maximal bronchodilatation to ipratropium but had a longer duration of action and a more constant bronchodilatory effect with no evidence of bronchodilator tolerance. It has been documented that 12-week treatment with formoterol Aerolizer 12 or 24 µg twice daily was significantly superior to ipratropium 40 µg four times daily [62]. However, a 12-week treatment with formoterol Turbuhaler 24 µg twice daily was not significantly different from that with ipratropium 80 µg three times daily [63]. Recently, salmeterol has been compared to tiotropium, a long-acting anticholinergic [64]. The FEV_1 measures were statistically significant in favour of long-acting anticholinergics compared to LABA.

Comparisons between LABA and theophylline in patients suffering from COPD are relatively scarce. Di Lorenzo *et al.* [65] compared the effects of salmeterol 50 µg twice daily for 3 months with oral dose-titrated theophylline twice daily in 178 patients with chronic bronchitis. The morning PEF increased from a baseline value of 324 l/min to 360.7 l/min 3 months after salmeterol and from a baseline value of 298.8 l/min to 325 l/min 3 months after theophylline ($p < 0.02$). There was a similar trend for evening PEF but differences were not statistically significant. A one-year Italian multicentre study [66] compared the effects of inhaled salmeterol (50 µg twice daily *via* Diskhaler) with those of oral dose-titrated slow release theophylline in 138 patients with reversible COPD. Salmeterol was found to be more effective than theophylline for the maximum value of morning PEF, but differences in FVC, FEV_1, and maximum value of evening PEF did not reach statistical significance although the effect of salmeterol was slightly superior to that of theophylline. However, it must be stressed that both asthmatic and COPD patients were enrolled in this study. ZuWallack *et al.* [67] enrolled 943 patients with COPD and compared salmeterol (50 µg twice daily) and theophylline for 12 weeks. In this study, the improvements in the salmeterol group were slightly greater than those in the theophylline group for both FEV_1 and FVC, but the differences were not significant. Rossi *et al.* [68] documented that compared to placebo, formoterol 12 µg and 24 µg, and theophylline both significantly improved the area under the curve for FEV_1 measured over a period of 12 h following the morning dose of study medication at 3 and 12 months. However, therapy with formoterol, 12 µg, was significantly more effective than that with theophylline.

IMPACT ON SYMPTOMS

The bronchodilation caused by LABAs can also reduce symptom scores [61, 62, 69]. Although several studies found no significant differences between these agents and placebo with regard to the reduction of breathlessness, one trial with the largest sample size [59] demonstrated that salmeterol reduces the degree of breathlessness produced by exercise.

By using a multidimensional instrument to measure changes in dyspnoea based on activities of daily living, Mahler *et al.* [60] showed that salmeterol reduced dyspnoea on the Transition Dyspnoea Index (TDI) after 2, 4, 8, and 10 weeks of treatment compared with placebo therapy. However, in a similarly designed study, Rennard *et al.* [61] observed no statistical differences in the TDI scores between salmeterol and placebo treatment groups. It must be highlighted that two subsequent randomised controlled trials [64, 66] with large sample sizes demonstrated a statistically significant difference with the use of LABAs in reducing dyspnoea. Formoterol, 24 µg bid, but not 12 µg bid, improved TDI focal scores compared with placebo over 3 months [70].

In the study of Mahler *et al.* [60], similar reductions in breathlessness (higher TDI scores) with both salmeterol and ipratropium were observed, which were evident at 2 weeks and were generally sustained over the entire 12-week period. The improvement in dyspnoea throughout the study was supported by the observed significant decrease in supplemental salbutamol use with both salmeterol and ipratropium. Salmeterol did not improve TDI focal scores even when compared with theophylline [67]. Formoterol has not yet been compared on TDI with other active treatments. However, in the study of Dahl *et al.* [62], formoterol 12 µg produced a significant improvement in mean total diary symptom score when compared with ipratropium, whereas formoterol 24 µg approached significance. On the contrary, Rossi *et al.* [68] were unable to record a statistically significant difference in the average symptom score between patients receiving formoterol 12 µg or formoterol 24 µg and those who received theophylline.

A second measure of COPD symptoms is patient use of 'reliever' short-acting β_2-agonists, since a treatment that effectively reduces symptoms should also reduce the need for rescue medication. Salmeterol at 50 µg and 100 µg reduced rescue medication use compared with placebo but not compared with ipratropium or theophylline [59, 60, 67, 71, 72]. In the study of Rossi *et al.* [68], the improvement in pulmonary function by formoterol was associated with a significant reduction in the use of rescue medication.

IMPACT ON HEALTH-RELATED QUALITY OF LIFE

It has been documented that LABAs significantly improved health-related quality of life (HRQoL), although a systematic review [69] demonstrated that there was variation in trial results for HRQoL. Three studies, two with salmeterol [61, 73] and one with formoterol [70], showed that LABAs significantly improved HRQoL using the St George's Respiratory Questionnaire (SGRQ). It is interesting to highlight that in another study [62], although the formoterol 24 µg dose achieved significant benefits, the magnitude of change was not as great as with the 12 µg dose. Rutten-van Molken [74] and Brusasco [64] did not find any statistically significant differences between salmeterol and placebo.

Other studies have used the Chronic Respiratory Disease Questionnaire (CRDQ) for measuring HRQoL. In a 12-week trial, the total score on the CRDQ was higher (better) for the salmeterol-treated group compared with the placebo group [60]. The proportion of patients who achieved an increase of ≥10 points in overall score (the minimum change indicative of an important difference) was significantly higher at week 12 in the salmeterol (46%) than in the placebo group (27%) in non-reversible patients. However, Rennard *et al.* [61] using the CRDQ showed that the proportion of patients who achieved a clinically significant change of 10 from the baseline was 46% in the salmeterol group and 38% in the placebo group.

Studies of salmeterol have not shown any significant effect on health status compared with either ipratropium [60, 61, 75], or theophylline [67]. Formoterol was superior on the SGRQ total score to ipratropium over 12 weeks [62], but not to theophylline over 12 months [68].

IMPACT ON EXERCISE PERFORMANCE

Although it has been shown that patients with COPD were able to walk a significantly greater distance on the treadmill after acute administration of salmeterol compared with placebo, Boyd et al. [59], Mahler et al. [60], Rennard et al. [61], and Grove et al. [76] found no differences in the 6-min walking distance with salmeterol compared with placebo therapy. In addition, formoterol did not improve shuttle walking test distances compared with placebo [70]. However, when the effect of one-week of treatment with formoterol 4.5, 9 or 18 µg twice daily, on exercise capacity was compared with that of ipratropium bromide, 80 µg tid, or placebo using a bicycle ergometer test [77], it was observed that all three doses of formoterol significantly prolonged the time to exhaustion, which was comparable to the effect of ipratropium. The maximum Borg dyspnoea scale was unaffected.

IMPACT ON EXACERBATIONS

The evaluation of the impact of LABAs on exacerbations has produced contrasting results. In a large multicentre trial, Calverley et al. [78] showed that compared with placebo, salmeterol reduced by 20% the rate of exacerbations per patient per year and by 29% the rate of exacerbations that needed treatment with oral corticosteroids. Another large multicentre trial over one year [68] found that formoterol was significantly superior to placebo for the mean percentages of bad days defined as 'mild COPD exacerbation'. Formoterol at 24 µg, but not lower doses, also reduced the number of exacerbations that were serious enough to require additional therapy compared with placebo [79, 80].

However, one systematic review [69] found that LABAs compared to placebo did not significantly affect the incidence of COPD exacerbations; in any case, this meta analysis was only based upon two RCTs [59, 71]. In two separate 12-week trials, there was no consistent effect of salmeterol on exacerbations of COPD compared with placebo [60, 61]. Three other trials [62, 64, 81] also found no significant difference in exacerbations.

Formoterol has been shown to reduce the number of bad days compared with theophylline [68], but not with ipratropium [62]. Salmeterol also does not seem to have a consistent effect on exacerbations compared with ipratropium [60, 61], and did not reduce the incidence of exacerbations compared with theophylline [67].

It is interesting to highlight that Dowling et al. [82, 83] reported that salmeterol reduced respiratory epithelial damage induced by Haemophilus influenzae and by Pseudomonas aeruginosa, probably by maintaining intracellular concentrations of cAMP. Moreover, in vitro studies have shown that β_2-agonists can reduce the chemotactic response of neutrophils to agents such as endotoxin without inhibiting their antibacterial activity [84]. If these in vitro observations can be extrapolated to the situation in COPD, long-acting inhaled β_2-agonists could interfere with the vicious circle underlying exacerbations, and thus have an important effect on the clinical outcome of the disease. However, the clinical impact of this 'cytoprotection' on the respiratory tract requires further investigation.

SPECIAL PROBLEMS RELATED TO THE USE OF LONG-ACTING β_2-AGONISTS

TOLERANCE TO BRONCHODILATING EFFECTS OF β-AGONISTS

Pharmacoepidemiological studies indicate a strong association between increased β_2-agonist use and β_2-adrenoceptor down-regulation and subsensitivity and consequent loss of airway control [85, 86]. In particular, Lipworth [87] advised that physicians should be aware of the airway subsensitivity that develops with LABA therapy. Patients should be warned that they might have to use higher than conventional dosages of short-acting β_2-agonists to relieve acute bronchoconstriction in order to overcome this effect.

While clinical evidence of tolerance has occurred in asthma and is generally well accepted, tolerance to chronic administration of inhaled β-agonists has not been adequately addressed in patients with COPD. Controlled clinical studies in patients with COPD examining up to 4 months treatment with formoterol or salmeterol have suggested that tolerance does not appear to occur, although specific analyses addressing the issue were not reported [62, 73]. Moreover, it has been shown that pre-treatment with a conventional dose of formoterol or salmeterol does not preclude the possibility of inducing a further bronchodilation with salbutamol in patients suffering from partially reversible COPD [88].

Bjermer and Larsson [89] have reviewed some data related to the debate warning against the use of LABAs and observed that the bronchodilatory effect seems to be fairly stable after regular treatment with these bronchodilators, even though some reports claim that this effect diminishes over time. Interestingly, Anderson *et al.* [90] have demonstrated the lack of loss of bronchodilator response to salmeterol after a 3-month period in patients with COPD, and this even in genotypes more susceptible to β_2-adrenoceptor down-regulation. However, a recent paper of Donohue *et al.* [91] has documented a relatively small diminishment of bronchodilator responses and duration of bronchodilation over time in patients with COPD during chronic administration of salmeterol $50 \mu g$ bid.

ADVERSE SIDE-EFFECTS

Side-effects of inhaled β-agonists are the result of activation of extrapulmonary β-ARs. Minor adverse effects such as palpitations, tremor, headache and metabolic effects are predictable and dose related. Cardiovascular adverse events are potentially the most serious. It must be highlighted that the impact of most bronchodilators on the heart is a very important point [92]. Cardiac arrhythmias are common in patients with respiratory failure due to COPD. Several factors are potentially arrhythmogenic in these patients, including hypoxaemia, hypercapnia, acid-base disturbances [93] and the use of β_2-agonists or theophylline [94]. In particular, patients with hypoxaemic COPD may have a subclinical autonomic neuropathy that has been associated with a prolonged electrocardiograph QTc interval and risk of ventricular arrhythmias and death [95]. It cannot be excluded that adverse cardiac events might occur in COPD patients with pre-existing cardiac arrhythmias and hypoxaemia [96].

β_2-Agonists are known to have several side-effects with potential effects on cardiac function as a result of direct stimulation of β_2-ARs in the atria and possibly β_1-ARs with higher doses of inhaled medication [97–99]. They include an increase in heart rate, an increase in contractile force, a decrease in peripheral vascular resistance with increased pulse pressure, an increase in cardiac output, as well as changes in serum potassium and magnesium levels which may affect conduction pathways in the heart [100]. Unequivocally, the chronotropic and electrophysiological effects of β_2-agonists are enhanced by conditions of hypoxaemia; in fact, mild hypoxaemia (90% O_2 saturation) has been demonstrated to extend the prolongation of the QTc interval caused by fenoterol [96]. Nonetheless, these effects are usually considered to be mild when these agents are given by inhalation at therapeutic dose [101]. A recent population-based epidemiological study found that short-acting β_2-agonists in any form did not increase the risk of acute myocardial infarction in a large cohort of patients (12,090 subjects) with COPD [102]. First time use, in particular, also did not increase the risk.

Also the impact of LABAs on the heart has been examined. We evaluated the acute effects of a single dose of salmeterol (50 µg) and two doses of formoterol (12 and 24 µg) in 12 patients with COPD who had pre-existing cardiac arrhythmias and hypoxemia [103]. We found slight increases in heart rate and in ventricular premature contractions with the LABAs compared with placebo. Moreover, the frequency of these cardiac effects was higher with the 24-µg dose of formoterol. Our conclusion was that salmeterol, 50 µg, is more favourable than formoterol, 12 µg, when we consider the bronchodilating effect and formoterol, 24 µg, when we consider the effect on the heart. A recent pooled analysis of cardiovascular safety data of randomised, double-blind, parallel group, multiple-dose studies, which included salmeterol, 50 µg bid, and placebo arms, showed no increased risk of cardiovascular adverse events compared with placebo. In particular, there were no episodes of sustained ventricular tachycardia, and no clinically significant differences were observed in the 24-h heart rate, ventricular and supraventricular ectopic events, qualitative electrocardiograms (ECGs), QT intervals, or vital signs between the salmeterol group and the placebo group. Similar findings were observed when patients were stratified for age of >65 years or the known presence of cardiovascular disease [104].

The administration of β_2-agonists to patients with airway obstruction often results in a transient decrease in oxygen partial pressure (PaO_2) despite concomitant bronchodilation [105]. This phenomenon, which is potentially dangerous in acute exacerbations of COPD, has been attributed to the pulmonary vasodilator action of these agents, increasing blood flow to poorly ventilated lung regions and thus increasing ventilation-perfusion inequality, and to a shunt-like effect [106, 107]. Both formoterol and salmeterol did not induce significant modifications in pulse oximetry (SpO_2) in patients suffering from acute exacerbation of COPD, although they were used at doses higher than that recommended in the treatment of airway obstruction [108–111]. However, considering that some patients presented a decrease in SpO_2 under 90%, the use of high doses of these two long-acting inhaled β_2-agonists must always be prudent.

Tremor can be induced by stimulation of β_2-ARs found in skeletal muscles. However, tremor did not occur more frequently with salmeterol compared with placebo in multi-centre trials [60, 61, 67], although the 100 µg dose (not recommended for use) was associated with a significantly higher incidence of tremor than the 50 µg dose [73]. Maconochie et al. [112] showed that tachyphylaxis occurred to the effects of salmeterol on tremor.

β_2-agonists can also cause hypokalemia because of shifting of potassium within cells [113]. In addition, these agents may increase levels of serum glucose, insulin, lactate, pyruvate, and free fatty acids when used in higher doses.

At least in asthmatic patients, formoterol shows tendency to more pronounced systemic side-effects, such as more pronounced decreased serum potassium and induced finger tremor, when compared to salmeterol [114]. It has been suggested that this is due to the different β-agonist intrinsic efficacy of the two agents [4].

β₂-AGONISTS AND GUIDELINES FOR THE PHARMACOLOGICAL TREATMENT OF STABLE COPD

Current best practice for the pharmacological treatment of COPD is based upon the guidelines issued by the Global Initiative for Chronic Obstructive Lung Disease (GOLD) [115], American Thoracic Society (ATS) [116], European Respiratory Society (ERS) [117], and British Thoracic Society (BTS) [118], and more recently, by ATS/ERS [119] and National Collaborating Centre for Chronic Conditions in the UK [120]. In general, there is a correlation between the type of suggested treatment and the disease severity, which has typically been determined using the degree of lung function (FEV_1 and FEV_1/FVC) impairment. However, the wisdom of this approach has been questioned, with the suggestion that factors such as arterial blood gas levels, time and distance walked, sensation of dyspnoea, and body mass index be included in this determination [121]. Methods of stratifying disease severity (also known as staging) vary between these guidelines. The latest GOLD criteria classify COPD into the following four stages: mild (FEV_1, ≥80% of predicted); moderate (FEV_1, ≥50 to <80% of predicted); severe (FEV_1, ≥30 to <50% of predicted); and very severe (FEV_1, <30% of predicted) [115].

Inhaled bronchodilators are considered as central to the symptomatic management of COPD, even for patients with few or intermittent symptoms, in all the four stages of severity. The most recent guidelines for the management of patients with COPD indicate that short-acting β₂-agonists should be the initial empirical treatment for the relief of breathlessness and exercise limitation [120], or for the control of intermittent symptoms (e.g., cough, wheeze, exertional dyspnoea) [119]. The effectiveness of bronchodilator therapy should not be assessed by lung function alone but should include a variety of other measures such as improvement in symptoms, activities of daily living, exercise capacity, and rapidity of symptom relief. Patients who remain symptomatic should have their inhaled treatment intensified to include long-acting bronchodilators or combined therapy with a short-acting β₂-agonist and a short-acting anticholinergic [119, 120].

LABAs should be used in patients who remain symptomatic despite treatment with short-acting bronchodilators because these drugs appear to have additional benefits over combinations of short-acting drugs [119, 120]. They should also be used in patients who have two or more exacerbations per year [119, 120]. In particular, GOLD guidelines [115] and ATS/ERS guidelines [119] recommend the use of long-acting bronchodilators for treating patients with moderate-to-very severe COPD.

Anyway, because patients with COPD with pre-existing cardiac arrhythmias receiving LABAs could be at special risk of developing new arrhythmias or of aggravating pre-existing ones, we have suggested the use of anticholinergic drugs in these patients with COPD [36, 37].

USE OF β₂-AGONISTS IN THE TREATMENT OF ACUTE EXACERBATIONS OF COPD

Symptoms of acute exacerbation of COPD occur frequently and are manifested as increased breathlessness, usually also with increased cough and sputum production. When airway obstruction increases, the therapeutic option is to add a short-acting

β_2-agonist, such as salbutamol or terbutaline, for rapid relief of bronchospasm [122, 123]. A small number of studies suggests that these agents, as a class, are of bene-fit in exacerbations of COPD, showing improvements in lung function and dyspnoea scores [124]. Unfortunately, their maximal effective dose in COPD exacerbation is not known. However, limited data from studies of COPD exacerbations indicate that 3–4 puffs of short-acting β_2-agonists produce significant (18–22%) levels of bronchodilation [125, 126]. Lloberes *et al.* [126] showed that in at least half of the patients the dose of salbutamol that elicited the maximal bronchodilatation was twice that currently employed. Obviously, these bronchodilators should be titrated to maximal effect when possible, monitoring closely for adverse effects of the larger-than-usual doses that are sometimes necessary to relieve airway obstruction.

These agents once were administered at a moderate dose every hour, but, unfortu-nately, the duration of the bronchodilator effect of short-acting, inhaled β_2-agonists is decreased in COPD exacerbation [127]. In order to overcome the reduced functional half-life of β_2-agonists, several authors suggest not only the use of larger-than-usual doses that are sometimes necessary to relieve airway obstruction, but also shortening the posologic interval [124, 125]. However, one study failed to demonstrate a significant advantage by giving salbutamol more frequently than once every 60 min [124]. Thus, when 3–4 puffs every 4 h have not been effective, 3–4 puffs of short-acting β_2-agonists should be administered every 1–2 h, if tolerated, under close supervision (including ECG monitoring) until clinical improvement occurs. In particular, the ATS recommen-dation for severe COPD exacerbation is 6–8 puffs every 2 h [116].

The use of LABAs formoterol and salmeterol should be another potential option to overcome the reduced functional half-life of β_2-agonists in exacerbation of COPD [128]. However, they are currently not approved for use in this pathologic condition because they must be intended for maintenance treatment and not immediate symptomatic relief. This opinion, however, contrasts with the evidence that at least formoterol produces dose-proportional bronchodilation in COPD patients with a reversible component [45].

Actually, when used for treating acute exacerbations of COPD, formoterol elicits a rapid and significant bronchodilation and can be used for as-needed medication in many patients [110]. A dose of 24 µg formoterol seems to induce clinically relevant effect in these subjects. However, since it has been documented that several patients benefited by a higher dose, it is advisable to administer at least a cumulative 36 µg dose of formoterol as rescue medication to cause rapid relief of bronchospasm in patients with acute exacerbation of COPD. This action will cause rapid relief of bronchospasm in these patients. In any case, it must be highlighted that each subject with COPD has his/her own best function that is regarded to be the best lung function that he/she can achieve either spontaneously or as a result of treatment. If the used agent has induced the maximum possible bronchodilation in our patient, a higher dose is clearly ineffec-tive. The documentation that formoterol induces a fast bronchodilation that is dose-dependent and not significantly different from that caused by salbutamol, at least in patients with mild acute exacerbation of COPD [108], corroborates the use of formoterol in the treatment of acute exacerbation of COPD.

There is a great deal of controversy regarding the timing and optimal dose of β_2-agonists in the treatment of acute exacerbations of COPD. This is also valid for LABAs. Recently, it has been documented that a high dose of formoterol (36 µg) is as effective as the same dose administered in a cumulative manner in patients with acute exacerbation of COPD [108]. This finding was unexpected considering that it has been suggested that the use of a cumulative technique to obtain bronchodilator dose–response curves will cause a greater response than a noncumulative technique, because sequential doses of drug will penetrate further into the lung [129, 130]. Nonetheless, it has important clinical implications with respect to the utilization of bronchodilators in the treatment of acute exacerbation of COPD. In fact, this posologic approach is preferable to prescription of the equivalent cumulative dose regimen when it does not involve additional risks because it simplifies the assumption of bronchodilator.

All these findings support the use of formoterol in the treatment of acute exacerbations of COPD. However, some clinicians avoid the use of this agent as relief medication in patients already taking it as regular treatment for the reasons that have previously been described. Luckily, it has been shown that regular treatment with formoterol does not compromise the bronchodilator response to further cumulative inhalations of formoterol [131]. Patients suffering from partially reversible COPD, who are taking this agent as regular maintenance therapy, can, therefore, also use formoterol as reliever medication.

NOVEL β_2-AGONISTS

Salbutamol is a racemic mixture containing equal parts of R and S salbutamol, which have different affinities for the β_2-AR. The S isomer may have some pro-inflammatory effects and binds to the β_2-receptor weakly, but for a longer period. The R isomer, or levalbuterol, is more active and produces greater bronchodilation over a longer period in both adults and children in long-term–dosing studies [132, 133]. Arformoterol [R,R-formoterol] is a single isomer form of the β_2-agonist formoterol. This isomer contains two chiral centres and is being developed as an inhaled preparation for the treatment of respiratory disorders [134].

Few studies are available and many are ongoing with levalbuterol as well as arformoterol for patients with COPD. Truitt *et al.* [135] reported a retrospective observational study of 125 hospitalised patients with asthma and/or COPD. Patients receiving levalbuterol required fewer β_2-agonist treatments and fewer doses of ipratropium. Patients receiving levalbuterol had a shorter length of stay, needed fewer rescue medications, and had fewer readmissions than those receiving racemic albuterol.

Earlier Phase II products include QAB149, an ultra LABA which has been shown to have a fast onset of action in lung function and offers a true once-daily dosing with a long duration of action [136]. This is being evaluated for treating COPD.

Sibenadet is a dual D2 dopamine receptor, β_2-adrenoceptor agonist that combines bronchodilator activity with the sensory afferent modulating effects associated with D2-receptor agonism [137]. Investigation in animal models of key COPD symptoms has demonstrated that sibenadet effectively inhibits sensory nerve activity, thereby reducing reflex cough, mucus production and tachypnoea [138]. However, the development of sibenadet has been dropped because trials proved that the drug has limited long-term benefit to patients. Phase III clinical trials of the drug failed to show that it was better than competing products in long-term treatment.

REFERENCES

1.   Lulich KM, Goldie RG, Paterson JW. β-Adrenoceptor function in asthmatic bronchial smooth muscle. *Gen Pharmacol* 1988; 19:307–311.
2.   Johnson M, Rennard S. Alternative mechanisms for long-acting β$_2$-adrenergic agonists in COPD. *Chest* 2001; 120:258–270.

3. Hanania NA, Moore RH, Dickey BF. The rational use of β_2-agonists in the management of asthma: maintenance, rescue, and emergency. *Sem Respir Crit Care Med* 1998; 19:613–633.
4. Hanania NA, Sharafkhaneh A, Barber R *et al*. β-agonist intrinsic efficacy: measurement and clinical significance. *Am J Respir Crit Care Med* 2002; 165:1353–1358.
5. Ferguson GT. Management of COPD. *Postgrad Med* 1998; 103:129–141.
6. Ikeda A, Nishimura K, Izumi T. Pharmacological treatment in acute exacerbations of chronic obstructive pulmonary disease. *Drugs Aging* 1998; 12:129–137.
7. Calverley PMA. Symptomatic bronchodilator treatment. In: Calverley PMA, Pride NB (eds) Chronic Obstructive Pulmonary Disease. Chapman & Hall, London, 1995, pp 419–445.
8. Tweedale PM, Alexander F, McHardy GJR. Short-term variability in FEV_1 and bronchodilator responsiveness in patients with obstructive ventilatory defects. *Thorax* 1987; 42:487–490.
9. Bellamy D, Hutchison DCS. The effects of salbutamol aerosol on lung function in patients with pulmonary emphysema. *Br J Dis Chest* 1981; 75:190–196.
10. Tucci M, Cazzola M, Granata A. L'azione del salbutamolo su alcuni dati spirometrici ed emogasometrici nelle sindromi broncoostruttive. *Rif Medica* 1975; 89:120–124.
11. Tucci M, Iodice F, Cazzola M *et al*. L'azione di un nuovo β_2-stimolante, la diidrossifenilorciprenalina (Th 1165a), sulla funzione respiratoria. *Rif Medica* 1976; 90:633–644.
12. Cazzola M, Iodice F, Tucci M *et al*. Valutazione degli effetti broncodilatanti e cardiovascolari e dell'influenza sui gas del sangue di un nuovo β_2 stimolante, la terbutalina, somministrato per aerosol a pazienti affetti da ostruzione bronchiale reversibile. *Min Pneumol* 1978; 17:215–222.
13. Tobin MJ, Hughes JA, Hutchinson DCS. Effects of ipratropium bromide and fenoterol aerosol on exercise tolerance. *Eur J Respir Dis* 1984; 65:441–446.
14. Dullinger D, Kronenberg R, Niewoehner DE. Efficacy of inhaled metaproterenol and orally-administered theophylline in patients with chronic airflow obstruction. *Chest* 1986; 89:171–173.
15. Leitch AG, Morgan A, Ellis DA *et al*. Effect of oral salbutamol and slow-release aminophylline on exercise tolerance in chronic bronchitis. *Thorax* 1981; 36:787–789.
16. Barclay J, Whiting B, Addis GJ. The influence of theophylline on maximal response to salbutamol in severe chronic obstructive pulmonary disease. *Eur J Clin Pharmacol* 1982; 22:389–393.
17. Prior JG, Cochrane GM. Assessment of optimum dose of inhaler terbutaline in patients with chronic asthma: the use of simple cumulative dose-response curves. *Br J Dis Chest* 1982; 72: 266–268.
18. Corris PA, Neville E, Nariman S *et al*. Dose-response study of inhaled salbutamol powder in chronic airflow obstruction. *Thorax* 1983; 38:292–296.
19. Cazzola M, Spina D, Matera MG. The use of bronchodilators in stable chronic obstructive pulmonary disease. *Pulm Pharmacol Ther* 1997; 10:129–144.
20. Ferguson GT. Update on pharmacologic therapy for chronic obstructive pulmonary disease. *Clin Chest Med* 2000; 21:723–738.
21. Sestini P, Renzoni E, Robinson S *et al*. Short-acting β_2 agonists for stable chronic obstructive pulmonary disease (Cochrane Review). In: *The Cochrane Library*, Issue 2, 2004.
22. Anthonisen NR, Wright EC, IPPB Trial Group. Bronchodilator response in chronic obstructive pulmonary disease. *Am Rev Respir Dis* 1986; 133:814–819.
23. Heffner JE. Chronic obstructive pulmonary disease: on an exponential curve of progress. *Resp Care* 2002; 47:586–607.
24. Mahler DA. The effect of inhaled β_2-agonists on clinical outcomes in chronic obstructive pulmonary disease. *J Allergy Clin Immunol* 2002; 110:S298–S303.
25. Leitch AG, Hopkin JM, Ellis DA *et al*. The effect of aerosol ipratropium bromide and salbutamol on exercise tolerance in chronic bronchitis. *Thorax* 1978; 33:711–713.
26. Calverley PMA. Modern treatment of chronic obstructive pulmonary disease. *Eur Respir J* 2001; 18(suppl 34):S60–S66.
27. Berger R, Smith D. Effect of inhaled metaproterenol on exercise performance in patients with stable 'fixed' airway obstruction. *Am Rev Respir Dis* 1988; 138:624–629.
28. Evald T, Keittelman S, Sindrup JH, Lange P. The effect of inhaled terbutaline on FEV_1, FVC, dyspnoea and walking distance in patients with chronic obstructive lung disease. *Respir Med* 1992; 86:93–96.
29. Heffner JE. Chronic obstructive pulmonary disease: on an exponential curve of progress. *Resp Care* 2002; 47:586–607.
30. Calverley PMA. COPD: early detection and intervention. *Chest* 2000; 117(suppl 2):S365–S371.

31. Belman MJ, Botnick WC, Shin JW. Inhaled bronchodilators reduce dynamic hyperinflation during exercise in patients with chronic obstructive pulmonary disease. *Am J Respir Crit Care Med* 1996; 153:967–975.
32. van Schayck CP, Dompeling E, van Herwaarden CLA *et al.* Bronchodilator treatment in moderate asthma or chronic bronchitis: continuous or on demand? *Br Med J* 1991; 303:1426–1431.
33. van Schayck CP, Cloosterman SGM, Hofland ID *et al.* How detrimental is chronic use of bronchodilators in asthma and chronic obstructive pulmonary disease? *Am J Respir Crit Care Med* 1995; 151:1317–1319.
34. van Schayck CP, Dompeling E, van Herwaarden CLA *et al.* Continuous use of bronchodilators versus use on demand in mild asthma and COPD [abstract]. *Am J Respir Crit Care Med* 1994; 149:A203.
35. Lipworth BJ, Clark RA, Dhillon DP *et al.* Comparison of β-adrenoceptor responsiveness following prolonged treatment with low and high doses of inhaled terbutaline in chronic obstructive lung disease. *Am Rev Respir Dis* 1990; 142:338–342.
36. Cazzola M, Matera MG. Should long-acting β$_2$-agonists be considered an alternative first choice option for the treatment of stable COPD? *Respir Med* 1999; 93:227–229.
37. Cazzola M, Donner CF. Long-acting β$_2$-agonists in the management of stable chronic obstructive pulmonary disease. *Drugs* 2000; 60:307–320.
38. Ullman A, Bergendal A, Linden A *et al.* Onset of action and duration of effect of formoterol and salmeterol compared to salbutamol in isolated guinea-pig trachea with or without epithelium. *Allergy* 1992; 47:384–387.
39. Jeppsson AB, Nilsson E, Waldeck B. Formoterol and salmeterol are both long acting compared to terbutaline in the isolated perfused and ventilated guinea-pig lung. *Eur J Pharmacol* 1994; 257:137–143.
40. Faulds D, Hollingshead LM, Goa KL. Formoterol. A review of its pharmacological properties and therapeutic potential in reversible obstructive airways disease. *Drugs* 1991; 42:115–137.
41. Ringdal N, Derom E, Wahlin-Boll E *et al.* Onset and duration of action of single doses of formoterol inhaled *via* Turbuhaler. *Respir Med* 1998; 92:1017–1021.
42. Cazzola M, Centanni S, Regolda S *et al.* Onset of action of single doses of formoterol administered *via* Turbuhaler in patients with stable COPD. *Pulm Pharmacol Ther* 2001; 14:41–45.
43. Naline E, Zhang Y, Qian Y *et al.* Relaxant effects and durations of action of formoterol and salmeterol on the isolated human bronchus. *Eur Respir J* 1994; 7:914–920.
44. Cazzola M, Santangelo G, Piccolo A *et al.* Effect of salmeterol and formoterol in patients with chronic obstructive pulmonary disease. *Pulm Pharmacol* 1994; 7:103–107.
45. Cazzola M, Matera MG, Santangelo G *et al.* Salmeterol and formoterol in partially reversible severe chronic obstructive pulmonary disease: a dose-response study. *Respir Med* 1995; 89:357–362.
46. Çelik G, Kayacan O, Beder S *et al.* Formoterol and salmeterol in partially reversible chronic obstructive pulmonary disease: a crossover, placebo-controlled comparison of onset and duration of action. *Respiration* 1999; 66:434–439.
47. Maesen BLP, Westermann CJJ, Duurkens VAM *et al.* Effects of formoterol in apparently poorly reversible chronic obstructive pulmonary disease. *Eur Respir J* 1999; 13:1103–1108.
48. Di Marco F, Milic-Emili J, Boveri B *et al.* Effect of inhaled bronchodilators on inspiratory capacity and dyspnoea at rest in COPD. *Eur Respir J* 2003; 21:86–94.
49. Ramirez-Venegas A, Ward J, Lentine T *et al.* Salmeterol reduces dyspnea and improves lung function in patients with COPD. *Chest* 1997; 112:336–340.
50. Johnson M, Rennard S. Alternative mechanisms for long-acting β$_2$-adrenergic agonists in COPD. *Chest* 2001; 120:258–270.
51. Bloeman PGM, Van den Tweek MC, Henricks PAJ *et al.* Increased cAMP levels in stimulated neutrophils inhibit their adhesion to human bronchial epithelial cells. *Am J Physiol* 1997; 272:L580–L587.
52. Eda R, Tanimoto Y, Marou H *et al.* Comparison of effect of formoterol and salbutamol on human neutrophil function *in vitro* [abstract]. *Allergy* 1997; 91:301.
53. Ottonello L, Morone P, Dapino P *et al.* Inhibitory effect of salmeterol on the respiratory burst of adherent human neutrophils. *Clin Exp Immunol* 1996; 106:97–102.
54. Ward C, Li X, Wang N *et al.* Salmeterol reduces BAL IL-8 levels in asthmatics on low dose inhaled corticosteroids [abstract]. *Eur Respir J* 1998; 12:S380.
55. Dentener MA, Buurman WA, Wouters EFM. Theophylline and the β-agonists salmeterol and salbutamol potently block neutrophil activation, as indicated by a reduced release of bacterial/permeability-increasing protein [abstract]. *Am J Respir Crit Care Med* 1998; 157:A602.
56. Johnson M. Effects of β$_2$-agonists on resident and infiltrating inflammatory cells. *J Allergy Clin Immunol* 2002; 110:S282–S290.

57. Bowden JJ, Sulakvelidze I, McDonald DM. Inhibition of neutrophil and eosinophil adhesion to venules of rat trachea by β_2-adrenergic agonist formoterol. *J Appl Physiol* 1994; 77:397–405.

58. Cazzola M, Matera MG. Long-acting bronchodilators are the first-choice option for the treatment of stable COPD. *Chest* 2004; 125:9–11.

59. Boyd G, Morice AH, Pounsford JC *et al.* An evaluation of salmeterol in the treatment of chronic obstructive pulmonary disease (COPD). *Eur Respir J* 1997; 10:815–821.

60. Mahler DA, Donohue JF, Barbee RA *et al.* Efficacy of salmeterol xinafoate in the treatment of COPD. *Chest* 1999; 115:957–965.

61. Rennard SI, Anderson W, ZuWallack R *et al.* Use of a long-acting inhaled β_2-adrenergic agonist, salmeterol xinafoate, in patients with chronic obstructive pulmonary disease. *Am J Respir Crit Care Med* 2001; 163:1087–1092.

62. Dahl R, Greefhorst LAPM, Nowak D *et al.* Inhaled formoterol dry powder versus ipratropium bromide in chronic obstructive pulmonary disease. *Am J Respir Crit Care Med* 2001; 164:778–784.

63. Wadbo M, Lofdahl CG, Larsson K *et al.* Effects of formoterol and ipratropium bromide in COPD: a 3-month placebo-controlled study. *Eur Respir J* 2002; 20:1138–1146.

64. Brusasco V, Hodder R, Miravitlles M *et al.* Health outcomes following treatment for six months with once daily tiotropium compared with twice daily salmeterol in patients with COPD. *Thorax* 2003; 58:399–404.

65. Di Lorenzo G, Morici G, Drago A *et al.* Tolerability and effects on quality of life of inhaled salmeterol 50 μg b.i.d. and oral twice daily dose-titrated theophylline in a patient population with mild to moderate chronic obstructive pulmonary disease. SLMT02 Italian Study Group. *Clin Ther* 1998; 20:1130–1148.

66. Taccola M, Bancalari L, Ghignoni G *et al.* Clinical efficacy of salmeterol in patients with reversible chronic pulmonary disease. Comparison with slow release theophylline. *Monaldi Arch Chest Dis* 1999; 54:302–306.

67. ZuWallack RL, Mahler DA, Reilly D *et al.* Salmeterol plus theophylline combination therapy in the treatment of COPD. *Chest* 2001; 119:1661–1670.

68. Rossi A, Kristufek P, Levine BE *et al.* Comparison of the efficacy, tolerability, and safety of formoterol dry powder and oral, slow-release theophylline in the treatment of COPD. *Chest* 2002; 121:1058–1069.

69. Appleton S, Smith B, Veale A *et al.* Long-acting β_2-agonists for chronic obstructive pulmonary disease. (Cochrane Review). In: *The Cochrane Library. Oxford: Update Software,* Issue 3, 2003.

70. Aalbers R, Ayres J, Backer V *et al.* Formoterol in patients with chronic obstructive pulmonary disease: A randomized, controlled, 3-month trial. *Eur Respir J* 2002; 19:936–943.

71. van Noord JA, de Munck DRAJ, Bantje T *et al.* Long-term treatment of chronic obstructive pulmonary disease with salmeterol and the additive effect of ipratropium. *Eur Respir J* 2000; 15:878–885.

72. Mahler DA, Wire P, Horstman D *et al.* Effectiveness of fluticasone propionate and salmeterol combination delivered *via* the diskus device in the treatment of chronic obstructive pulmonary disease. *Am J Respir Crit Care Med* 2002; 166:1084–1091.

73. Jones PW, Bosh TK. Quality of life changes in COPD patients treated with salmeterol. *Am J Respir Crit Care Med* 1997; 155:1283–1289.

74. Rutten-van Molken M, Roos B, Van Noord JA. An empirical comparison of the St George's Respiratory Questionnaire (SGRQ) and the Chronic Respiratory Disease Questionnaire (CRDQ) in a clinical trial setting. *Thorax.* 1999; 54:995–1003.

75. Patakas D, Andreadis D, Mavrofridis E *et al.* Comparison of the effects of salmeterol and ipratropium bromide on exercise performance and breathlessness in patients with stable chronic obstructive pulmonary disease. *Respir Med* 1998; 92:1116–1121.

76. Grove A, Lipworth BJ, Reid P *et al.* Effects of regular salmeterol on lung function and exercise capacity in patients with chronic obstructive airways disease. *Thorax* 1996; 51:689–693.

77. Liesker JJ, Van De Velde V, Meysman M *et al.* Effects of formoterol (Oxis Turbuhaler) and ipratropium on exercise capacity in patients with COPD. *Respir Med* 2002; 96:559–566.

78. Calverley P, Pauwels R, Vestbo J *et al.* Combined salmeterol and fluticasone in the treatment of chronic obstructive pulmonary disease: A randomised controlled trial. *Lancet* 2003; 361:449–456.

79. D'Urzo AD, De Salvo MC, Ramirez-Rivera A *et al.* In patients with COPD, treatment with a combination of formoterol and ipratropium is more effective than a combination of salbutamol and ipratropium: a 3-week, randomized, double-blind, within-patient, multicenter study. *Chest* 2001; 119:1347–1356.

80. Szafranski W, Cukier A, Ramirez A et al. Efficacy and safety of budesonide/formoterol in the management of chronic obstructive disease. Eur Respir J 2003; 21:74–81.

81. Ulrik CS. Efficacy of inhaled salmeterol in the management of smokers with chronic obstructive pulmonary disease: a single centre randomised, double blind, placebo controlled, crossover study. Thorax 1995; 50:750–754.

82. Dowling RB, Johnson M, Cole PJ et al. Effect of salmeterol on Haemophilus influenzae infection of respiratory mucosa in vitro. Eur Respir J 1998; 11:86–90.

83. Dowling RB, Rayner CFJ, Rutman A et al. Effect of salmeterol on Pseudomonas aeruginosa infection of respiratory mucosa. Am J Respir Crit Care Med 1997; 155;327–336.

84. Silvestri M, Oddera S, Lantero S et al. β₂-agonist-induced inhibition of neutrophil chemotaxis is not associated with modification of LFA-1 and Mac-l expression or with impairment of polymorphonuclear leukocyte antibacterial activity. Respir Med 1999; 93:416–423.

85. Cazzola M. Valutazione critica dell'effetto paradosso dei β-adrenergici nell'asma bronchiale. Rass Pat App Respir 1994; 9:238–248.

86. Taylor DR, Sears MR, Cockcroft DW. The β agonist controversy. Med Clin North Am 1996; 80:719–748.

87. Lipworth BJ. Airway subsensitivity with long-acting β₂-agonists. Is there cause for concern? Drug Saf 1997; 16:295–308.

88. Cazzola M, Di Perna F, Noschese P et al. Effects of a pre-treatment with conventional doses of formoterol, salmeterol or oxitropium bromide on the dose-response curves to salbutamol in patients suffering from partially reversible COPD. Eur Respir J 1998; 11:1337–1341.

89. Bjermer L, Larsson L. Long-acting β₂-agonists: how are they used in an optimal way? Respir Med 1997; 91:578–591.

90. Anderson W, Fling M, Xue Z et al. The lack of effect of β₂-adrenoceptor polymorphisms on response to salmeterol in COPD [abstract]. Am J Respir Crit Care Med 2000; 161:A571.

91. Donohue F, Menjoge S, Kesten S. Tolerance to bronchodilating effects of salmeterol in COPD. Respir Med 2003; 97:1014–1020.

92. Costello J. Cardiac effects of β-agonists in patients with COPD. Chest 1998; 114:353–354.

93. Sarubbi B, Esposito V, Ducceschi V et al. Effect of blood gas derangement on QTc dispersion in severe chronic obstructive pulmonary disease: evidence of an electropathy? Int J Cardiol 1997; 58:287–292.

94. Conradson TB, Eklundh G, Olofsson B et al. Cardiac arrhythmias in patients with mild-to-moderate obstructive pulmonary disease: comparison of β-agonist therapy alone and in combination with a xanthine derivative, enprophylline or theophylline. Chest 1985; 88:537–542.

95. Stewart AG, Waterhouse JC, Howard T. The QTc interval, autonomic neuropathy and mortality in hypoxaemic COPD. Respir Med 1995; 89:79–84.

96. Bremner P, Burgess CD, Crane J et al. Cardiovascular effects of fenoterol under conditions of hypoxaemia. Thorax 1992; 47:814–817.

97. Burgess CD, Flatt A, Siebers R et al. A comparison of the extent and duration of hypokalaemia following three nebulized β₂-adrenoceptor agonists. Eur J Clin Pharmacol 1989; 36:415–417.

98. Kiely DG, Cargill RI, Grove A et al. Abnormal myocardial repolarisation in response to hypoxaemia and fenoterol. Thorax 1995; 50:1062–1066.

99. Salpeter SR, Ormiston TM, Salpeter EE. Cardiovascular effects of β-agonists in patients with asthma and COPD: a meta-analysis. Chest 2004; 125:2309–2321.

100. Lipworth BJ. Risks versus benefits of inhaled β₂-agonists in the management of asthma. Drug Saf 1992; 7:54–70.

101. Maesen FPV, Costongs R, Smeets JJ et al. The effect of maximal doses of formoterol and salbutamol from a metered dose inhaler on pulse rates, ECG, and serum potassium concentrations. Chest 1991; 99:1367–1373.

102. Suissa S, Assimes T, Ernst P. Inhaled short acting β agonist use in COPD and the risk of acute myocardial infarction. Thorax 2003; 58:43–46.

103. Cazzola M, Imperatore F, Salzillo A et al. Cardiac effects of formoterol and salmeterol in patients suffering from COPD with preexisting cardiac arrhythmias and hypoxemia. Chest 1998; 114:411–415.

104. Ferguson GT, Funck-Brentano C, Fischer T et al. Cardiovascular safety of salmeterol in COPD. Chest 2003; 123:1817–1824.

105. Khoukaz G, Gross NJ. Effects of salmeterol on arterial blood gases in patients with stable chronic obstructive pulmonary disease comparison with albuterol and ipratropium. Am J Respir Crit Care Med 1999; 160:1028–1030.

106. Ingram Jr. RH, Krumpe PE, Duffel GM *et al.* Ventilation-perfusion changes after aerosolized isoproterenol in asthma. *Am Rev Respir Dis* 1970; 101:364–370.

107. Wagner PD, Dantzker DR, Iacovoni VE *et al.* Ventilation-perfusion inequality in asymptomatic asthma. *Am Rev Respir Dis* 1978; 118:511–524.

108. Cazzola M, D'Amato M, Califano C *et al.* Formoterol as dry powder oral inhalation in comparison with salbutamol metered dose inhaler in acute exacerbations of chronic obstructive pulmonary disease. *Clin Ther* 2002; 24:595–604.

109. Cazzola M, Santus P, Matera MG *et al.* A single high dose of fomoterol is as effective as the same dose administered in a cumulative manner in patients with acute exacerbation of COPD. *Respir Med* 2003; 97:458–462.

110. Cazzola M, Califano C, Di Perna F *et al.* Acute effects of higher than customary doses of salmeterol and salbutamol in patients with acute exacerbation of COPD. *Respir Med* 2002; 96:790–795.

111. Cazzola M, Matera MG, D'Amato M *et al.* Long-acting β_2 agonists in the treatment of acute exacerbations of COPD. *Clin Drug Invest* 2002; 22:369–376.

112. Maconochie JG, Minton NA, Chilton JE *et al.* Does tachyphylaxis occur to the non-pulmonary effects of salmeterol? *Br J Clin Pharmacol* 1994; 37:199–204.

113. Gelmont DM, Balms JR, Vee A. Hypokalemia induced by inhaled bronchodilators. *Chest* 1988; 94:763–766.

114. Palmqvist M, Ibsen T, Mellen A *et al.* Comparison of the relative efficacy of formoterol and salmeterol in asthmatic patients. *Am J Respir Crit Care Med* 1999; 160:244–249.

115. Global Initiative for Chronic Obstructive Lung Disease: Global Strategy for the Diagnosis, Management and Prevention of Chronic Obstructive Pulmonary Disease. *NHLBI/WHO workshop report.* Bethesda, National Heart, Lung and Blood Institute, April 2001; Update of the Management Sections; GOLD website (www.goldcopd.com). Date updated: July 2003.

116. American Thoracic Society. Standards for the diagnosis and care of patients with chronic obstructive pulmonary disease. *Am J Respir Crit Care Med* 1995; 152:S77–S121.

117. Siafakas NM, Vermeire P, Pride NB *et al.* Optimal assessment and management of chronic obstructive pulmonary disease (COPD). The European Respiratory Society Task Force. *Eur Respir J* 1995; 8:1398–1420.

118. The COPD Guideline Group of the Standards of Care Committee of the BTS. BTS guidelines for the management of chronic obstructive pulmonary disease. *Thorax* 1997; 52(suppl 5):S1–S28.

119. American Thoracic Society and European Respiratory Society. Standards for the diagnosis and management of patients with COPD. http://www.thoracic.org/copd/.

120. Chronic Obstructive Pulmonary Disease. National Collaborating Centre for Chronic Conditions. National clinical guideline on management of chronic obstructive pulmonary disease in adults in primary and secondary care. *Thorax* 2004; 59(suppl 1):1–232.

121. Mannino DM. COPD: epidemiology, prevalence, morbidity and mortality, and disease heterogeneity. *Chest* 2002; 121(Suppl 5):S6–S121.

122. Kuhl DA, Agiri OA, Mauro LS. β-agonists in the treatment of acute exacerbation of chronic obstructive pulmonary disease. *Ann Pharmacother* 1994; 28:1379–1388.

123. Fromm Jr. RE, Varon J. Acute exacerbations of obstructive lung disease. What to do when immediate care is crucial. *Postgrad Med* 1994; 95:101–106.

124. Emerman CL, Cydulka RK. Effect of different albuterol dosing regimens in the treatment of acute exacerbation of chronic obstructive pulmonary disease. *Ann Emerg Med* 1997; 29:474–478.

125. Karpel JP, Pesin J, Greenberg D *et al.* A comparison of the effects of ipratropium bromide and metaproterenol sulfate in acute exacerbations of COPD. *Chest* 1990; 98:835–839.

126. Lloberes P, Ramis L, Montserrat JM *et al.* Effect of three different bronchodilators during an exacerbation of chronic obstructive pulmonary disease. *Eur Respir J* 1988; 1:536–539.

127. Bernasconi M, Brandolese R, Poggi R *et al.* Dose–response effects and time course of effects of inhaled fenoterol on respiratory mechanics and arterial oxygen tension in mechanically ventilated patients with chronic airflow obstruction. *Intensive Care Med* 1990; 16:108–114.

128. Cazzola M, Matera MG. Long-acting β_2-agonists as potential option in the treatment of acute exacerbations of COPD. *Pulm Pharmacol Ther* 2003; 16:197–201.

129. Heimer D, Shim C, Williams M. The effect of sequential inhalations of metaproterenol aerosol in asthma. *J Allergy Clin Immunol* 1980; 66:75–77.

130. Britton J, Tattersfield A. Comparison of cumulative and noncumulative techniques to measure dose-response curves for β-agonists in patients with asthma. *Thorax* 1984; 39:597–599.

131. Cazzola M, Matera MG, D'Amato M *et al.* Bronchodilator response to formoterol Turbuhaler in patients with COPD under regular treatment with formoterol Turbuhaler. *Pulm Pharmacol Ther* 2003; 16:105–109.
132. Nelson HS, Bensch G, Pleskow WW *et al.* Improved bronchodilation with levalbuterol compared with racemic albuterol in patients with asthma. *J Allergy Clin Immunol* 1998; 102:943–952.
133. Gawchik SM, Saccar CL, Noonan M *et al.* The safety and efficacy of nebulized levalbuterol compared with racemic albuterol and placebo in the treatment of asthma in pediatric patients. *J Allergy Clin Immunol* 1999; 103:615–621.
134. Handley DA, Senanayake CH, Dutczak W *et al.* Biological actions of formoterol isomers. *Pulm Pharmacol Ther* 2002; 15:135–145.
135. Truitt T, Witko J, Halpern M. Levalbuterol compared to racemic albuterol: efficacy and outcomes in patients hospitalized with COPD or asthma. *Chest* 2003; 123:128–135.
136. Garaud J-J. Attractive projects in important public health issues. http://www.novartis.com/downloads_new/investors/j_g_rnd_day_2003.pdf
137. Bonnert RV, Brown RC, Chapman D *et al.* Dual D2-receptor and β_2-adrenoceptor agonists for the treatment of airway diseases. 1. Discovery and biological evaluation of some 7-(2-aminoethyl)-4-hydroxybenzothiazol-2(3H)-one analogues. *J Med Chem* 1998; 41:4915–4917.
138. Dougall IG, Young A, Ince F *et al.* Dual dopamine D2 receptor and β_2-adrenoceptor agonists for the treatment of chronic obstructive pulmonary disease: the pre-clinical rationale. *Respir Med* 2003; 97(suppl A):S3–S7.

5

Anticholinergics: basic pharmacology

M. G. Belvisi, H. J. Patel

INTRODUCTION

The parasympathetic cholinergic nerves play a major role in the control and regulation of airway tone and mucus secretion in man and in animals [1, 2]. Acetylcholine (ACh) released from these nerves activates muscarinic receptors on smooth muscle to contract and maintain airway tone, on submucosal glands to stimulate mucus secretion, on blood vessels to cause vasodilation and on cholinergic nerve terminals to inhibit further ACh release. Muscarinic receptor antagonists (anticholinergics) are used as bronchodilators and are central to the management of patients with chronic obstructive pulmonary disease (COPD). Since the 1970s the anticholinergic ipratropium bromide has been widely used for the treatment of patients with regular symptoms. Ipratropium bromide is a non-selective muscarinic antagonist and therefore blocks M_2 as well as M_1 and M_3 receptors, so that the increased ACh release *via* M_2 receptor blockade may overcome the blockade of muscarinic M_3 receptors. This has prompted a search for selective muscarinic receptors that block M_3 or M_1/M_3 receptors and for drugs that have a longer duration of action in order to achieve a once-a-day therapy.

PARASYMPATHETIC INNERVATION TO THE AIRWAYS

The parasympathetic efferent nerves provide the dominant neural bronchoconstrictor mechanism in all species. It is evident that in most species, including man, there is a degree of basal cholinergic activity providing a resting level of bronchomotor tone since it can be abolished by antimuscarinic agents such as atropine or by vagal section [2–4].

Pre-ganglionic cholinergic nerves arising from the vagal nuclei of the medulla travel down the vagus nerve to the airways where they synapse in parasympathetic ganglia in the airway wall. Short post-ganglionic fibres pass from the ganglia and form a dense nerve plexus over target cells such as airway smooth muscle [5] and submucosal glands [6]. The density of cholinergic innervation is greatest proximally and diminishes peripherally [1, 7].

Stimulation of parasympathetic pathways leads to bronchoconstriction, mucus secretion and bronchial vasodilation *via* the activation of muscarinic receptors by ACh released from the nerve terminals by exocytosis. ACh rapidly diffuses the relatively short distance to muscarinic receptors on the target cell and is subject to rapid degradation by the enzyme acetylcholine esterase (AChE), which is concentrated in the synaptic cleft.

Maria G. Belvisi, BSc, PhD, Professor of Respiratory Pharmacology, Respiratory Pharmacology Group, Airway Disease Section, National Heart & Lung Institute, Imperial College School of Medicine, London, UK.

Hema J. Patel, BSc, PhD, Respiratory Pharmacology Group, Airway Disease Section, Imperial College School of Medicine at the National Heart & Lung Institute, London, UK.

MUSCARINIC RECEPTORS IN THE AIRWAYS

Pharmacological characterisation of these receptors has been problematic due to the lack of selective agonists and antagonists that have a high selectivity for any single receptor [8]. There are no selective muscarinic receptor agonists with a high selectivity for an individual muscarinic receptor subtype. However, receptor characterisation has been achieved supported by the use of radioligand binding techniques with ligands such as [³H] pirenzepine and [³H]N-methylscopolamine and membrane preparations from cells transfected with the gene for a particular receptor. Antagonist affinity estimates obtained using these techniques have been comparable to those obtained in isolated tissue studies using Arunlakshana-Schild analysis [8] (see Table 5.1). However, it seems clear from Table 5.1 that, because of the lack of high subtype selectivity of any single antagonist listed, it is necessary to distinguish the involvement of a particular receptor subtype using more than one antagonist (a possible exception being the selectivity of MT7 toxin for the M_1 receptor). Therefore, experimental design is of critical importance in receptor classification.

Muscarinic receptors are present throughout the airways of a variety of species including humans [9–11]. Five types of muscarinic receptor genes have been identified (M_1–M_5, [12]), three of which (M_1, M_2 and M_3) have been identified in the lung pharmacologically [13]. M_4 muscarinic receptors are present in rabbit lung [14, 15] but their function remains unknown. There is little data regarding the functional expression of the M_5 receptor in peripheral tisues [8, 16] (Figure 5.1).

MUSCARINIC M_1 RECEPTORS

M_1 receptors have been localised by functional studies to parasympathetic ganglia of animals [17] and humans [18] and on sympathetic nerves. M_1 receptor activation on parasympathetic ganglia inhibits the opening of K^+ channels; resulting in depolarisation of parasympathetic ganglion cells and a facilitatory effect on neurotransmission through airway ganglia [19–22]. In addition to ACh, many other neurotransmitters and mediators may be released near the ganglia that affect the excitability of pre-ganglionic and post-ganglionic membranes [23].

Submucosal glands are known to express both M_1 and M_3 muscarinic receptors [24]. While the M_3 receptors are the most abundant and mediate mucus, water and electrolyte secretion, the M_1 receptor only appears to be involved in the regulation of water and electrolyte secretion [25].

Table 5.1 Antagonist affinity constants

	Receptor			
Antagonist	M_1	M_2	M_3	M_4
Pirenzepine	7.8–8.5	6.3–6.7	6.7–7.1	7.1–8.1
Methoctramine	7.1–7.8	7.8–8.3	6.3–6.9	7.4–8.1
4-DAMP	8.6–9.2	7.8–8.4	8.9–9.3	8.4–9.4
AF-DX 384	7.3–7.5	8.2–9.0	7.2–7.8	8.0–8.1
Tripitramine	8.4–8.8	9.4–9.6	7.1–7.4	7.8–8.2
Darifenacin	7.5–7.8	7.0–7.4	8.4–8.9	7.7–8.0
MT3	7.1	<6	<6	<6
MT7	9.8	<6	<6	<6

The values listed are log affinity constants or pKB values for mammalian muscarinic receptors adapted from Caulfield and Birdsall, 1998 [8].

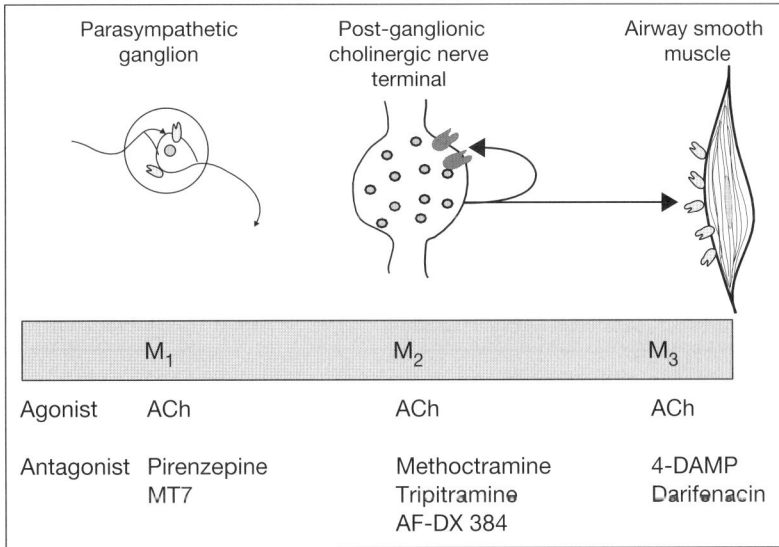

Parasympathetic ganglion	Post-ganglionic cholinergic nerve terminal	Airway smooth muscle
M$_1$	M$_2$	M$_3$
Agonist ACh	ACh	ACh
Antagonist Pirenzepine MT7	Methoctramine Tripitramine AF-DX 384	4-DAMP Darifenacin

Figure 5.1 Three types of muscarinic receptor genes have been identified in the lung pharmacologically using a range of receptor antagonists. M$_1$ receptors have been localised by functional studies to parasympathetic ganglia of animals and on sympathetic nerves, where they may have a facilitatory effect on neurotransmission through airway ganglia. M$_2$ receptors (autoreceptors) are located on cholinergic pre-junctional nerve terminals. ACh released from these terminals can act back on the pre-junctional M$_2$ receptors to inhibit further release of ACh. M$_3$ muscarinic receptors are present in guinea-pig and human airway smooth muscle and have been localised to submucosal glands. Activation of M$_3$ receptors results in smooth muscle contraction and mucus secretion.

MUSCARINIC M$_2$ RECEPTORS

ACh released from cholinergic nerve terminals is modulated by pre-synaptic M$_2$-receptors (autoreceptors) located on cholinergic post-ganglionic, pre-junctional nerve terminals. ACh released from these terminals can act back on the pre-junctional M$_2$ receptors to inhibit further release of ACh [26]. *In vitro* isolated tissue studies where cholinergic neuronally-mediated contractile responses are compared to contractions of similar magnitude to exogenous ACh have described M$_2$-receptors on post-ganglionic pre-junctional cholinergic nerve terminals in a number of species and this has been confirmed by direct measurement of ACh release *in vitro* in both guinea-pig [27, 28] and human trachea [28–30]. M$_2$ receptors are also expressed on parasympathetic ganglia where they also act to inhibit ACh release [31]. RT-PCR, Western analysis and immunocytochemical techniques have also demonstrated functional M$_2$ muscarinic receptors in guinea-pig primary cultures of parasympathetic nerves [32] (Figure 5.2).

The majority of the muscarinic receptors on the airway smooth muscle are of the M$_2$ receptor subtype [33]. However, the relative proportions of M$_2$ and M$_3$ muscarinic receptors in airway tissue may vary depending upon whether central, peripheral or whole lung tissue is used as well as the age of the animal [34]. M$_2$ and M$_3$ receptor mRNAs and functional M$_2$ and M$_3$ receptors have been detected in cultured human airway smooth muscle [35, 36]. The M$_2$ receptors do not directly contract airway smooth muscle, but appear to functionally antagonise airway smooth muscle relaxation mediated by β_2-adrenoceptor activation *via* its opposing actions on adenylyl cyclase activity and Ca^{2+}-dependant K$^+$ channels [37–41]. Interestingly, a recent study by Matsui *et al.* [42] demonstrated that the relaxant effects of forskolin on muscarinic agonist-induced contractions were significantly

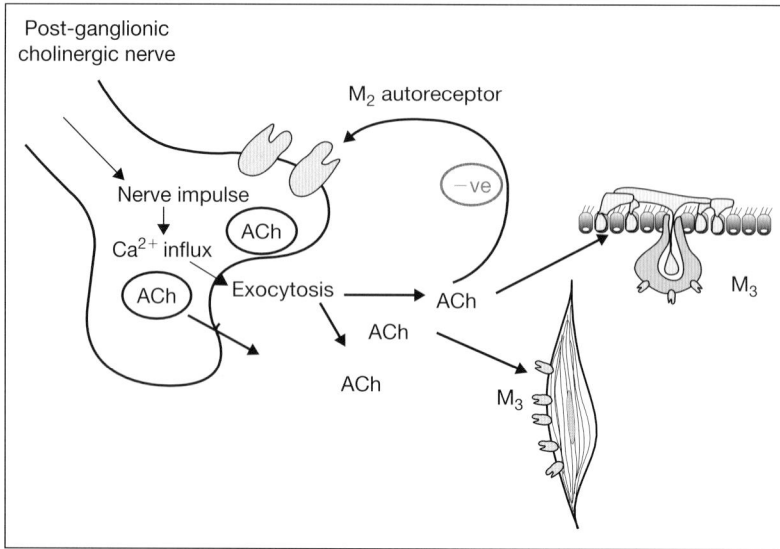

Figure 5.2 Post-ganglionic, parasympathetic nerves innervate the airway smooth muscle and glands. ACh released from cholinergic nerve terminals activates M_3 muscarinic receptors on muscle and glands to produce contraction and mucus secretion. ACh release from post-ganglionic, parasympathetic nerve endings can act on pre-junctional M_2 receptors to inhibit the further release of ACh.

greater in tracheal preparations from mACHR2$^{-/-}$ mice than in the corresponding preparations from wild-type mice, suggesting that a component of the muscarinic agonist-induced contraction response in the tracheal smooth muscle involves an M_2 receptor-mediated functional antagonism of airway smooth muscle relaxation mediated by agents that increase cAMP levels [42].

MUSCARINIC M_3 RECEPTORS

M_3 muscarinic receptors are present in guinea-pig and human airway smooth muscle and have been localised to submucosal glands by autoradiographic [10, 35] and *in situ* hybridisation studies with M_3-selective cDNA probes [35]. Binding studies indicate that in guinea-pig lung membranes the M_3 receptor subtype predominates, whereas in human lung the M_3 receptor subtype makes up less than half of the receptors [43]. Activation of M_3 receptors results in smooth muscle contraction [44–47], mucus secretion [25, 48, 49] and vasodilation of blood vessels in the tracheobronchial circulation [50]. Stimulation of M_3 muscarinic receptors by ACh activates inositol triphosphate- and phosphoinositide-specific phospholipase C, increasing intracellular Ca^{2+} and causing contraction of airway smooth muscle [45, 51, 52]. These effects can be blocked by anti-muscarinic agents such as atropine or ipratropium bromide as well as M_3-selective muscarinic antagonists such as 4-DAMP.

Although previous work suggests that the muscarinic constriction of tracheal smooth muscle and main bronchi is predominantly mediated by the M_3 receptor subtype [45, 53, 54], it is not clear which muscarinic receptors are involved in eliciting this response in the smaller intrapulmonary airways. An understanding of which muscarinic receptors mediate ACh-induced contractile responses is important given that airway resistance is determined largely by the diameter of the small intrapulmonary airways [55, 56]. Interestingly, recent studies in receptor-deficient mice have suggested that cholinergic constriction of murine peripheral airways is mediated by the concerted action of the M_2 and M_3 receptor subtypes.

These data also suggest the existence of pulmonary M_1 receptors, the activation of which counteracts this bronchoconstrictor activity [57].

SIGNAL TRANSDUCTION MECHANISMS

The muscarinic acetylcholine receptors (mAChR) are prototypical members of the G-protein-coupled receptor superfamily characterised by seven transmembrane domains. Agonist binding triggers conformational changes within the helical bundle, which are then transmitted to the cytoplasmic face where the interaction with specific G-proteins occur.

It is generally presumed that muscarinic receptors can be generally classed into two major categories [8]. The M_2 and M_4 muscarinic receptor subtypes preferentially couple to inhibition of adenylyl cyclase *via* pertussis toxin-sensitive G_i/G_o [58–60]; however, M_2 receptors may also couple to inhibition of adenylyl cyclase activity *via* the PTX-resistant G-protein, G_z [58]. The M_1, M_3 and M_5 muscarinic receptor subtypes predominantly stimulate phospholipase Cß (PLCß) *via* pertussis toxin-insensitive G_q/G_{11} class [61, 62]. Activation of muscarinic M_3 receptors results in IP_3 and DAG production *via* activation of PLC. IP_3 increases intracellular calcium concentrations that ultimately promotes the rapid phase of smooth muscle contraction. Activation of PKC by DAG is thought to mediate the sustained phase of smooth muscle contraction [63].

While this general distinction still holds, muscarinic receptors can also couple to other signal transduction pathways, including phospholipases A_2 and D, tyrosine kinases and calcium and potassium channels [8, 64]. Muscarinic agonists can stimulate large conductance calcium-activated potassium channels (BK_{Ca}) in airway smooth muscle cells. These channels are implicated in the functional antagonism between cholinergic agonist-induced contraction and β-adrenoceptors-mediated relaxation, where activation of post-juctional M_2 receptors leads to inhibition of adenylyl cyclase, a decrease in cAMP and an inhibition of BK_{Ca} channel activity [39].

CHOLINERGIC REFLEXES

Cholinergic responses such as bronchoconstriction, mucus secretion [65–67] and bronchial vasodilation [68] can be elicited by mechanical or chemical stimulation of sensory neural pathways *via* central reflex pathways. As well as mechanical stimulation of sensory nerves, a wide variety of chemical stimuli including gastroeosophageal reflux (GER, [69]) are able to elicit cholinergic reflexes by activation of sensory nerves. Stimulation of the nasal mucosa, larynx, central and peripheral chemoreceptors, baroceptors and the oesophagus may cause reflex bronchoconstriction. Reflex cholinergic bronchoconstriction can be demonstrated *in vivo* by activation of afferent vagal fibre (sensory) endings in the airways, since it can be blocked by vagal section, administration of a muscarinic antagonist, or by the administration of the nicotinic antagonist, hexamethonium [2] to block ganglionic transmission at cholinergic ganglia. *In vivo*, electrical stimulation of the vagus nerve in anaesthetised animals causes rapid bronchoconstriction, which can be potentiated in the presence of AChE inhibitors and reversed by the muscarinic antgonist atropine [2]. The rapid onset and reversibility of the bronchoconstriction suggests that it is due to constriction of airway smooth muscle rather than mucosal oedema or obstruction of the airway lumen by mucus. The extent of cholinergic reflex is species- and maybe stimulus-dependent and demonstration of this response relies on the degree of attenuation by vagal section, antimuscarinics or hexamethonium.

It is assumed that methacholine, a regularly used muscarinic agonist to assess airway responsiveness in clinical settings, causes bronchoconstriction exclusively by acting directly on airway smooth muscle. Studies have shown that cholinergic agonists can increase sensory nerve activity in the lungs [70] and that vagotomy significantly reduces bronchoconstriction induced by methacholine infused directly into the bronchial artery in sheep [71, 72]. The authors conclude that there is a substantial reflex effect of cholinergic agonists and therefore a response to methacholine in humans or animals should not be assumed to be solely *via* a direct action on smooth muscle.

In man, evidence for such a reflex depends primarily on the inhibitory efficiency of anti-cholinergics such as atropine. There is some disagreement over the relative importance of reflex mechanisms in bronchoconstrictor responses because there are variations between subjects, provoking stimuli and the degree of the cholinergic reflex. Anticholinergics are generally effective against bronchoconstriction induced by sulphur dioxide [73, 74], carbon dust [75, 76], ozone [77] and acid challenge to the oesophagus [78] but are less effective against allergen-induced bronchoconstriction [79]. This may be because the inflammatory mediators released during allergen challenge have more impact on airway smooth muscle than on the afferent nerve endings. Evidence for reflex mechanisms induced by histamine in man is also conflicting [80], although the majority of studies show that the bronchoconstriction is due to a direct effect of histamine on airway smooth muscle [81, 82].

M_2 RECEPTOR DYSFUNCTION

The existence of muscarinic auto-inhibitory receptors on cholinergic nerve terminals in human airways has important implications in view of the fact that these receptors may represent an important mechanism by which vagal control of the airways may be regulated. Loss of neural M_2-muscarinic receptor function has been implicated in asthmatic patients [83, 84]. Furthermore, neurally evoked cholinergic responses *in vitro* of airways from mild asthmatics also appear to be greater than that from airways from normal patients [85]. M_2 autoreceptor dysfunction may also be a factor which contributes to airway hyperresponsiveness [30] and enhanced cholinergic reflex bronchoconstriction [26]. Airway hyperresponsiveness is an important feature of asthma in humans and is occasionally seen in COPD patients.

Several *in vivo* animal models have been described which demonstrate increased activity of the parasympathetic nerves, such as infection with parainfluenza virus [86, 87], sensitisation and challenge with antigen [30, 88–89], acute exposure to ozone [90] and vitamin A deficiency [91]. Furthermore, increased basal tone in the airways and airway hyperreactivity in humans with asthma and COPD may also be as a result of increased parasympathetic nerve activity. There is no evidence that the number or function of M_3 muscarinic receptors on airway smooth muscle is altered in the above animal models or in human asthma or COPD, whereas there are several lines of evidence which demonstrate M_2 receptor dysfunction. Compromised neuronal M_2 muscarinic receptor function increases the concentration of ACh released in the vicinity of the airway smooth muscle and results in an enhanced bronchoconstrictor response to vagal stimulation.

Possible hypotheses for M_2 receptor dysfunction have arisen from a number of studies in these animal models [89, 91–94]. Firstly, the loss of M_2 muscarinic receptor function in the sensitised and antigen-challenged guinea-pig model would appear to be due to the presence of activated eosinophils [94–97]. Activated eosinophils release preformed proteins, including the cationic protein major basic protein (MBP) and it is thought that this can act as an allosteric antagonist of the muscarinic M_2 receptor. Evidence for this hypothesis stems from experiments demonstrating that M_2 muscarinic receptor dysfunction and airway hyperreactivity in antigen-challenged, sensitised guinea-pigs can be prevented by blockade of MBP with a selective antibody [98] or reversed by the polyanionic molecule heparin [99]. Other mechanisms appear to play a role in this dysfunction following viral infection. In non-sensitised animals viruses can act to induce M_2 receptor dysfunction by (a) producing neuraminidase, which cleaves sialic acid residues from M_2 receptors, decreasing the affinity of agonists for the receptor by 10-fold [100], (b) the release of an unidentified mediator from activated macrophages as depletion of macrophages with liposome-encapsulated clodronate protects receptor function and prevents airway hyperreactivity [101] or through (c) the activation of inflammatory cells and the release of Th1-type cytokines (e.g., interferons). However, on a background of atopy, virus-induced M_2 receptor dysfunction may be due to the activation of eosinophils and the release of MBP *via* a mechanism that may involve $CD8^+$ T-lymphocytes [101, 102].

Interestingly, M_2 muscarinic receptors are functional in patients with stable COPD [103]. However, the role for neuronal M_2 muscarinic receptors in acute exacerbations of COPD is not yet known (Figure 5.3).

NON-NEURONAL ACh

Although ACh has historically been regarded as a classical neurotransmitter, it is increasingly being recognised that ACh may also serve as an autocrine and paracrine signalling molecule. Non-neuronal ACh is implicated in regulating a wide range of basic cell functions such as proliferation, differentiation, cell–cell contact, secretion, absorption [104], trophic and immune functions and the release of mediators.

The non-neuronal cholinergic system is widely expressed in human airways, and in particular in epithelial and immune (lymphocytes) cells which play an important role in inflammation. ACh-synthesising enzyme, choline acetyl transferase (ChAT) and/or ACh is present in human epithelial surface cells including goblet cells, ciliated cells and basal cells [105–107]. Epithelial cells also express both muscarinic (M_1 and M_3 subtypes) and nicotinic receptors [35, 107, 108].

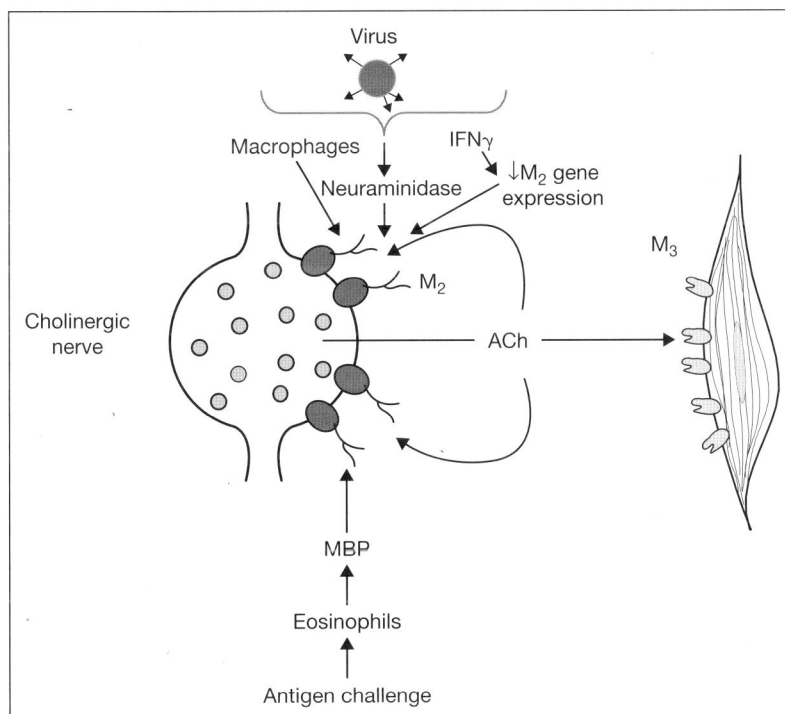

Figure 5.3 Mechanisms involved in neuronal M_2 muscarinic receptor dysfunction. Antigen challenge in a guinea-pig animal model leads to M_2 receptor dysfunction *via* the activation of eosinophils and the release of MBP, resulting in increased ACh release and enhanced bronchoconstrictor responses. Virus infection is thought to elicit receptor dysfunction *via* activation of macrophages and the release of interferons and also *via* the action of viral neuraminidase which cleaves sialic acid residues from the M_2 receptor, thereby compromising its functionality.

Immune cells which invade the airway mucosa, for example lymphocytes, alveolar macrophages and granulocytes, can synthesise and release ACh and may release inappropriate amounts of ACh under inflammatory conditions [107, 109–111]. ACh and ACh-sensitive receptors have been detected on many of the individual components of the immune system: lymphocytes (CD4$^+$ > CD8$^+$ > B cells), monocytes, macrophages, mast cells, thymus and spleen [for reviews, see 104, 112]. Evidence suggests that ACh mediates its actions *via* both muscarinic and nicotinic receptors on lymphocytes [112]; however, the exact muscarinic receptor subtype that is involved is not clear and may involve some or all subtypes depending on the lymphocyte sub-population. Interestingly, data from bovine and insect tissue suggest the existence of a chimeric nicotinic receptor responding to both nicotine and muscarinic agonists and appears to be a target for non-neuronal ACh [113, 114].

ACh also modulates immune function indirectly *via* the release of cytokines. For example, ACh or nicotine stimulates the release of pro-inflammatory chemotactic activity from bronchial epithelial cells and macrophages [115–117]. Hence, it is becoming increasingly apparent that non-neuronal ACh contributes to both the non-specific and specific host defence system and is involved in modulating the inflammatory response [107, 112, 118].

ANTICHOLINERGICS IN ASTHMA AND COPD

Chronic COPD encompasses a number of diseases, including chronic bronchitis and emphysema. COPD is characterised by airflow limitation that is not fully reversible and is usually progressive and associated with an abnormal inflammatory response of the lungs to noxious particles and gases [119]. Prevention and relief of symptoms by regular use of bronchodilators is central to the management of patients with COPD. It is now well established that cholinergic neural mechanisms contribute to airway narrowing and increased mucus secretion. Similarly, anticholinergics decrease airway hyperreactivity in patients with COPD [120]. Furthermore, the role of this pathway in COPD is evidenced by the effectiveness of antimuscarinic agents. In fact, anticholinergics are the bronchodilators of choice [81] and have proved to be of particular value in the treatment of COPD as cholinergic vagal tone appears to be the only reversible element of airway narrowing. Anticholinergics are also effective in reducing neurogenic control of mucus hypersecretion in chronic bronchitis [121].

Since the 1970s the anticholinergic ipratropium bromide has been widely used for the treatment of patients with regular symptoms. Ipatropium bromide is a non-selective muscarinic antagonist and therefore blocks M_2 as well as M_1 and M_3 receptors, so that the increased ACh release *via* M_2 receptor blockade may overcome some of the blockade of the muscarinic M_3 receptors. This has prompted a search for selective muscarinic receptors that block M_3 or M_1/M_3 receptors. In lieu of genuinely selective M_3 muscarinic receptor compounds, a therapeutic approach for selective blockade of M_3 muscarinic receptors has been to exploit differences in receptor kinetics. One such compound is tiotropium bromide (Spiriva).

A series of pharmacological studies have shown that tiotropium shows kinetic selectivity for M_1 and M_3 receptors over M_2 receptors, and is a potent muscarinic receptor antagonist with a prolonged duration of action [122]. Tiotropium binds with equal affinity to human cloned (Hm1, Hm2, and Hm3) muscarinic receptors [123, 124] but with greater affinity than ipratropium bromide. Importantly, however, kinetic studies demonstrate that tiotropium bromide dissociates very slowly in comparison with ipratropium bromide [33] but also more rapidly from M_2 receptors than from M_1 or M_3 receptors, thus achieving a prolonged effect and subtype selectivity through a kinetic mechanism [123]. Tiotropium bromide inhibits exogenous ACh-induced bronchospasm three times more potently than ipratropium bromide and has a markedly longer duration of action than an equipotent dose of ipratropium bromide in the dog *in vivo* [123]. Comparable *in vivo* and *in vitro* results have been obtained in rabbits and guinea-pigs [123, 125]. In guinea-pig trachea *in vitro*, tiotropium potently inhibits EFS-evoked cholinergic contractions five times more potently than ipatropium bromide or atropine. Although the onset of action of tiotropium bromide was slower than atropine or ipatropium bromide, after wash out, tiotropium was still effective for a considerably greater period, with a half-life of 540 min compared with 18 min for ipatropium. Similar effects were seen in human bronchi [125]. Experiments involving the measurement of ACh release have confirmed the non-selective action of these muscarinic antagonists as ACh release is increased *via* M_2-receptor blockade as expected. However, 2 h after wash out, the facilitatory effect of tiotropium on ACh release *via* activation of M_2 receptors is lost, while the inhibitory action of tiotropium on cholinergic contractile responses *via* blockade of the M_3 receptors is maintained for a prolonged period.

Clinical studies with inhaled tiotropium bromide confirm that it is a potent and long-lasting bronchodilator in COPD, protecting against cholinergic bronchoconstriction for up to 24 h [126–128]. It is more effective when given once daily by inhalation than ipatropium given four times daily [129]. Tiotropium bromide has been developed as a dry powder inhaler for COPD patients and has already been introduced in some countries. Evidence suggests that once-daily treatment with tiotropium (Spiriva) is the most effective therapy for COPD patients currently available. Patients demonstrated improved lung function and health status with a reduction in symptoms and number of exacerbations [130, 131]. The drug appears to be well tolerated with a dryness of the mouth being the only notable side effect and does not usually warrant discontinuation.

CONCLUSIONS

The parasympathetic nerves provide the dominant autonomic control and regulation of airway tone and mucus secretion in man and in animals. Muscarinic receptor antagonists (anticholinergics) are used as bronchodilators and are central to the management of patients with COPD. Currently, the anticholinergic medications used in the treatment of airway diseases are not selective for the M_3 muscarinic receptor subtype. New compounds that exhibit increased selectivity for this receptor subtype over the M_2 receptor are becoming available and may have advantages over other non-selective compounds by blocking the contractile activity of ACh without increasing the neuronal release of ACh.

REFERENCES

1. Richardson JB. Nerve supply to the lungs. *Am Rev Respir Dis* 1979; 119:785–802.
2. Nadel JA, Barnes PJ. Autonomic regulation of the airways. *Annu Rev Med* 1984; 35:451–467.
3. Carlyle RF. The responses of the guinea-pig isolated intact trachea to transmural stimulation and the release of an acetylcholine-like substance under conditions of rest and stimulation. *Br J Pharmacol* 1964; 22:126–136.
4. De Troyer AJ, Yernault C, Rodenstein D. Effects of vagal blockade on lung mechanics in normal man. *J Appl Physiol* 1979; 46:217–226.
5. Baker DG. Parasympathetic motor pathways to the trachea: recent morphologic and electrophysiologic studies. *Clin Chest Med* 1986; 7:223–229.
6. Barnes PJ. Neural control of human airways in health and disease. *Am Rev Respir Dis* 1986; 134:1289–1314.
7. Kalia M, Mesulam MM. Brain stem projections of sensory and motor components of the vagus complex in the cat: II. Laryngeal, tracheobronchial, pulmonary, cardiac, and gastrointestinal branches. *J Comp Neurol* 1980; 193:467–508.
8. Caulfield MP, Birdsall NJ. International Union of Pharmacology. XVII. Classification of muscarinic acetylcholine receptors. *Pharmacol Rev* 1998; 50:279–290.
9. Barnes PJ, Nadel JA, Roberts JM, Basbaum CB. Muscarinic receptors in lung and trachea: autoradiographic localization using [3H]quinuclidinyl benzilate. *Eur J Pharmacol* 1982; 86:103–106.
10. Mak JC, Barnes PJ. Autoradiographic visualization of muscarinic receptor subtypes in human and guinea-pig lung. *Am Rev Respir Dis* 1990; 141:1559–1568.

11. van Koppen CJ, Blankesteijn WM, Klaassen AB, Rodrigues de Miranda JF, Beld AJ, van Ginneken CA. Autoradiographic visualization of muscarinic receptors in pulmonary nerves and ganglia. *Neurosci Lett* 1987; 83:237–240.

12. Hulme EC, Birdsall NJ, Buckley NJ. Muscarinic receptor subtypes. *Annu Rev Pharmacol Toxicol* 1990; 30:633–673.

13. Maclagan J, Barnes PJ. Muscarinic pharmacology of the airways. *Trends Pharmacol Sci* 1989; (suppl):88–92.

14. Mak JC, Haddad EB, Buckley NJ, Barnes PJ. Visualization of muscarinic m4 mRNA and M4 receptor subtype in rabbit lung. *Life Sci* 1993; 53:1501–1508.

15. Dorje F, Levey AI, Brann MR. Immunological detection of muscarinic receptor subtype proteins (m1-m5) in rabbit peripheral tissues. *Mol Pharmacol* 1991; 40:459–462.

16. Eglen RM, Nahorski SR. The muscarinic M(5) receptor: a silent or emerging subtype? *Br J Pharmacol* 2000; 130:13–21.

17. Bloom JW, Yamamura HI, Baumgartener C, Halonen M. A muscarinic receptor with high affinity for pirenzepine mediates vagally induced bronchoconstriction. *Eur J Pharmacol* 1987; 133:21–27.

18. Lammers JW, Minette P, McCusker M, Barnes PJ. The role of pirenzepine-sensitive (M1) muscarinic receptors in vagally mediated bronchoconstriction in humans. *Am Rev Respir Dis* 1989; 139:446–449.

19. Maclagan J, Fryer AD, Faulkner D. Identification of M1 muscarinic receptors in pulmonary sympathetic nerves in the guinea-pig by use of pirenzepine. *Br J Pharmacol* 1989; 97:499–505.

20. Maclagan J, Faulkner D. Effect of pirenzepine and gallamine on cardiac and pulmonary muscarinic receptors in the rabbit. *Br J Pharmacol* 1989; 97:506–512.

21. Yang ZJ, Biggs DF. Muscarinic receptors and parasympathetic neurotransmission in guinea-pig trachea. *Eur J Pharmacol* 1991; 193:301–308.

22. Barnes PJ. Muscarinic receptor subtypes in airways. *Life Sci* 1993; 52:521–527.

23. Myers AC. Transmission in autonomic ganglia. *Respir Physiol* 2001; 125:99–111.

24. Rogers DF. Motor control of airway goblet cells and glands. *Respir Physiol* 2001; 125:129–144.

25. Ramnarine SI, Haddad EB, Khawaja AM, Mak JC, Rogers DF. On muscarinic control of neurogenic mucus secretion in ferret trachea. *J Physiol* 1996; 494:577–586.

26. Barnes PJ. Muscarinic autoreceptors in airways. Their possible role in airway disease. *Chest* 1989; 96:1220–1221.

27. Kilbinger HR, Schneider R, Siefken H, Wolf D, D'Agostino G. Characterization of prejunctional muscarinic autoreceptors in the guinea-pig trachea. *Br J Pharmacol* 1991; 103:1757–1763.

28. Patel HJ, Barnes PJ, Takahashi T, Tadjkarimi S, Yacoub MH, Belvisi MG. Evidence for prejunctional muscarinic autoreceptors in human and guinea-pig trachea. *Am J Respir Crit Care Med* 1995; 152:872–878.

29. Wessler I, Bender H, Harle P, Hohle KD, Kirdorf G, Klapproth H *et al.* Release of [3H]acetylcholine in human isolated bronchi. Effect of indomethacin on muscarinic autoinhibition. *Am J Respir Crit Care Med* 1995; 151:1040–1046.

30. ten Berge RE, Santing RE, Hamstra JJ, Roffel AF, Zaagsma J. Dysfunction of muscarinic M2 receptors after the early allergic reaction: possible contribution to bronchial hyperresponsiveness in allergic guinea-pigs. *Br J Pharmacol* 1995; 114:881–887.

31. Myers AC, Undem BJ. Muscarinic receptor regulation of synaptic transmission in airway parasympathetic ganglia. *Am J Physiol* 1996; 270:L630–L636.

32. Fryer AD, Elbon CL, Kim AL, Xiao HQ, Levey AI, Jacoby DB. Cultures of airway parasympathetic nerves express functional M2 muscarinic receptors. *Am J Respir Cell Mol Biol* 1996; 15:716–725.

33. Haddad EB, Landry Y, Gies JP. Muscarinic receptor subtypes in guinea-pig airways. *Am J Physiol* 1991; 261:L327–L333.

34. Wills-Karp M. Effects of age on muscarinic agonist-induced contraction and IP accumulation in airway smooth muscle. *Life Sci* 1991; 49:1039–1045.

35. Mak JC, Baraniuk JN, Barnes PJ. Localization of muscarinic receptor subtype mRNAs in human lung. *Am J Respir Cell Mol Biol* 1992; 7:344–348.

36. Widdop S, Daykin K, Hall IP. Expression of muscarinic M2 receptors in cultured human airway smooth muscle cells. *Am J Respir Cell Mol Biol* 1993; 9:541–546.

37. Watson N, Eglen RM. Effects of muscarinic M2 and M3 receptor stimulation and antagonism on responses to isoprenaline of guinea-pig trachea *in vitro*. *Br J Pharmacol* 1994; 112:179–187.

38. Fernandes LB, Fryer AD, Hirshman CA. M2 muscarinic receptors inhibit isoproterenol-induced relaxation of canine airway smooth muscle. *J Pharmacol Exp Ther* 1992; 262:119–126.
39. Kume H, Kotlikoff MI. Muscarinic inhibition of single KCa channels in smooth muscle cells by a pertussis-sensitive G protein. *Am J Physiol* 1998; 261:C1204–C1209.
40. Schramm CM, Arjona NC, Grunstein MM. Role of muscarinic M2 receptors in regulating beta-adrenergic responsiveness in maturing rabbit airway smooth muscle. *Am J Physiol* 1995; 269:L783–L790.
41. Mitchell RW, Koenig SM, Popovich KJ, Kelly E, Tallet J, Leff AR. Pertussis toxin augments beta-adrenergic relaxation of muscarinic contraction in canine trachealis. *Am Rev Respir Dis* 1993; 147:327–331.
42. Matsui M, Griffin MT, Shehnaz D, Taketo MM, Ehlert FJ. Increased relaxant action of forskolin and isoproterenol against muscarinic agonist-induced contractions in smooth muscle from M2 receptor knockout mice. *J Pharmacol Exp Ther* 2003; 305:106–113.
43. Mak JC, Barnes PJ. Muscarinic receptor subtypes in human and guinea-pig lung. *Eur J Pharmacol* 1989; 164:223–230.
44. Blaber LC, Fryer AD, Maclagan J. Neuronal muscarinic receptors attenuate vagally-induced contraction of feline bronchial smooth muscle. *Br J Pharmacol* 1985; 86:723–728.
45. Roffel AF, Elzinga CR, Zaagsma J. Muscarinic M3 receptors mediate contraction of human central and peripheral airway smooth muscle. *Pulm Pharmacol* 1990; 3:47–51.
46. Minette PA, Barnes PJ. Prejunctional inhibitory muscarinic receptors on cholinergic nerves in human and guinea-pig airways. *J Appl Physiol* 1988; 64:2532–2537.
47. Howell RE, Laemont K, Gaudette R, Raynor M, Warner A, Noronha-Blob L. Characterization of the airway smooth muscle muscarinic receptor *in vivo*. *Eur J Pharmacol* 1991; 197:109–112.
48. Yang CM, Farley JM, Dwyer TM. Muscarinic stimulation of submucosal glands in swine trachea. *J Appl Physiol* 1988; 64:200–209.
49. Gater PR, Alabaster VA, Piper I. A study of the muscarinic receptor subtype mediating mucus secretion in the cat trachea *in vitro*. *Pulm Pharmacol* 1989; 2:87–92.
50. Matran R, Alving K, Lundberg JM. Differential bronchial and pulmonary vascular responses to vagal stimulation in the pig. *Acta Physiol Scand* 1991; 143:387–393.
51. Chilvers ER, Batty IH, Barnes PJ, Nahorski SR. Formation of inositol polyphosphates in airway smooth muscle after muscarinic receptor stimulation. *J Pharmacol Exp Ther* 1990; 252:786–791.
52. Grandordy BM, Cuss FM, Sampson AS, Palmer JB, Barnes PJ. Phosphatidylinositol response to cholinergic agonists in airway smooth muscle: relationship to contraction and muscarinic receptor occupancy. *J Pharmacol Exp Ther* 1986; 238:273–279.
53. Stengel PW, Gomeza J, Wess J, Cohen ML. M(2) and M(4) receptor knockout mice: muscarinic receptor function in cardiac and smooth muscle *in vitro*. *J Pharmacol Exp Ther* 2000; 292:877–885.
54. Stengel PW, Yamada M, Wess J, Cohen ML. M(3)-receptor knockout mice: muscarinic receptor function in atria, stomach fundus, urinary bladder, and trachea. *Am J Physiol Regul Integr Comp Physiol* 2002; 282:R1443–R1449.
55. Martin RJ. Therapeutic significance of distal airway inflammation in asthma. *J Allergy Clin Immunol* 2002; 109:S447–S460.
56. Escolar JD, Escolar MA, Guzman J, Roques M. Morphological hysteresis of the small airways. *Histol Histopathol* 2003; 18:19–26.
57. Struckmann N, Schwering S, Wiegand S, Gschnell A, Yamada M, Kummer W et al. Role of muscarinic receptor subtypes in the constriction of peripheral airways: studies on receptor-deficient mice. *Mol Pharmacol* 2003; 64:1444–1451.
58. Parker EM, Kameyama K, Higashijima T, Ross EM. Reconstitutively active G protein-coupled receptors purified from baculovirus-infected insect cells. *J Biol Chem* 1991; 266:519–527.
59. Caulfield MP. Muscarinic receptors—characterization, coupling and function. *Pharmacol Ther* 1993; 58:319–379.
60. Rumenapp U, Asmus M, Schablowski H, Woznicki M, Han L, Jakobs KH et al. The M3 muscarinic acetylcholine receptor expressed in HEK-293 cells signals to phospholipase D *via* G12 but not Gq-type G proteins: regulators of G proteins as tools to dissect pertussis toxin-resistant G proteins in receptor-effector coupling. *J Biol Chem* 2001; 276:2474–2479.
61. Smrcka AV, Hepler JR, Brown KO, Sternweis PC. Regulation of polyphosphoinositide-specific phospholipase C activity by purified Gq. *Science* 1991; 251:804–807.
62. Berstein G, Blank JL, Smrcka AV, Higashijima T, Sternweis PC, Exton JH, Ross EM. Reconstitution of agonist-stimulated phosphatidylinositol 4,5-bisphosphate hydrolysis using purified m1 muscarinic receptor, Gq/11, and phospholipase C-beta 1. *J Biol Chem* 1992; 267:8081–8088.

63. Schramm CM, Grunstein MM. Assessment of signal transduction mechanisms regulating airway smooth muscle contractility. *Am J Physiol* 1992; 262:L119–L139.

64. Felder CC. Muscarinic acetylcholine receptors: signal transduction through multiple effectors. *FASEB J* 1995; 9:619–625.

65. Coleridge HM, Coleridge JC. Pulmonary reflexes: neural mechanisms of pulmonary defense. *Annu Rev Physiol* 1994; 56:69–91.

66. Eljamal M, Wong LB, Yeates DB. Capsaicin-activated bronchial- and alveolar-initiated pathways regulating tracheal ciliary beat frequency. *J Appl Physiol* 1994; 77:1239–1245.

67. Lee LY, Pisarri TE. Afferent properties and reflex functions of bronchopulmonary C-fibers. *Respir Physiol* 2001; 125:47–65.

68. Coleridge HM, Coleridge JC, Green JF, Parsons GH. Pulmonary C-fiber stimulation by capsaicin evokes reflex cholinergic bronchial vasodilation in sheep. *J Appl Physiol* 1992; 72:770–778.

69. Stein MR. Possible mechanisms of influence of esophageal acid on airway hyperresponsiveness. *Am J Med* 2003; 115(suppl 3A):55S–59S.

70. Dixon M, Jackson DM, Richards IM. The effects of histamine, acetylcholine and 5-hydroxytryptamine on lung mechanics and irritant receptors in the dog. *J Physiol* 1979; 287:393–403.

71. Wagner EM, Mitzner WA. Contribution of pulmonary versus systemic perfusion of airway smooth muscle. *J Appl Physiol* 1995; 78:403–409.

72. Wagner EM, Jacoby DB. Methacholine causes reflex bronchoconstriction. *J Appl Physiol* 1999; 86:294–297.

73. Nadel JA, Salem H, Tamplin B, Tokiwa Y. Mechanism of bronchoconstriction during inhalation of sulfur dioxide. *J Appl Physiol* 1965; 20:164–167.

74. Snashall PD, Baldwin C. Mechanisms of sulphur dioxide induced bronchoconstriction in normal and asthmatic man. *Thorax* 1982; 37:118–123.

75. Simonsson BG, Jacobs FM, Nadel JA. Role of autonomic nervous system and the cough reflex in the increased responsiveness of airways in patients with obstructive airway disease. *J Clin Invest* 1967; 46:1812–1818.

76. Widdicombe JG, Kent DC, Nadel JA. Mechanism of bronchoconstriction during inhalation of dust. *J Appl Physiol* 1962; 17:613–616.

77. Holtzman MJ, Cunningham JH, Sheller JR, Irsigler GB, Nadel JA, Boushey HA. Effect of ozone on bronchial reactivity in atopic and nonatopic subjects. *Am Rev Respir Dis* 1979; 120:1059–1067.

78. Mansfield LE, Hameister HH, Spaulding HS, Smith NJ, Glab N. The role of the vagus nerve in airway narrowing caused by intraesophageal hydrochloric acid provocation and esophageal distention. *Ann Allergy* 1981; 47:431–434.

79. Fish JE, Rosenthal RR, Summer WR, Menkes H, Norman PS, Permutt S. The effect of atropine on acute antigen-mediated airway constriction in subjects with allergic asthma. *Am Rev Respir Dis* 1977; 115:371–379.

80. Holtzman MJ, Sheller JR, Dimeo M, Nadel JA, Boushey HA. Effect of ganglionic blockade on bronchial reactivity in atopic subjects. *Am Rev Respir Dis* 1980; 122:17–25.

81. Gross NJ, Skorodin MS. Anticholinergic, antimuscarinic bronchodilators. *Am Rev Respir Dis* 1984; 129:856–870.

82. Mann JS, George CF. Anticholinergic drugs in the treatment of airways disease. *Br J Dis Chest* 1985; 79:209–228.

83. Minette PA, Lammers JW, Dixon CM, McCusker MT, Barnes PJ. A muscarinic agonist inhibits reflex bronchoconstriction in normal but not in asthmatic subjects. *J Appl Physiol* 1989; 67:2461–2465.

84. Ayala LE, Ahmed T. Is there loss of protective muscarinic receptor mechanism in asthma? *Chest* 1989; 96:1285–1291.

85. Haddad EB, Mak JC, Belvisi MG, Nishikawa M, Rousell J, Barnes PJ. Muscarinic and beta-adrenergic receptor expression in peripheral lung from normal and asthmatic patients. *Am J Physiol* 1996; 270:L947–L953.

86. Fryer AD, Jacoby DB. Parainfluenza virus infection damages inhibitory M2 muscarinic receptors on pulmonary parasympathetic nerves in the guinea-pig. *Br J Pharmacol* 1991; 102:267–271.

87. Sorkness R, Clough JJ, Castleman WL, Lemanske RF Jr. Virus-induced airway obstruction and parasympathetic hyperresponsiveness in adult rats. *Am J Respir Crit Care Med* 1994; 150:28–34.

88. Fryer AD, Wills-Karp M. Dysfunction of M2-muscarinic receptors in pulmonary parasympathetic nerves after antigen challenge. *J Appl Physiol* 1991; 71:2255–2261.

89. Fryer AD, Adamko DJ, Yost BL, Jacoby DB. Effects of inflammatory cells on neuronal M2 muscarinic receptor function in the lung. *Life Sci* 1999; 64:449–455.

90. Schultheis AH, Bassett DJ, Fryer AD. Ozone-induced airway hyperresponsiveness and loss of neuronal M2 muscarinic receptor function. *J Appl Physiol* 1994; 76:1088–1097.

91. McGowan SE, Smith J, Holmes AJ, Smith LA, Businga TR, Madsen MT *et al*. Vitamin A deficiency promotes bronchial hyperreactivity in rats by altering muscarinic M(2) receptor function. *Am J Physiol Lung Cell Mol Physiol* 2002; 282:L1031–L1039.

92. Coulson FR, Fryer AD. Muscarinic acetylcholine receptors and airway diseases. *Pharmacol Ther* 2003; 98:59–69.

93. Jacoby DB, Fryer AD. Interaction of viral infections with muscarinic receptors. *Clin Exp Allergy* 1999; 29(suppl 2):59–64.

94. Costello RW, Schofield BH, Kephart GM, Gleich GJ, Jacoby DB, Fryer AD. Localization of eosinophils to airway nerves and effect on neuronal M2 muscarinic receptor function. *Am J Physiol* 1997; 273:L93–L103.

95. Elbon CL, Jacoby DB, Fryer AD. Pretreatment with an antibody to interleukin-5 prevents loss of pulmonary M2 muscarinic receptor function in antigen-challenged guinea-pigs. *Am J Respir Cell Mol Biol* 1995; 12:320–328.

96. Fryer AD, Costello RW, Yost BL, Lobb RR, Tedder TF, Steeber DA, Bochner BS. Antibody to VLA-4, but not to L-selectin, protects neuronal M2 muscarinic receptors in antigen-challenged guinea-pig airways. *J Clin Invest* 1997; 99:2036–2044.

97. Belmonte KE, Fryer AD, Costello RW. Role of insulin in antigen-induced airway eosinophilia and neuronal M2 muscarinic receptor dysfunction. *J Appl Physiol* 1998; 85:1708–1718.

98. Evans CM, Fryer AD, Jacoby DB, Gleich GJ, Costello RW. Pretreatment with antibody to eosinophil major basic protein prevents hyperresponsiveness by protecting neuronal M2 muscarinic receptors in antigen-challenged guinea-pigs. *J Clin Invest* 1997; 100:2254–2262.

99. Fryer AD, Jacoby DB. Function of pulmonary M2 muscarinic receptors in antigen-challenged guinea-pigs is restored by heparin and poly-L-glutamate. *J Clin Invest* 1992; 90:2292–2298.

100. Fryer AD, el Fakahany EE, Jacoby DB. Parainfluenza virus type 1 reduces the affinity of agonists for muscarinic receptors in guinea-pig lung and heart. *Eur J Pharmacol* 1990; 181:51–58.

101. Adamko DJ, Yost BL, Gleich GJ, Fryer AD, Jacoby DB. Ovalbumin sensitization changes the inflammatory response to subsequent parainfluenza infection. Eosinophils mediate airway hyperresponsiveness, m(2) muscarinic receptor dysfunction, and antiviral effects. *J Exp Med* 1999; 190:1465–1478.

102. Adamko DJ, Fryer AD, Bochner BS, Jacoby DB. CD8+ T lymphocytes in viral hyperreactivity and M2 muscarinic receptor dysfunction. *Am J Respir Crit Care Med* 2003; 167:550–556.

103. On LS, Boonyongsunchai P, Webb S, Davies L, Calverley PM, Costello RW. Function of pulmonary neuronal M(2) muscarinic receptors in stable chronic obstructive pulmonary disease. *Am J Respir Crit Care Med* 2001; 163:1320–1325.

104. Wessler I, Kirkpatrick CJ, Racke K. The cholinergic 'pitfall': acetylcholine, a universal cell molecule in biological systems, including humans. *Clin Exp Pharmacol Physiol* 1999; 26:198–205.

105. Klapproth H, Reinheimer T, Metzen J, Munch M, Bittinger F, Kirkpatrick CJ *et al*. Non-neuronal acetylcholine, a signalling molecule synthesized by surface cells of rat and man. *Naunyn Schmiedebergs Arch Pharmacol* 1997; 355:515–523.

106. Wessler I, Kirkpatrick CJ, Racke K. Non-neuronal acetylcholine, a locally acting molecule, widely distributed in biological systems: expression and function in humans. *Pharmacol Ther* 1998; 77:59–79.

107. Wessler IK, Kirkpatrick CJ. The non-neuronal cholinergic system: an emerging drug target in the airways. *Pulm Pharmacol Ther* 2001; 14:423–434.

108. Maus AD, Pereira EF, Karachunski PI, Horton RM, Navaneetham D, Macklin K *et al*. Human and rodent bronchial epithelial cells express functional nicotinic acetylcholine receptors. *Mol Pharmacol* 1998; 54:779–788.

109. Kawashima K, Fujii T, Watanabe Y, Misawa H. Acetylcholine synthesis and muscarinic receptor subtype mRNA expression in T-lymphocytes. *Life Sci* 1998; 62:1701–1705.

110. Fujii T, Tsuchiya T, Yamada S, Fujimoto K, Suzuki T, Kasahara T, Kawashima K. Localization and synthesis of acetylcholine in human leukemic T cell lines. *J Neurosci Res* 1996; 44:66–72.

111. Fujii T, Yamada S, Watanabe Y, Misawa H, Tajima S, Fujimoto K *et al*. Induction of choline acetyltransferase mRNA in human mononuclear leukocytes stimulated by phytohemagglutinin, a T-cell activator. *J Neuroimmunol* 1998; 82:101–107.

112. Kawashima K, Fujii T. Extraneuronal cholinergic system in lymphocytes. *Pharmacol Ther* 2000; 86:29–48.
113. Shirvan MH, Pollard HB, Heldman E. Mixed nicotinic and muscarinic features of cholinergic receptor coupled to secretion in bovine chromaffin cells. *Proc Natl Acad Sci USA* 1991; 88:4860–4864.
114. Lapied B, Le Corronc H, Hue B. Sensitive nicotinic and mixed nicotinic-muscarinic receptors in insect neurosecretory cells. *Brain Res* 1990; 533:132–136.
115. Koyama S, Rennard SI, Robbins RA. Acetylcholine stimulates bronchial epithelial cells to release neutrophil and monocyte chemotactic activity. *Am J Physiol* 1992; 262:L466–L471.
116. Klapproth H, Racke K, Wessler I. Acetylcholine and nicotine stimulate the release of granulocyte-macrophage colony stimulating factor from cultured human bronchial epithelial cells. *Naunyn Schmiedebergs Arch Pharmacol* 1998; 357:472–475.
117. Sato E, Koyama S, Okubo Y, Kubo K, Sekiguchi M. Acetylcholine stimulates alveolar macrophages to release inflammatory cell chemotactic activity. *Am J Physiol* 1998; 274:L970–L979.
118. Wessler I, Kilbinger H, Bittinger F, Unger R, Kirkpatrick CJ. The non-neuronal cholinergic system in humans: expression, function and pathophysiology. *Life Sci* 2003; 72:2055–2061.
119. Pauwels RA, Buist AS, Calverley PM, Jenkins CR, Hurd SS. Global strategy for the diagnosis, management, and prevention of chronic obstructive pulmonary disease. NHLBI/WHO Global Initiative for Chronic Obstructive Lung Disease (GOLD) Workshop summary. *Am J Respir Crit Care Med* 2001; 163:1256–1276.
120. Cazzola M, Matera MG, Di Perna F, Calderaro F, Califano C, Vinciguerra A. A comparison of bronchodilating effects of salmeterol and oxitropium bromide in stable chronic obstructive pulmonary disease. *Respir Med* 1998; 92:354–357.
121. Tamaoki J, Chiyotani A, Tagaya E, Sakai N, Konno K. Effect of long term treatment with oxitropium bromide on airway secretion in chronic bronchitis and diffuse panbronchiolitis. *Thorax* 1994; 49:545–548.
122. Barnes PJ. The pharmacological properties of tiotropium. *Chest* 2000; 117:63S–66S.
123. Disse B, Reichl R, Speck G, Traunecker W, Ludwig Rominger KL, Hammer R. Ba 679 BR, a novel long-acting anticholinergic bronchodilator. *Life Sci* 1993; 52:537–544.
124. Haddad EB, Mak JC, Barnes PJ. Characterization of [3H]Ba 679 BR, a slowly dissociating muscarinic antagonist, in human lung: radioligand binding and autoradiographic mapping. *Mol Pharmacol* 1994; 45:899–907.
125. Takahashi T, Belvisi MG, Patel H, Ward JK, Tadjkarimi S, Yacoub MH, Barnes PJ. Effect of Ba 679 BR, a novel long-acting anticholinergic agent, on cholinergic neurotransmission in guinea-pig and human airways. *Am J Respir Crit Care Med* 1994; 150:1640–1645.
126. Maesen FP, Smeets JJ, Costongs MA, Wald FD, Cornelissen PJ. Ba 679 Br, a new long-acting antimuscarinic bronchodilator: a pilot dose-escalation study in COPD. *Eur Respir J* 1993; 6:1031–1036.
127. Maesen FP, Smeets JJ, Sledsens TJ, Wald FD, Cornelissen PJ. Tiotropium bromide, a new long-acting antimuscarinic bronchodilator: a pharmacodynamic study in patients with chronic obstructive pulmonary disease (COPD). Dutch Study Group. *Eur Respir J* 1995; 8:1506–1513.
128. Cazzola M, Marco FD, Santus P, Boveri B, Verga M, Matera MG, Centanni S. The pharmacodynamic effects of single inhaled doses of formoterol, tiotropium and their combination in patients with COPD. *Pulm Pharmacol Ther* 2004; 17:35–39.
129. van Noord JA, Bantje TA, Eland ME, Korducki L, Cornelissen PJ. A randomised controlled comparison of tiotropium and ipratropium in the treatment of chronic obstructive pulmonary disease. The Dutch Tiotropium Study Group. *Thorax* 2000; 55:289–294.
130. Vincken W, van Noord JA, Greefhorst AP, Bantje TA, Kesten S, Korducki L, Cornelissen PJ. Improved health outcomes in patients with COPD during 1 yr's treatment with tiotropium. *Eur Respir J* 2002; 19:209–216.
131. Casaburi R, Mahler DA, Jones PW, Wanner A, San PG, ZuWallack RL *et al.* A long-term evaluation of once-daily inhaled tiotropium in chronic obstructive pulmonary disease. *Eur Respir J* 2002; 19:217–224.

6

The clinical use of anticholinergics

B. R. Celli

INTRODUCTION

The American Thoracic and the European Respiratory Societies have recently defined chronic obstructive pulmonary disease (COPD) as a *preventable* and *treatable* disease state characterised by airflow limitation that is not fully reversible [1]. The airflow limitation is usually progressive and is associated with an abnormal inflammatory response of the lungs to noxious particles or gases, primarily caused by cigarette smoking. In some areas of the world where biomass fuel is used as a source of energy primarily for cooking, persons exposed to the particles can develop airflow obstruction that is indistinguishable from that characteristic of COPD [2]. Although COPD primarily affects the lungs, it also produces significant systemic consequences that are very important because their presence is associated with significant morbidity and mortality and also because some of them are amenable to therapy.

The new statements of COPD being *preventable* and *treatable* stress the importance of carefully organising therapy and optimising the treatment of the patients afflicted by the disease. Indeed, over the last two decades, our armamentarium has grown considerably. Our understanding of outcome measures other than the degree of airflow limitation and the consequent planning of studies addressing patient-centred outcomes have provided us with information that is useful to the treating health care provider and the treated patient. The increased number of pharmacological agents provide us with more choices and their understanding is crucial to our decision-making process.

Within this framework, anticholinergics are very useful bronchodilators in the management of COPD and work by blocking muscarinic receptors in airway smooth muscle as has been described in the previous chapter. The discovery of different subtypes of muscarinic receptor has led to the development of more selective anticholinergics. One of them, tiotropium bromine, which has kinetic selectivity for M_3 receptors in airway smooth muscle, also has a very long duration of action. Once daily administration of tiotropium bromide has shown significant advantages over placebo and even over four times daily ipratropium bromide. This chapter will review the evidence that anticholinergics constitute the cornerstone of pharmacological therapy in COPD.

Currently available anticholinergic drugs include ipratropium bromide, oxitropium bromide and more recently tiotropium bromide. As antagonists of muscarinic receptors they do promote bronchodilation with the added advantage of having minimal side-effects when used in therapeutic doses. In healthy animals and man there is a small degree of resting bronchomotor tone due to tonic vagal nerve impulses which release acetylcholine around

Bartolome R. Celli, MD, Professor of Medicine, Tufts University, Chief, Pulmonary and Critical Care Medicine, Caritas St Elizabeth's Medical Center, Boston, MA, USA.

airway smooth muscle. This can be blocked by section of the vagal nerve in animals and also by anticholinergic drugs in humans. COPD-enhanced cholinergic tone and response to inflammatory events render anticholinergics even more important. Indeed, anticholinergics are very effective bronchodilators in COPD [3]. Vagal cholinergic tone appears to be the most important reversible element of airway obstruction in COPD and its effects are exaggerated by geometric factors due to the already narrowed airway. Since cholinergic nerves cause mucus secretion, in addition to bronchoconstriction, anticholinergics may reduce airway mucus secretion and clearance. The clinical relevance of this finding remains to be of limited importance even though oxitropium bromide has been shown to reduce mucus hypersecretion in a small trial of patients with COPD [4].

As we have seen in the previous chapter, ipratropium and oxitropium bromide are non-selective blockers and therefore block M_1, M_2 and M_3-receptors [5]. In practice, the major side-effects of anticholinergics, including dry mouth, glaucoma and urinary retention are all mediated by M_3 receptors, so that it is difficult to reduce the side-effects if dosed systemically. In practice these side-effects are not a problem with currently available anti-cholinergics since they are inhaled and not absorbed. In contrast, tiotropium bromide dissociates more slowly from M_1- and M_3-receptors than from M_2-receptors [6–8].

Bronchodilators in general are the mainstay of current therapy in COPD and while providing less improvement in the degree of airflow obstruction compared to asthma, they significantly reduce symptoms of dyspnoea, and improve exercise tolerance [9, 10]. It has been customary to judge the beneficial effect of bronchodilators by their impact on short- or long-term effect on the degree of airflow limitation as measured by the forced expiratory volume in one second (FEV_1) and indeed we will evaluate that as one important outcome. However, the impact of bronchodilators on other physiologic outcomes such as reduction in lung volume and improved exercise performance as well as on non-physiological ones such as dyspnoea and health-related quality of life will also be explored. The abundant data on these important outcomes has made therapy all the more valuable.

ANTICHOLINERGICS: AIRFLOW LIMITATION

The bronchodilator effect of ipratropium bromide has been well studied. Administration of an inhaled dose of 36 μg results in a 5–23% increase in FEV_1 within one hour with the effects maintained for 4–6 h [11, 12]. In the study by Mahler *et al.* [12] the bronchodilator response appeared to be similar after 84 days of therapy, indicating no development of tolerance. The most extensive review of the topic was provided by Rennard *et al.* [13] who pooled the data from seven clinical trials designed to compare the 90-day effect of ipratropium to that of the β-agonist agents metaproterenol or albuterol. The entry criteria included patients older than 40 years of age, smoking history of at least 10-pack years and stable, moderate airflow obstruction. Patients with a history of asthma, allergic rhinitis or atopy, and an elevated eosinophil count were excluded. Likewise, patients on more than 10 mg of prednisone or equivalent were not allowed to enter the studies. Pulmonary functions were conducted for a total of 8 h after study drug administration and the examinations repeated 90 days after the initiation of therapy. Out of 1,836 patients, 1,445 completed the trials and were included in the analysis. The 744 patients who received ipratropium consisted primarily of men (65%) and had a baseline FEV_1 around one litre. After the 90 days, the mean FEV_1 had increased by 28 ml and the forced vital capacity (FVC) by 131 ml. Incidentally, this compared favourably to the change observed in the group receiving β-agonists in whom there was a decrease of 1 ml in the FEV_1 and an increase of 20 ml in FVC. In the study, there was also a small, but significant, improvement in quality of life measured with the Chronic Respiratory Disease Questionnaire.

As a result of these early studies ipratropium bromide became the first-line agent for the treatment of symptomatic patients with COPD [14]. The use of ipratropium combined with β-agonist agents received a significant boost when the result of several trials showed that the combination was more effective than either agent alone [15–17]. In the combivent trial [15], the 182 patients receiving the combination had an increase in FEV_1 of 31–33% compared to 24% for the 179 patients receiving ipratropium alone and 24–27% for the 173 patients receiving albuterol alone for all 4 days tested. The area under the curve for the same days was 21–44% greater for the combination than for ipratropium alone and 30–46% geater than that for albuterol alone. In the formoterol trial [16], the patients receiving formoterol plus ipratropium had a larger improvement in airflow than those receiving salbutamol and ipratropium. However, the increase in FEV_1 for the two arms of the trial were within the 20% described above.

The best conducted study on the effect of bronchodilators on airflow obstruction was the Lung Health Study [18]. In that study, the effect of an aggressive smoking cessation program and administration of inhaled ipratropium at a dose of 36 μg four times per day on the FEV_1, were evaluated against placebo in a total of 5,887 patients with mild COPD (mean FEV_1 was 2.65 l). The patients were followed over 5 years. The study is a landmark one because it demonstrated that smoking cessation is associated not only with an increase in FEV_1 of 57 ml in the first year after cessation, but also with a lower rate of decline in lung function compared to that of the patients who continued to smoke. In addition, the use of ipratropium resulted in an increase in FEV_1 of 40 ml (18%). However, the rate of decline in FEV_1 did not differ among the different groups. In addition, the gain in lung function was lost once the medication was stopped.

The other short-acting anticholinergic agent oxitropium has received less clinical attention and most of the studies comprise a small number of patients. As ipratropium bromide, oxitropium bromide has a 4–6 h effect. Ikeda et al. [19] studied 14 patients with a mean FEV_1 of 0.85 l before and 90 min after the administration of 800 μg of oxitropium. The FEV_1 increased a mean of 25%, a finding that was actually smaller than previous studies with the same agent [20, 21]. As was the experience with ipratropium, the combination of oxitropium with β-agonists produces a larger change in the FEV_1 compared with either agent alone. Cazzola et al. [22] studied 16 outpatients with COPD in 4 consecutive days. The patients received 24 mg of formoterol, 50 μg of salmeterol, 200 μg of oxitropium or placebo. After the baseline determination, the patients received ascending doses of salbutamol. The FEV_1 increased approximately 22% after oxitropium and it further increased another 20% after salbutamol.

The most recent anticholinergic agent tiotropium bromide is a long-lasting bronchodilator [23]. Single doses of inhaled tiotropium bromide have been investigated in clinical studies in patients with COPD and asthma. In asthmatic patients, there is a prolonged bronchodilator effect after a single dose, lasting for up to 36 h [24]. There is also a prolonged dose-dependent protection against inhaled methacholine challenge [25]. In patients with COPD tiotropium bromide provides a dose-related bronchodilatation that persists for over 24 h [26, 27]. The actual degree of bronchodilation at one hour after the administration of the medication is very similar to that observed for the shorter-acting anticholinergics. An average of the studies here cited shows an increase in FEV_1 of close to 19%. The difference in favour of the tiotropium is that the trough FEV_1 prior to the morning dose once the patient has been receiving the medication for one week is a staggering 16%. As shown in Figure 6.1, this is significantly better than the trough in FEV_1 in patients receiving placebo. These studies demonstrated that tiotropium is suitable for once daily dosing and that at the lower doses where most improvement is seen there are unlikely to be significant side-effects. Once daily tiotropium is significantly more effective than four times daily ipratropium bromide at recommended doses [28]. The reasons for this remain speculative but they include: first, the increased potency of tiotropium bromide may mean that there is more effective blockade of muscarinic receptors. Dose-ranging studies have demonstrates a maximal effect at relatively low doses, whereas this may not be achieved at the recommended doses of

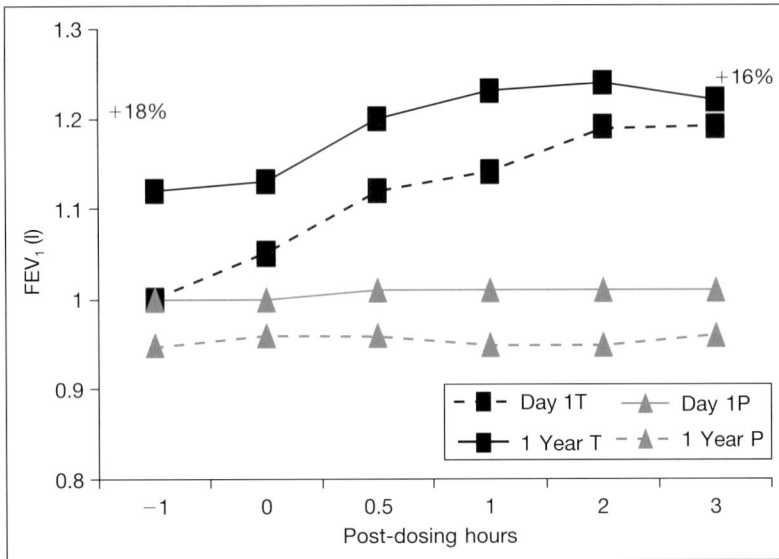

Figure 6.1   Inhaled tiotropium not only improves the FEV_1 within hours of its administration by an average of 16% but also induces prolonged bronchodilation (185 compared to baseline) that is seen after 24 h and before the following day's dose [modified with permission from reference 44].

ipratropium or oxitropium [29]. Secondly, the prolonged duration of action may have a better long-term bronchodilator effect than repeated doses of short-acting drugs. Long-acting bronchodilators appear to have a much better controlling effect than short-acting drugs and this has been well illustrated by the superiority of long-acting inhaled β_2-agonists (salmeterol, formoterol), compared to short-acting β_2-agonists (albuterol, terbutaline) [30]. It is possible that by maintaining a prolonged bronchodilator effect in airway smooth muscle cells, they behave in a different way to recurrent bronchodilatation with constant forming and reforming of latch-bridges [31]. Whatever the mechanism, the once a day regimen of an effective bronchodilator is a major step forward in achieving longer lasting effects [32] and better symptoms control as we shall see below. In addition, improved compliance may be a factor not to be forgotten when dealing with patients with a chronic condition such as COPD.

In summary, in contrast to the perceived notion that the airflow obstruction of COPD is irreversible, anticholinergics do induce a bronchodilation of around 20% that is maintained over time. However, as demonstrated in the Lung Health Trial [18], regular use of short-acting ipratropium did not alter the rate of decline of lung function as measured by the FEV_1. Some of the studies where the major end point was the change in FEV_1 in response to anticholinergics made the interesting observation that the change in other outcomes, such as decreased dyspnoea [33] or increased exercise performance [19] did not seem to correlate with the improvement in FEV_1 alone. The mechanism that explained this paradox was clarified by the important study of Belman et al. [34]. Using albuterol as the bronchodilator, they showed that the improvement in exercise-induced dyspnoea after treatment correlated better with less dynamic hyperinflation than with the improvement in FEV_1. This opened the door to the concept that the FEV_1 is only one of several parameters that describe the complex picture of COPD and that lung volumes could be very important lung function variables to study. Indeed, the end expiratory volume to total lung capacity ratio (EELV/TLC) decreased from

80% to 76% (p < 0.05) and this change had the best correlation with the change in Borg dyspnoea score (r = 0.771, p < 0.01).

ANTICHOLINERGICS: EXERCISE PERFORMANCE AND LUNG VOLUME

Following the study by Belman et al. [34], O'Donnell et al. [35] explored the role of dynamic hyperinflation with exercise before and after inhaled ipratropium. They studied 29 patients with stable COPD (FEV$_1$ of 40% predicted) in a double-blind placebo-controlled crossover design. The patients performed a constant load exercise before and after receiving 50 μg of nebulised ipratropium and compared the results with those obtained after inhalation of saline. In this study, instead of reporting the complex EELV/TLC ratio, the authors reported the inspiratory capacity (IC), a much easier variable to measure and one that represents the same physiological expression, namely, the available capacity to inhale. The IC describes the operational maximal reserve for patients during exercise. A drop in that value implies a decrease in the reserve to breathe due to air-trapping. In this study, the increase in FEV$_1$ one hour after ipratropium was 7%, whereas the FVC had increased by 10% and the IC by 14%. The exercise endurance to a submaximal load increased by 32% and the slope for Borg dyspnoea scale decreased by 11%. As Belman et al. [34] had reported for albuterol, the change in dyspnoea correlated better with the change in IC than with FEV$_1$. The authors concluded that IC decreases during exercise and it should be considered an important and different outcome to measure in our assessment of the effect of medications for COPD, independent from the changes in FEV$_1$.

Although no similar study has been conducted with oxitropium, the study by Ikeda et al. [19] reported an increase in exercise performance as evidenced by an increase in maximal power (94 compared to 87 watts) after oxitropium. In addition, these authors observed an increase in minute ventilation and oxygen uptake with a positive correlation between the change in FEV$_1$ and the maximal work load (r = 0.625, p < 0.01). Although resting lung volumes were only measured at baseline, there was a 425-ml increase in the FVC, suggesting a significant decrease in residual volume (RV) in the patients after oxitropium. In the study by Hay et al. [33], no mention is made of lung volumes. Once again, a closer look at their data shows a significant increase in FVC and also in the 6-minute walk distance (7%) or a distance of 27 m over a baseline of 401 m. This was associated with a decrease in breathlessness score. Finally, Oga et al. [36] reported the results of a double-blind, randomised crossover study of 30 men who were treated with oxitropium versus placebo and the effect tested on three forms of exercise, maximal cardiopulmonary ergometry, submaximal constant load exercise and the 6-minute walk distance. Oxitropium increased the exercise endurance by 19% and the 6-minute walk distance by 1%, both statistically significant with no changes in maximal oxygen consumption.

The effect of tiotropium on lung volume and exercise is only beginning to be reported. As improbable as it may sound, there have been very few studies designed to evaluate the effect of any inhaled anticholinergics, or for that matter any bronchodilator, on resting lung volume over time. The first one specifically designed to do so is the one by Celli et al. [37] who examined the effect of tiotropium compared to placebo in a group of 94 patients with COPD. In that study, the administration of 18 μg of tiotropium given once daily over 4 weeks was compared with that observed for placebo in: IC, FEV$_1$, FVC, slow vital capacity (SVC) and thoracic gas volume (TGV). The mean FEV$_1$ at baseline was 1.21l and the TGV was 171% of predicted, indicating important hyperinflation. After treatment there were significant changes in the tiotropium group with improvement in FEV$_1$ of 220 ml, of 300 ml for the IC and of 700 ml in the TGV. The changes for the tiotropium and placebo are seen in Figure 6.2. The magnitude of the decrease in resting lung volume is even larger than that described after succesful lung volume reduction surgery [38]. Interestingly, the volumes reported in the study by Flaminiano and Celli [39] decreased progressively over the 4 weeks

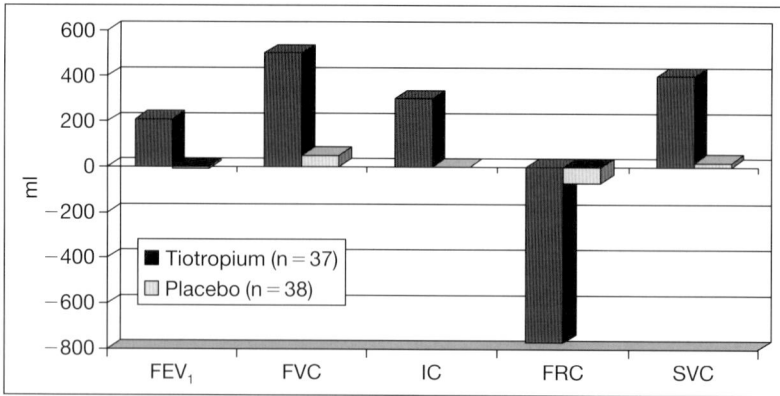

Figure 6.2   The administration of once-a-day inhaled tiotropium was effective in improving not only the resting forced expiratory volume in one second (FEV$_1$) and forced vital capacity (FVC), but also the inspiratory capacity (IC), slow vital capacity (SVC) and functional residual capacity (FRC) [modified with permission from reference 37].

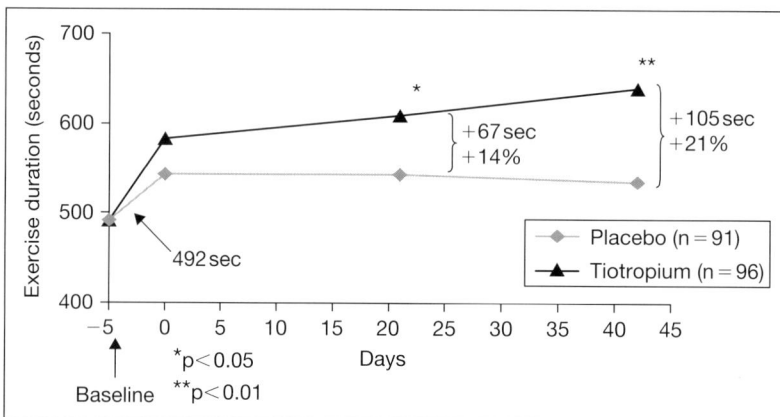

Figure 6.3   Exercise endurance during a submaximal load exercise test was 20% longer in patients receiving tiotropium compared with patients receiving placebo [modified with permission from reference 40].

of the study and the changes seemed not to have reached a plateau at the end of the study. This is important as a decrease in lung volume results in improved chest wall mechanics and places the foreshortened respiratory muscles in a better contractile position and a continued improvement may actually occur over more prolonged treatment.

More recently, O'Donnell *et al.* [40] have reported the results of a multicentre, double-blind trial comparing the effect of tiotropium and placebo on exercise endurance and lung volume. Throughout the study (Figure 6.3), exercise endurance was increased in the tiotropium group compared to placebo with the difference reaching a value of 20% at 12 weeks. The change in resting lung volume and IC was very similar to that described by Celli *et al.* [37] in their study. In addition, there was improvement in functional dyspnoea and health status associated with the physiological changes described above. The evidence indicates that the effect of tiotropium is physiologically similar to that reported by other anticholinergics but of a longer duration.

ANTICHOLINERGICS: DYSPNOEA, HEALTH STATUS AND EXACERBATION

Over the last 15 years, there has been increased interest in evaluating the effect of medications not only on their capacity to induce physiological improvements but also on their effect on patient centred outcomes such as their functional dyspnoea and health status. In addition, the interest has extended to the evaluation of the effect of therapy on important health outcomes such as exacerbations, a cause of great morbidity and mortality [41]. Although inhaled anticholinergics have a long history in the treatment of airway disease, drugs such as atropine and strammonium fell out of favour because of the problem with anticholinergic side-effects, and particularly central nervous system effects that included hallucinations. The effect on dyspnoea and health status were never evaluated in those initial trials. Anticholinergics only came back into fashion when quaternary ammonium derivatives, such as ipratropium bromide, were found to have none of these side-effects.

Ipratropium and oxitropium are effective bronchodilators, the action of which can persist for at least 90 days [13] and likely, more. As we have reviewed above, these agents do increase exercise endurance, likely, through decreased dynamic hyperinflation. However, their effect on other outcomes is less well documented. A close analysis of the seven trials reviewed by Rennard et al. [13] shows that there were significant improvements in shortness of breath score (p = 0.005) in ex-smoking patients receiving ipratropium. In addition, there was small, but statistically significant, improvement in health status as measured with the chronic respiratory quality of life questionnaire (CRQ). The actual change of 0.35 units on a seven point scale is below the 0.5 deemed clinically significant. That the effect of ipratropium on health status may be rather modest is borne out by the study of Dahl et al. [42] who compared the effect of ipratropium and formoterol in 780 patients randomised to either treatment over a 12-week period. Although treatment with 40 µg of ipratropium in the 194 patients randomised to this treatment provoked an increase in FEV_1 of 137 ml over placebo, the improvement in health status measured with the St. George's disease specific questionnaire was only of 2 units (p > 0.3). This was in contrast to the comparator, formoterol, the administration of which resulted in a clinically significant improvement of 5 units (p < 0.001). On the other hand, using the baseline and transitional dyspnoea scale, Mahler et al. [12] compared the effect of ipratropium and salmeterol over 6 months in 361 patients randomised to placebo or either of the two medications for a total of 12 weeks. At the usual dose of 36 µg, regular use of ipratropium resulted in an improvement in the dyspnoea index of over 1 unit which was statistically and clinically significant [43]. This improvement was of a similar magnitude to that seen in the salmeterol group. In this study, the poorly defined exacerbation rate was lower in the ipratropium group than in placebo (30 vs. 31%) but lower still in the salmeterol group (20%). Finally, the study by Vincken et al. [28] comparing the effect of ipratropium and that of tiotropium on health status and dyspnoea is also very instructive. With the longest follow up period of one year and the largest number of patients yet reported (179 in the ipratropium group vs. 356 in the tiotropium group), the data can only be inferred from the graphs presented. Ipratropium improved the TDI some 0.5 units at 100 days (9 weeks) compared to baseline, a finding consistent with the previous studies of shorter duration, but at one year the functional dyspnoea score was actually 0.3 units below baseline, indicating a deterioration in the score over this time. Indeed, only 18% of patients reported a clinically significant increase of 1 unit in TDI over that time. Interestingly, the improvement in health-related quality of life was also transient with a drop in 2 units over the first 200 days to return toward baseline at one year and the difference in health status values were significantly better in a larger proportion of patients in the tiotropium compared with the ipratropium group (Figure 6.4). From these studies, we can conclude that

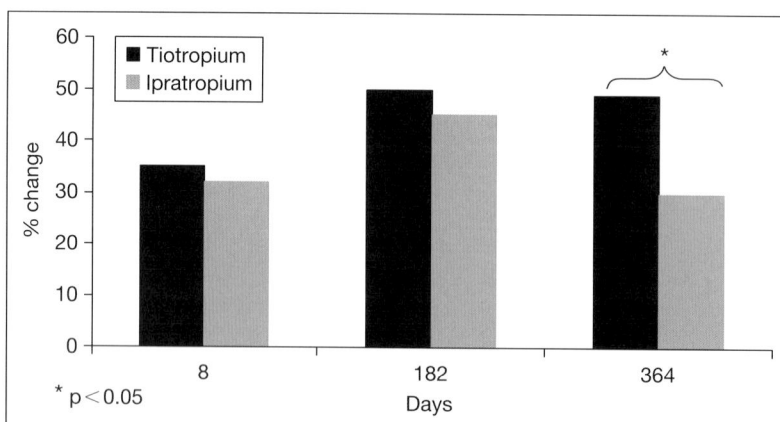

Figure 6.4 The percentage of patients with a clinically significant (4 units) improvement in the St. George's questionnaire was higher at all time points in patients receiving tiotropium compared with placebo. The difference was significant at one year [modified with permission from reference 28].

ipratropium does induce improved exercise dyspnoea, modest improvement in functional dyspnoea and health status lasting up to 3 months but the effects seem to disappear after one year of follow up. However, the natural history of the disease is to worsen over time and one would expect those outcomes to worsen over time. Whether the rate of change over time is different between ipratropium and no treatment has never been studied, and they probably will never be because of the more favourable results observed after the development and clinical use of tiotropium.

Perhaps the most important study of any bronchodilator in COPD to date is the one-year randomised double-blind multicentre trial reported by Casaburi et al. [44]. In that study reporting the result from two separate identical studies, the authors evaluated the effect of tiotropium compared with placebo in 921 patients where the randomised design resulted in 550 patients receiving tiotropium and 371, the placebo. The patients had the typical age for patients with COPD, close to 65 years with an average FEV_1 around one litre. At one year there were significant differences in pre-dosing (110 ml in favour of tiotropium compared with placebo) and post-dosing FEV_1 (120 ml in favour of tiotropium) as shown in Figure 6.1. In that study, functional dyspnoea as measured by the transitional dyspnoea index increased by 1.2 units over the 12 months, whereas the placebo group did not change after one year (Figure 6.5). The change was clinically significant for tiotropium. The quality of life scores as judged by the St. George's questionnaire was also improved in the tiotropium group with a mean change for the total score of 3.7 units, statistically significant but slightly below the 4 units described as being clinically significant (Figure 6.6). However, the results seem more impressive when compared to the worsened value of one unit seen in the placebo group. The findings were very similar in the parallel study comparing tiotropium with ipratropium (28).

Finally Niewoehner et al. [45] have just reported in an abstract form the results of a 6-month randomised trial evaluating the effect of once daily tiotropium compared with usual care in 1,200 patients with COPD followed over 6 months. The outcome was the incidence of exacerbations and hospitalisations. Tiotropium resulted in a decrease in the number of exacerbations and a similar decrease in the number of hospital days [45]. Thus, tiotropium can be added to the list of bronchodilators that have been shown to decrease exacerbation rates.

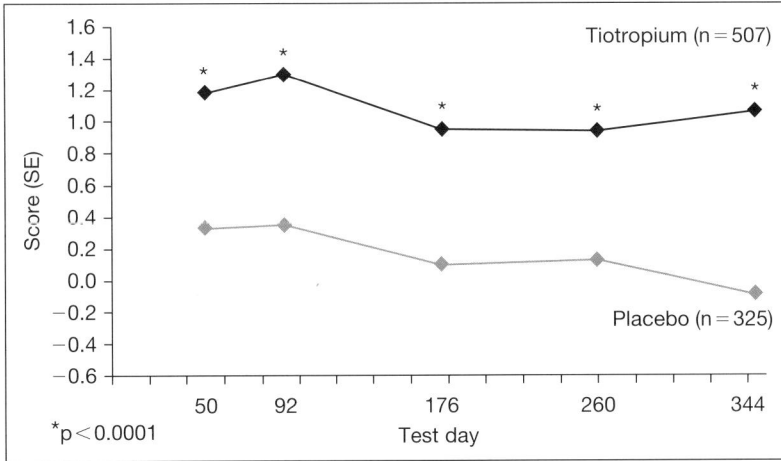

Figure 6.5 The sensation of dyspnoea as measured by the transitional dyspnoea index improved significantly and remained so throughout the study in patients receiving tiotropium compared with placebo [modified with permission from reference 44].

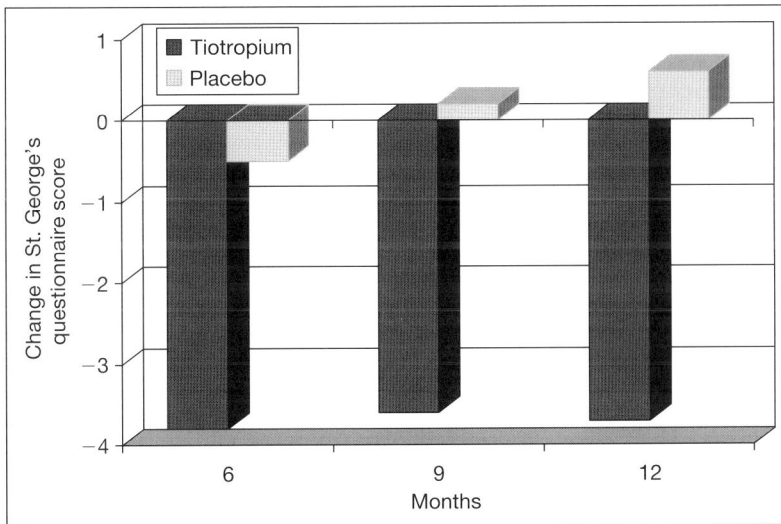

Figure 6.6 The change in health status as measured with the St. George's questionnaire was significantly better in the group receiving tiotropium compared with placebo [modified with permission from reference 44].

SIDE-EFFECTS

Inhaled anticholinergic drugs are usually well tolerated and there are almost no side-effects with either ipratropium or oxitropium bromide because there is virtually no systemic absorption of these positively charged quaternary ammonium compounds. The expected side-effects of anticholinergic drugs are dryness of the mouth, urinary retention, glaucoma (secondary to mydriasis). However, these have not proved to be a problem in clinical practice, even in an elderly population. These side-effects are all mediated *via* blockade of M_3-receptors and therefore development of more selective drugs is unlikely to provide any clinical benefit. Reports of paradoxical bronchoconstriction with ipratropium bromide, particularly when given by nebuliser, were largely explained by the hypotonicity of the nebuliser solution. Nebuliser solutions free of these problems are less likely to cause bronchoconstriction. Occasionally, bronchoconstriction may occur with ipratropium bromide given by a metered dose inhaler. One theoretical concern with anticholinergics has been that inhibition of mucus secretion might slow mucus clearance or may make the mucus more viscous and difficult to expectorate. In clinical practice this does not appear to be a problem, perhaps indicating that cholinergic mechanisms are not important for basal mucus secretion but only in the mucus hypersecretion that occurs in COPD.

Tiotropium bromide is well tolerated. There are no local side-effects reported and no effects have been reported on sputum production, consistent with previous experience with regular doses of inhaled ipratropium bromide, even when high doses are used. There is a potential danger of induction of glaucoma in susceptible patients after accidental topical administration, but this is not a possibility with the dry powder inhaler formulation currently in the market. In trials that have involved chronic treatment with inhaled tiotropium bromide in patients with COPD, there is a low incidence of anticholinergic side-effects. Approximately 18% of patients experience dryness of the mouth, but this is not of sufficient magnitude to cause withdrawal from the trial [44]. There are no other consistent side-effects that can be attributed to systemic effects of anticholinergics. In the study that compared tiotropium once daily with ipratropium four times daily, there was a 15% incidence of dry mouth compared to a 10% incidence with ipratropium [28].

FUTURE DIRECTIONS

Inhaled anticholinergics are very important bronchodilators in the management of COPD and currently bronchodilators are the most effective drug therapy available for COPD. As the worldwide prevalence of COPD is increasing, it is likely that the use of anticholinergic drugs will increase, particularly as the diagnosis and treatment become more widely disseminated through international treatment guidelines [1, 2]. In addition, there is a large multicentre randomised trial testing the hypothesis that tiotropium may actually alter the faster rate of decline in FEV_1 that is characteristic of patients with COPD. This international trial is named 'Understanding Potential Long-term Impacts on Function with Tiotropium' or the UPLIFT trial. Six thousand patients from around the world have been enrolled and the primary outcome will be the trough FEV_1 after 3 years. The results of this study will not only provide information about the value of long-acting anticholinergics in altering the course of COPD but also, as the largest study ever on COPD, provide insight about the phenotypic presentation, regional differences and course of the disease.

Tiotropium bromide is likely to be an important advance in the management of COPD as once daily medication is effective and this will improve compliance with long-term therapy. Indeed, the long duration of action of tiotropium bromide means that even if occasional daily doses are missed this will not affect symptom control, as it takes 2 weeks for the effects of the drug to disappear.

Anticholinergics are much less effective than β_2-agonists in patients with asthma and therefore have only a minor role as an additional bronchodilator [46]. Whether tiotropium bromide will have a role in asthma remains to be determined, but it may be useful as an additional bronchodilator in patients with fixed airflow obstruction and patients with severe disease.

Finally, the combination with other bronchodilator classes or inhaled or oral anti-inflammatory agents is very likely to become routine. As this topic is being addressed in a different chapter in this book I would only like to stress the concept that combination therapy has been highly effective in other chronic diseases such as hypertension, congestive heart failure and diabetes. It makes perfect sense that the same will hold true for pharmacological agents in COPD.

REFERENCES

1. Celli BR, MacNee W. Standards for the diagnosis and treatment of COPD. *Eur Respir J* 2004; 23:932–946.
2. Pauwels RA, Buist AS, Calverley PM, Jenkins CR, Hurd SS, the GOLD Scientific Committee. Global strategy for the diagnosis, management, and prevention of chronic obstructive pulmonary disease. NHLBI/WHO Global Initiative for Chronic Obstructive Lung Disease (GOLD) Workshop summary. *Am J Respir Crit Care Med* 2001; 163:1256–1276.
3. Gross N. Ipratropium bromide. *N Engl J Med* 1988; 319:486–494.
4. Tamaoki J, Chiyotani A, Tagaya E, Sakai N, Konno K. Effect of long term treatment with oxitropium bromide on airway secretion in chronic bronchitis and diffuse panbronchiolitis. *Thorax* 1994; 49:545–548.
5. Patel HJ, Barnes PJ, Takahashi T, Tadjkarimi S, Yacoub MH, Belvisi MG. Characterization of prejunctional muscarinic autoreceptors in human and guinea-pig trachea *in vitro*. *Am J Resp Crit Care Med* 1995; 152:872–878.
6. Disse B, Speck GA, Rominger KL, Witek TJ, Hammer R. Tiotropium (Spiriva): Mechanistic considerations and clinical profile in obstructive lung disease. *Life Sci* 1999; 64:457–464.
7. Haddad E-B, Patel H, Keeling JE, Yacoub MH, Barnes PJ, Belvisi MG. Pharmacological characterization of the muscarinic receptor antagonist, glycopyrrolate, in human and guinea-pig airways. *Br J Pharmacol* 1999; 127:413–420.
8. Disse B, Reichal R, Speck G, Travnecker W, Rominger KL, Hammer R: Ba679BR, a novel anticholinergic bronchodilator: preclinical and clinical aspects. *Life Sci* 1993; 52:537–544.
9. Barnes PJ. Chronic obstructive pulmonary disease. *N Engl J Med* 2000; 343:269–280.
10. Disse B. Antimuscarinic treatment for lung diseases from research to clinical practice. *Life Sci* 2001; 68:2557–2564.
11. Tashkin D, Ashutosh K, Bleecker E *et al*. Comparisons of the anticholinergic bronchodilator ipratropium bromide with metaproterenol in chronic obstructive pulmonary disease. *Am J Med* 1986; 81:81–89.
12. Mahler D, Donohue J, Barbee R, Goldman M, Gross N, Wisniewski M *et al*. Efficacy of salmeterol xinafoate in the treatment of COPD. *Chest* 1999; 115:957–965.
13. Rennard SI, Serby CW, Ghafouri M, Johnson PA, Friedman M. Extended therapy with ipratropium is associated with improved lung function in patients with COPD. A retrospective analysis of data from seven clinical trials. *Chest* 1996; 110:62–70.
14. Standards for the diagnosis and care of patients with COPD. *Am J Respir Crit Care Med* 1995; 152:S77–S121.
15. Combivent Inhalation Aerosol Study Group. Chronic obstructive pulmonary disease, a combination of ipratropium and albuterol is more effective than either agent alone. *Chest* 1994; 105:1411–1419.
16. D'Urzo A, De Salvo M, Ramirez-Rivera A, Almeida J, Sichletidis L, Guenter R, Kottakis J, FOR-INT-03 Study Group. In patients with COPD, treatment with a combination of formoterol and ipratropium is more effective than a combination of salbutamol and ipratropium. *Chest* 2001; 119:1347–1356.
17. van Noord JA, de Munck DR, Bantje TA, Hop WC, Akveld ML, Bommer AM. Long-term treatment of chronic obstructive pulmonary disease with salmeterol and the additive effect of ipratropium. *Eur Respir J* 2000; 15:878–885.
18. Anthonisen N, Connett J, Kiley J, Altose M, Bailey W, Buist AS *et al*. Effect of smoking intervention and the use of an inhaled anticholinergic bronchodilator on the rate of decline of FEV_1. *JAMA* 1994; 272:1497–1505.
19. Ikeda A, Nishimura K, Koyama H, Sugiura N, Izumi T. Oxitropium bromide improves exercise performance in patients with COPD. *Chest* 1994; 106:1740–1745.
20. Peel E, Anderson G. A dose response study of oxitropium bromide in chronic bronchitis. *Thorax* 1984; 39:453–456.

21. Frith P, Jenner B, Dangerfield R, Atkinson J, Drennan C. Oxitropium bromide: dose and time response study of a new anticholinergic bronchodilator drug. *Chest* 1986; 89:249–253.
22. Cazzola M, Di Perna F, Noschese P, Vinciguerra A, Calderaro F, Girbino G, Matera M. Effects of formoterol, salmeterol or oxitropium bromide on airway responses to salbutamol in COPD. *Eur Repir J* 1998; 11:1337–1341.
23. Haddad E-B, Mak JC, Barnes PJ. Characterization of [³H]Ba 679, a slow-dissociating muscarinic receptor antagonist in human lung: radioligand binding and autoradiographic mapping. *Mol Pharmacol* 1994; 45:899–907.
24. Maesen FPV, Smeets JJ, Costongs MAL, Wald FDM, Cornelissen PJG. BA 679 Br, a new long-acting antimuscarinic bronchodilator; a pilot dose-escalation study. *Eur Resp J* 1993; 6:1031–1036.
25. O'Connor B, Towse L, Barnes P. Prolonged effect of tiotropium bromide on methacoline induced bronchoconstriction in asthma. *Am J Respir Crit Care Med* 1996; 154:876–880.
26. Littner MR, Ilowite JS, Tashkin DP, Friedman M, Serby CW, Menjoge SS, Witek TJ. Long-acting bronchodilation with once-daily dosing of tiotropium (Spiriva) in stable chronic obstructive pulmonary disease. *Am J Respir Crit Care Med* 2000; 161:1136–1142.
27. van Noord JA, Bantje TA, Eland ME, Korducki L, Cornelissen PJ. A randomised controlled comparison of tiotropium and ipratropium in the treatment of chronic obstructive pulmonary disease. The Dutch Tiotropium Study Group. *Thorax* 2000; 55:289–294.
28. Vincken W, van Noord J, Greefhorst A, Bantje TA, Kesten S, Korducki L, Cornelissen P, Dutch/Belgium Tiotropium Study Group. Improved health outcomes in patients with COPD during 1 year's treatment with tiotropium. *Eur Respir J* 2002; 19:209–216.
29. Casaburi R, Briggs DDJ, Donohue JF, Serby CW, Menjoge SS, Witek TJJ. The spirometric efficacy of once-daily dosing with tiotropium in stable COPD: A 13-week multicenter trial. *Chest* 2000; 118:1294–1302.
30. Kesten S, Chapman KR, Broder I, Cartier A, Hyland RH, Knight A *et al*. A 3 month comparison of twice daily inhaled formoterol versus four times daily inhaled albuterol in the management of stable asthma. *Am Rev Respir Dis* 1991; 144:622–625.
31. Fredberg JJ, Inouye DS, Mijailovich SM, Butler JP. Perturbed equilibrium of myosin binding in airway smooth muscle and its implications in bronchospasm. *Am J Respir Crit Care Med* 1999; 159:959–967.
32. Calverley P, Lee A, Towse L, van Noord J, Witek T, Kesten S. Effect of tiotropium bromide on circadian variation in airflow limitation in chronic obstructive pulmonary disease. *Thorax* 2003; 58:855–860.
33. Hay J, Stone P, Carter J, Church S, Eyre-Brock A, Pearson M, Woodcock A, Calverley P. Bronchodilator reversibility, exercise performance and breathlessness in stable chronic obstructive pulmonary disease. *Eur Respir J* 1992; 5:659–664.
34. Belman M, Botnick W, Shin J. Inhaled bronchodilators reduce dynamic hyperinflation during exercise in patients with chronic obstructive pulmonary disease. *Am J Respir Crit Care Med* 1996; 153:967–975.
35. O'Donnell D, Lam M, Webb K. Spirometric correlates of improvement in exercise performance after anticholinergic therapy in chronic obstructive pulmonary disease. *Am J Respir Crit Care Med* 1999; 160:542–549.
36. Oga T, Nishimura K, Tsukino M, Hajiro T, Ikeda A, Izumi T. The effects of oxitropium bromide on exercise performance in patients with stable chronic obstructive pulmonary disease. *Am J Respir Crit Care Med* 2000; 161:1897–1901.
37. Celli B, ZuWallack R, Wang S, Kesten S. Improvement of inspiratory capacity and hyperinflation with tiotropium in COPD patients with severe hyperinflation. *Chest* 2003; 124:1743–1748.
38. National Emphysema Treatment Trial Research Group. A randomized trial comparing lung-volume-reduction surgery with medical therapy for severe emphysema. *N Engl J Med* 2003; 348:2059–2073.
39. Flaminiano L, Celli BR. Respiratory muscle testing. *Clin Chest Med* 2001; 22:661–677.
40. O'Donnell D, Fluge T, Gerken F, Hamilton A, Webb K, Agulaniu B *et al*. Effects of tiotropium on lung hyperinflation, dyspnea and exercise tolerance in COPD. *Eur Respir J* 2004; 23:832–840.
41. Higgins MW, Thom T. Incidence, prevalence and mortality: intra- and inter-country difference. In: Hensley MJ, Saunders NA (eds) Clinical Epidemiology of Chronic Obstructive Pulmonary Disease. Marcel Dekker, New York, 1990, pp 23–43.
42. Dahl R, Greefhorst L, Nonikov V, Byrne A, Thomson M, Till D, DellaCioppa G. The formoterol in chronic obstructive pulmonary disease study group. *Am J Respir Crit Care Med* 2001; 164:778–784.
43. Witek T, Mahler D. Minimal important difference of the transitional dyspnea index in a multinational clinical trial. *Eur Respir J* 2003; 21:267–272.

44. Casaburi R, Mahler D, Jones P, Wanner A, San Pedro G, ZuWallack R *et al*. A long-term evaluation of once-daily inhaled tiotropium in chronic obstructive pulmonary disease. *Eur Respir J* 2002; 19:217–224.

45. Niewoehner D, Rice K, Cote C, Paulson D, Cooper J, Korducki L *et al*. Reduced COPD exacerbation and associated health care utilization with once-daily tiotropium in the VA medical system. *Am J Respir Crit Care Med* 2004; 169:A207.

46. Qureshi F, Pestian J, Paris B, Zaritsky A. Effect of nebulized ipratropium on the hospitalization rates of children with asthma. *N Engl J Med* 1998; 339:1030–1035.

7

Pharmacology of phosphodiesterase inhibitors

V. Boswell-Smith, C. P. Page

INTRODUCTION

Cyclic 3', 5' adenosine monophosphate (cAMP) is pivotal in modulating physiological responses and elevation of this ubiquitous second messenger has been demonstrated to be broadly anti-inflammatory. Phosphodiesterases (PDE), hydrolyse the catalytic breakdown of both cAMP and cyclic 3', 5' guanosine monophosphate (cGMP), to their inactive mono-nucleotides, 5'-AMP and 5'-GMP which are unable to activate cyclic nucleotide-dependent protein kinase cascades. Consequently, they play a vital role in regulating intracellular levels of cyclic nucleotides. Advances in molecular pharmacology have identified 11 PDE families and the success of sidenafil, a PDE5 selective inhibitor, in treating erectile dysfunction has invigorated research into the therapeutic potential of selective PDE inhibitors in other diseases. Non-selective PDE inhibitors such as theophylline have been in use since the 1950s for the treatment of inflammatory airways diseases, although use has been limited due to their narrow therapeutic index and side-effect profile. As a result, there have been attempts to improve the therapeutic window and the PDE4 isoenzyme, expressed in the majority of leukocytes, has been identified as an important target in the treatment of asthma and COPD and a number of inhibitors, which are at least 30-fold selective for PDE4, are undergoing clinical development and are discussed later in this chapter. This part of the chapter will discuss the role of PDEs in modulating inflammation, with particular reference to COPD and highlight how our increasing understanding of the molecular biology of PDE4 is assisting in the development of potent, new drugs.

CLASSIFICATION OF PDE

Eleven PDE families, encompassing 50 separate isoforms [1], have now been identified. They have been characterised by their substrate specificity, whether they can hydrolyse either or both cAMP and cGMP, regulatory actions, inhibitor potency, enzyme kinetics and genetic homology [1]. PDE4, PDE7 and PDE8 are highly selective for cAMP, whereas PDE5, PDE6 and PDE9 favour cGMP. PDE1, PDE2 and PDE3 are promiscuous and can hydrolyse both cyclic nucleotides. The characteristics of the PDE family are summarised in Table 7.1.

All the PDE isoenzymes are made of between one and four gene products (designated by letters A, B, C and D, e.g., PDE4D) which each have a characteristic structure encompassing three functional domains: a central catalytic domain, a regulatory NH$_2$ terminal and

Victoria Boswell-Smith, BSc, Sackler Institute of Pulmonary Pharmacology, Guy's, King's and St Thomas' School of Biomedical Sciences, Kings College London, London, UK.

Clive Peter Page, BSc, PhD, Professor of Pharmacology, Sackler Institute of Pulmonary Pharmacology, Guy's, King's and St Thomas' School of Biomedical Sciences, Kings College London, London, UK.

Table 7.1   The characteristics of the PDE isoenzyme family

Family	No. of isoforms identified	Substrate	Km cAMP (>1,000 not shown)	Km GMP (>1,000 not shown)	Tissue expression	Specific inhibitors
1 (4 genes)	8	Ca^{2+}/ Calmodulin- stimulated	1–30	3	Heart, brain, lung, smooth muscle	KS-505a Vinpocetine
2 (1 gene)		cGMP- stimulated	50	50	Adrenal gland, heart, lung, liver, platelets	EHNA (MEP-1)
3 (2 genes)	4	cGMP- inhibited, cAMP- selective	0.2	0.3	Heart, lung, liver, platelets, adipose tissue, inflammatory cells	Cilostamide Milrinone Siguazodan
4 (4 genes)	16	cAMP- specific	4		Sertoli cells, kidney, brain, liver, lung, inflammatory cells	Rolipram, Roflumilast Cilomilast
5 (1 gene)	3	cGMP- specific	150	1	Lung, platelets, vascular smooth muscle	Sildenafil Zaprinast
6 (3 genes)		cGMP- specific		60	Photoreceptors	Dipyridamole Zaprinast
7 (2 genes)	3	cAMP-specific, high- affinity	0.2		Skeletal muscle, heart, kidney, brain, pancreas, T-lymphocytes	None
8 (2 genes)		cAMP- selective	0.06		Testes, eye, liver, skeletal muscle, heart, kidney, ovary, brain, T-lymphocytes	None
9 (1 gene)	4	cGMP-specific		0.17	Kidney, liver, lung, brain	SCH51866
10 (1 gene)	2	cGMP-sensitive, cAMP-selective	0.05	3.0	Testes, brain	None
11 (1 gene)	4	cGMP-sensitive dual specificity	0.7	0.6	Skeletal muscle, prostate, kidney, liver, pituitary and salivary glands, testes	None

a regulatory COOH terminal. The N-terminal region is involved in allosteric regulation *via* phosphorylation, calmodulin and cyclic nucleotide binding, and intracellular membrane targeting and the C-terminal is thought to posses PDE specific kinase docking sites [2]. The catalytic domains are highly conserved, both within and between families, and contain histidine residues which are essential for their catalytic activity. Both the N and C termini have proportional homology (approximately 70%) within families, although mRNA splicing of the termini results in the numerous isoforms of these enzymes.

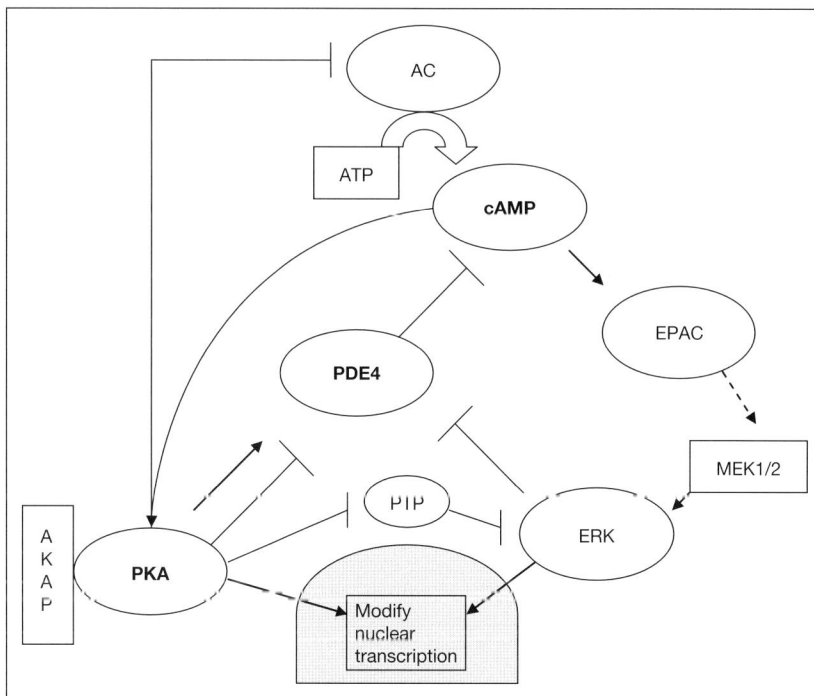

Figure 7.1 A schematic diagram of the role of PDE4 in intracellular signalling. PKA= Phosphokinase A, PDE= phosphodiesterase, AKAP= A Kinase anchor protein, cAMP= cyclic adenosine monophosphate, ATP= adenosine triphosphate, AC= adenylyl cyclase, EPAC= exchange protein activated by cAMP, ERK= extracellular signal related protein kinase, PTP= protein tyrosine phosphatase.

It is now evident that individual PDE isoforms are differentially expressed in tissues and are also compartmentalised within the subcellular apparatus. cAMP is generated from ATP by the actions of adenylyl cyclase and its signalling primarily regulated by protein kinase A (PKA) [3], as well as *via* the GTP exchange protein, EPAC and cyclic nucleotide gated ion channels which regulate levels of the accessory protein calmodulin [4]. PKA modulates cAMP levels by phosphorylation of both adenylyl cyclase and PDEs and its distribution within cells is controlled by A kinase anchoring proteins (AKAPs) which anchor PKA to distinct sites within cells [5]. Compartmentalisation of adenylyl cyclase, PDE isoenzymes and PKA results in tightly regulated cAMP gradients throughout the cellular compartments and allows tailored cAMP intracellular signalling [6]. It has been proposed that the discrete expression of PDE isoforms within subcellular compartments regulates the level of cyclic nucleotides in the vicinity of PKA and consequently plays a key role in the regulation of cell function [7]. A schematic diagram of the role of PDE in cell signalling is described in Figure 7.1.

PHOSPHODIESTERASE 4

The advent of highly selective inhibitors has enabled the modulation of different PDEs in specific tissues to be studied in great detail. Attention has focused on the PDE4 isoenzyme as a possible therapeutic target in airway diseases as it is the predominant isoenzyme in most inflammatory cells including neutrophils, macrophages and eosinophils [8], and alongside PDE3 is widely distributed in airways and vascular smooth muscle. A number of

Table 7.2   PDE4 inhibitors in development for the treatment of inflammatory airways disease

Compound	Manufacturer	Development stage	Reference
Cilomilast	GSK	Phase III	[90]
Roflumilast	Altana/Pfizer	Phase III	[91]
L-791,943	Merck	Preclinical	[92]
CDP840	Celltech	Preclinical	[78]
AWD12-281	Elbion		[93]
GRC-3015	Glenmark	Patent applied for	[94]
SCH 351591	Schering-plough	Preclinical	[62]
BAY-19-8004	Bayer	Phase 11	[95]
VMX-554	Vernalis	Preclinical	[85]

selective PDE4 isoenzyme inhibitors are in development for the treatment of inflammatory airways disease. A list of these is shown in Table 7.2.

The four gene products of PDE4 are defined as PDE4A, 4B, 4C and 4D and have been localised and characterised in humans, rats and mice. In humans, they are distributed on 3 different chromosomes (PDE4A and 4C on chromosome 19, 4B on chromosome 1 and 4D on chromosome 5) [7]. Sequence analysis of the PDE4 structure has identified 3 conserved regions within the family termed the catalytic domain, upstream conserved region 1 and upstream conserved region 2 (UCR1 and 2). mRNA post transitional splicing of the 4 gene products adds further diversity and 18 different PDE4 isoforms, each with a unique N-terminal, have now been characterised. Functional consequences of N-terminal modifications include alterations in subcellular localisation [9] and activation and targeting by isoenzyme-specific inhibitors [10]. As the genetic PDE4 structure in humans and mice is highly conserved, the diversity of isoforms probably has functional significance and is unlikely to be evolutionarily redundant, although this remains to be determined [6]. The splice variants are divided into 3 different types according to where splicing has occurred. These are known as long, short and supershort isoforms. Long isoforms contain both UCR1 and 2, short isoforms lack UCR1 and in the supershort isoforms UCR1 is absent and UCR2 is only present in a shortened form. Truncation affects the ability of isoforms to undergo phosphorylation, their enzyme activity and subcellular positioning. Indeed all PDE4 isoforms exhibit cAMP activity except the widely expressed supershort isoform PDE4A7 which has no discernable PDE activity, the functional significance of which remains unclear. The catalytic activity and inhibitor potency of PDE4 can be modulated by PKA phosphorylation of UCR1 [7] and in the case of PDE4B, 4C and 4D, ERK2 (p42^{MAPK}) phosphorylation [11] of the catalytic domain, thereby providing integration between the cAMP and ERK MAP kinase signalling pathways. The ability of PDE4 to activate signalling pathways can also be modulated by alterations in levels of extracellular stimuli including Mg^{2+} ions, cytokines and lipopolysaccharide [7]. This may have functional significance in times of stress, including inflammation, as the capacity of the enzyme to degrade cAMP may be altered, and consequently the ability of inhibitors to modulate actions of PDE.

PDE4 EXPRESSION

PDE4 isoenzyme expression has been identified in all inflammatory cells except platelets. Significantly, it predominates in neutrophils and is highly expressed in alveolar macrophages and CD8+ lymphocytes [12]. As shown in Table 7.3, PDE4A, 4B and 4D are widely distributed in inflammatory cells whilst significant PDE4C expression has been limited to the epithelium

Table 7.3 The expression of PDE4 subtypes in human inflammatory cells

Cell type	A	B	C	D	Reference
CD4 T cell	+	++ (B2)		Weak	[86]
Th1 cells	++	++	−	−	[87]
Th2 cells	++	++	−	++	[87]
CD8 T cell	++	++ (B2)	+	++	[13, 14, 86]
Monocyte	+	++ (B2)	+	Weak	[13, 14, 16, 86]
Eosinophil	++	++	−	++	[86]
Neutrophil	±	++ (B2)	+	±	[13, 14, 16, 88]
Macrophage	++	+		++	[13, 89]

in the adult lung and it has therefore not been considered an important therapeutic target. This may prove to be premature as latest investigations into isoform expression within inflammatory cells have also reported the presence of PDE4C mRNA within these cells [13, 14].

ANTI-INFLAMMATORY EFFECTS OF PDE4 INHIBITION

The effects of PDE4 inhibition have been thoroughly investigated in an extensive array of *in vitro* and *in vivo* assays and they have been shown to have a potent anti-inflammatory effect on a wide range of cellular functions which are summarised in Figure 7.2. The following section will highlight the role of PDE4 in regulating the cellular effects of neutrophils, macrophages, monocytes and CD8+ lymphocytes, the primary infiltrating inflammatory cells in COPD, and the epithelium and airway smooth muscle, both of which undergo remodelling in COPD [15]. Neuronal dysfunction has also been suggested to contribute to the development of COPD and therefore the potential role of PDE4 inhibitors in modulating sensory nerve function will also be examined.

Neutrophil
The neutrophil is one of the predominant infiltrating leukocytes in COPD. PDE4 has been repeatedly demonstrated to be the predominant isoenzyme in human neutrophils [12–14] with the principal isoform being PDE4B [16]. No significant difference in PDE4 isoform expression between COPD patients, smokers and nonsmokers has been detected [13, 14]. Recent studies have also demonstrated high expression of the PDE7 isoenzyme in this cell type [13, 14], although the functional significance of this is yet to be fully explored as the selective PDE7 isoenzyme inhibitor PF0332040 failed to suppress formyl-methionyl-leucinephenylalanine-induced neutrophil activation [14]. In contrast, PDE4 inhibitors can attenuate numerous neutrophil functions including degranulation [17, 18], respiratory burst [19, 20], apoptosis [21], chemotaxis, leukotriene biosynthesis [20, 22] and IL-8 release [23]. *In vivo* PDE4 inhibitors can suppress LPS-induced neutrophilia in rats [24, 25] and in a model of tobacco smoke-induced inflammation in the guinea-pig, the PDE4 inhibitor, BAY-19-8004 ablated the inflammatory cell influx, including neutrophils induced by the tobacco. Rolipram also inhibited the retention of activated neutrophils in the rabbit lung *in vivo* by suppressing CDIIb up-regulation and reducing deformity changes associated with neutrophil sequestration [26, 27]. The failure of selective PDE3 inhibitors, including milrinone and amrinone, to suppress neutrophil function [19, 28] has been attributed to the lack of expression of this isoenzyme within neutrophils. However, using RT-PCR, Barber et al. [13] detected expression of this enzyme within neutrophils. Consequently, the role of this enzyme in modulating cAMP in neutrophils needs further investigation. These data demonstrate that PDE4 inhibitors can suppress a wide range of neutrophil functions both *in vitro* and *in vivo*,

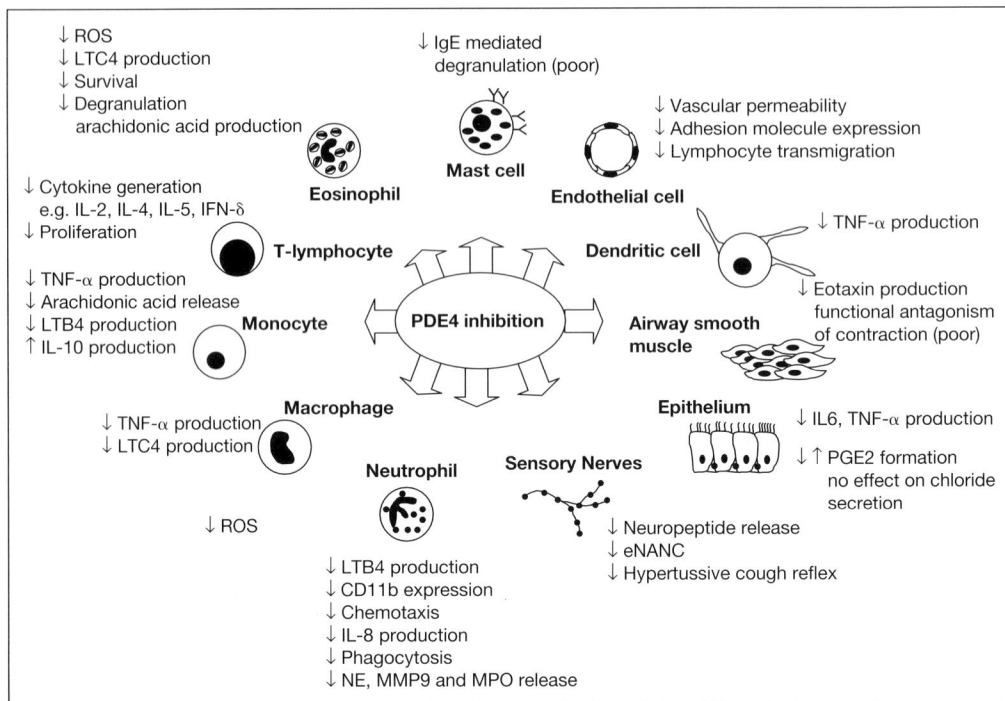

Figure 7.2   The effect of phosphodiesterase 4 inhibition in modulating airways cellular function (adapted from [55] with permission).

suggesting that some of the clinical effects of these drugs may manifest through inhibition of neutrophil function.

Monocyte

PDE4 has been shown to be the predominant isoenzyme in human monocytes [29]. PDE4A, 4B and 4D isoform transcripts have been demonstrated consistently in these cells with PDE4A being the predominant isoform [12, 30]. PDE4C expression has been rarely documented in monocytes, although recent studies have described its presence within these cells. Small quantities of membrane bound PDE3 and PDE7A and 7B have also been detected in monocytes [13, 31]. PDE4 inhibitors including rolipram, roflumilast and cilomilast can attenuate a number of monocyte functions including LPS-induced TNF-α release [17, 32, 33], LTB4 release [34], GM-CSF release [35] and arachidonic acid release [36]. The ability of PDE4 inhibitors to attenuate IL-1β release is conflicting with some studies demonstrating inhibition [37, 38] and others demonstrating no effect [39]. Rolipram was also shown to enhance the release of the pro-inflammatory cytokine IL-10, which may contribute to the anti-inflammatory effects of this class of drug [40]. Overall, PDE4 inhibitors are effective in suppressing pro-inflammatory mediator release which may contribute to some of their clinical effects in COPD.

Alveolar Macrophages

The PDE profile changes upon differentiation of monocytes to macrophages. The predominant isoenzyme present in mature macrophages is the cGMP hydrolysing enzyme PDE1, 3 (primarily 3B) and PDE4 are expressed in equivalent amounts, although the PDE4 activity is significantly lower than in monocytes [13, 29]. The PDE4D5 isoform present in monocytes is absent in mature macrophages, whereas PDE5 and 7 are also expressed in macrophages [13, 31]. Interestingly, PDE4A4 expression is up-regulated in macrophages in patients with COPD [13], although the functional significance of this observation remains to be determined. Functional studies with PDE4 inhibitors have demonstrated their ability to attenuate TNF-α release [32, 41], LPS-induced NO release [42] and to elevate IL-10 release [43] from human alveolar macrophages. Rolipram has also been shown to attenuate LPS-induced leukotriene C_4 release from murine peritoneal macrophages. These data demonstrate that although macrophages express both PDE3 and PDE4, inhibition of the latter isoenzyme can significantly modulate macrophage activity.

CD8+ Lymphocytes

PDE4 and PDE3 are the predominant isoenzymes present in CD8+ lymphocytes. PDE4A, 4B and 4D subtypes have been consistently demonstrated to be present in the cytosol of lymphocytes [12, 13, 44]. A recent study has also detected the presence of low levels of PDE4C [14]. Other isoenzymes reported to be present include PDE1, 2, 5 and 7 [31, 44]. Cellular functions inhibited by PDE4 inhibitors include phytohaemagglutinin (PHA) and anti CD3 induced proliferation [15], and these effects are enhanced in the presence of both PDE3 and PDE7 inhibitors [41, 46]. This suggests that alongside PDE4, 3 and 7 may play a role in regulating T-lymphocyte proliferation. In clinical trials, 12-week treatment with cilomilast has been demonstrated to suppress the number of CD8+ lymphocytes as assessed by bronchial biopsy, suggesting that some of the clinical effects of cilomilast are through modulating CD8+ lymphocyte infiltration [47].

Epithelium

It is now evident that in severe COPD there is up-regulation of a number of inflammatory mediators including IL-8, MPO, and MIP-1 from the epithelium [48, 49]. PDE1, 3, 4, 5, and 7 have all been localised to the human airways epithelium [50, 51]. The PDE4 isoenzyme is the major cAMP metabolising enzyme, with PDE4A5, 4C1, 4D1, 4D2 and 4D3 isoforms being characterised in the epithelium [50]. However, PDE4 inhibitors have shown varied effects in epithelial functional assays *in vitro*. PGE$_2$, IL-8 and 15-HETE release are unaffected by rolipram, rofumilast, GRC 3566 and GRC 3884 [50, 51, 52], although rolipram did suppress bacterial-induced epithelial damage of the bronchial mucosa [53] and cilomilast significantly reduced TNF-α release from epithelial cells from both COPD patients and smokers. KF19514, rofumilast, GRC 3566 and GRC 3884 also inhibited TNF-α-induced release of GM-CSF from a human bronchial epithelial cell line *in vitro*. In addition, in a murine model of asthma, rofumilast suppressed eosinophil accumulation in the epithelium and reversed both sub-epithelial fibrosis and hypertrophy, demonstrating that PDE4 inhibition ameliorates pathological changes associated with inflammatory airways disease [54]. *In vivo* pre-treatment with BAY-19-8004 significantly suppressed LPS-induced mucin hypersecretion from guinea-pigs [27], a key index of epithelial dysfunction. These data demonstrate the ability of PDE4 inhibitors to attenuate epithelial function, which may contribute to their clinical effects.

Airway Smooth Muscle

PDE3 and 4 are the major isoenzymes expressed in airways smooth muscle alongside PDE1, 2, 5 and 7 [31, 55]. *In vitro*, PDE4 inhibitors have been documented to suppress spontaneous tone, mediated by leukotrienes and histamine [56]. However, they only weakly suppress spasmogen, including allergen, LTC4 and histamine-induced contractions in isolated human airways smooth muscle and this effect is only significant when combined with a PDE3 inhibitor [57, 58]. These data suggest that RDE4 inhibitors have enough efficacy to suppress endogenous tone, although it is not sufficient to overcome spasmogen-induced contraction. This is further evident in clinical trials with rofumilast and CDP840, which have reported a failure to suppress allergen-induced bronchoconstriction in asthmatics [59, 60]. These studies suggest that the PDE4 inhibitors do not predominantly mediate their effects through direct actions on airways smooth muscle and therefore their actions may be a consequence of other cell types in the airways. However, PDE4 inhibitors were demonstrated to be equally efficacious in suppressing allergen and LTC_4-induced constriction *in vitro* implying that suppression of leukotriene release from mast cells is not a major action of these drugs [58]. Significantly, PDE4 inhibitors are generally superior in animal models, compared to human subjects, both *in vitro* and *in vivo* at suppressing spasmogen and allergen-induced bronchoconstriction [61, 62]. This may be a consequence of the propensity of guinea-pig airways to synthesise prostanoids in comparison with human airways and it is postulated that in these species PDE4 inhibitors exert their effects by potentiating the action of endogenous prostaglandins [63]. This is evident from investigations with cilomilast which demonstrated an inability to reverse histamine-induced tone in the presence of indomethacin [62] and in studies with PDE4D knockout murine models which showed that in the absence of the PDE4D isoform, endogenous generation of PGE_2 functionally antagonised contraction of smooth muscle *in vitro* and *in vivo* [64]. In conclusion, these data suggest that the clinical actions of phosphodiesterase 4 inhibitors are unlikely to be a sole consequence of a direct action on airways smooth muscle nor do they exert their actions primarily through suppression of mast cell degranulation.

Airways Nerves

There is a paucity of information concerning the effect of PDE4 inhibitors in modulating sensory nerves in the airways. However, there is evidence both circumstantial and direct that indicates that some of the effects of these drugs may be a consequence of neuronal modulation. An improvement in lung function in asthmatics is observed within 24 h of administration of rofumilast (500 μg od) [65] which has been proven not to be a consequence of direct smooth muscle contraction [59]. This could be a result of immuno-modulation but could equally be a result of sensory nerve modulation. Ro 20-1724 and rolipram can suppress excitatory non-adrenergic non-cholinergic (eNANC) contraction in the isolated guinea-pig bronchus [66], whilst *in vivo*, CDP840 and rolipram can potently suppress vagally-induced non cholinergic bronchoconstriction, mediated by tachykinins in guinea-pigs [67]. The PDE4 inhibitor SCN 351591 also significantly suppressed hyper-ventilation-induced bronchospasm [62], a stimulus proposed to be mediated by the release of tachykinins from C-fibres [68]. These data suggest that PDE4 inhibitors can modulate tackykinin release from sensory nerve endings. Studies with cilomilast have also demonstrated that this PDE4 inhibitor can normalise the hypertussive state in sensitised guinea-pigs [69]. PDE4D has been localised in the nodose ganglia of squirrel monkeys giving rise to the possibility of a role for PDE4 inhibitors in modulating sensory nerves activity originating from here [70]. In clinical trials, 500 μg of roflumilast resulted in a significant increase in FEV_1 within 24 h of the first oral dose, which is a much quicker effect than you would expect if roflumilast was modulating inflammation alone [71]. Consequently, the modulatory effect of roflumilast and other PDE4 inhibitors on sensory nerves requires further investigation.

IMPROVING THE SIDE-EFFECT PROFILE OF PDE4 INHIBITORS

The major side-effects of PDE4 inhibitors include emesis, nausea and headache. Improving their side-effect profile is of prime importance in the development of novel PDE4 inhibitors, as the currently most clinically advanced inhibitors, roflumilast and cilomilast, whilst attenuating characteristic features of airways disease, and exhibiting a lower emetogenic potential, are not free from such side-effects. This effectively limits the dose which can be administered to patients, and thus limits the potential gain from these compounds. A number of different development strategies have been undertaken in the pursuit of side-effect free compounds.

The catalytic domain of PDE4 isoforms can exist in at least 2 conformationally distinct states which have different affinities to bind the archetypal PDE4 inhibitor, rolipram [7]. Therefore, sensitivity of rolipram can be altered under different conditions, dependent on the conformational state of the isoenzyme. These states have been termed the high affinity and low affinity rolipram conformers [72]. Investigations with competitive PDE4 inhibitors have demonstrated a positive correlation between rolipram displacement and gastric acid secretion [73] and emesis [74], both undesirable side-effects of PDE4 inhibitors. In contrast, PDE4 inhibitor affinity for the low affinity conformer is generally associated with the anti-inflammatory effects of PDE4 inhibition including suppression of LPS-induced TNF-α release from monocytes [75] and IL-2 release from murine splenocytes [76]. Selective targeting of the low affinity rolipram conformer by inhibitors has therefore been attempted in order to improve the side-effect profile of these drugs [75]. Cilomilast and CDP840 are both more selective for the low-affinity binding site and do exhibit an improved side-effect profile, whilst maintaining their anti-inflammatory capacities [77, 78]. AWD12-281 exhibits very little affinity for the high-affinity binding rolipram conformer and *in vivo* appears to be less emetogenic than both cilomilast and roflumilast, although the clinical effect of this drug has yet to be determined [25]. However, the high-affinity conformer is still associated with some cellular functions including MPO release from human neutrophils, a key marker of neutrophil degranulation. The conformational state can also be altered by PKA phosphorylation and therefore conformational switching may alter catalytic activity and inhibitor sensitivity under inflammatory conditions [7]. Consequently, it remains to be determined whether selectively targeting one conformer over another will result in a clinically efficacious compound with a better side-effect profile [75] and results from ongoing clinical studies are anticipated with interest.

Generating novel compounds with subtype selectivity has been another strategy in an attempt to improve the side-effect profile of PDE4 inhibitors. Of the compounds that have undergone clinical evaluation, none have been reported to exhibit subtype selectivity, yet have a markedly improved side-effect profile compared with rolipram, whilst cilomilast is marginally more selective for PDE4D than PDE4A and 4B. Investigations with a PDE4D knockout mouse have associated this subtype with emesis [79]. PDE4D is also expressed in the area postrema and the vagal afferent nerves innervating the gut [69, 80]. These data suggest the PDE4D subtype may be involved in the gastrointestinal side-effects associated with PDE4 inhibition, which may account for the inferior side-effect profile of cilomilast compared with rofumilast, even though it is selective for the low affinity conformer. In contrast, studies with PDE4B knockout mice have shown the PDE4B isoform is required for LPS-induced TNF-α responses [81] and therefore selective targeting of PDE4B over PDE4D may provide an advantageous therapeutic index. A number of therapeutic compounds that demonstrate selectivity towards either PDE4A/B or PDE4D have been developed [30, 82]. A strong correlation between PDE4A/B inhibition, but not PDE4D inhibition, and the suppression of TNF-α release from monocytes and T-cell proliferation has been observed. This is consistent with weak expression of this isoform in these cells (see Table 7.3). In contrast, a correlation between both PDE4A/B and D inhibition and eosinophil function was seen, reflecting the strong expression of all three subtypes in these cells [83]. Further knowledge of the role of the individual isoforms in different cell types is required before it can be determined whether selective targeting of PDE4 isoforms will result in an improved side-effect profile, whilst remaining effective modulators of inflammatory cell function.

Another approach being actively pursued to reduce the incidence of side-effects with PDE4 inhibitors is to administer the drugs *via* inhalation rather than orally. There is a well established precedence of administering drugs such as bronchodilators and anti-inflammatory glucocorticosteroids *via* inhalation and administering PDE4 inhibitors by this route is an alternative way to reduce systemic exposure and therefore unwanted side-effects. Since a considerable proportion of an inhaled drug is swallowed, this approach alone does not guarantee success as the inhalation of zardaverine, a mixed PDE3/4 inhibitor, still produced gastrointestinal disturbances at doses improving FEV_1 [84]. Nonetheless, a number of PDE4 inhibitors in development are being formulated for inhaled administration including AWD-12-281, which when administered intratracheally produced no emesis in an *in vivo* canine model [25] and VMX-554, a long acting mixed PDE3/4 isoenzyme inhibitor [85].

CONCLUSION

Increasing our understanding of the biology of the extensive PDE family is providing further appreciation into the key regulatory role of PDEs, especially the role PDE4 plays in modulating the ubiquitous cAMP intracellular signalling pathway. Whilst early selective PDE4 inhibitors were potent anti-inflammatory agents *in vitro* and in animal models, their clinical use was tempered as a result of unwanted side-effects such as emesis and nausea. Increasing knowledge of PDE4 isoforms, along with a greater understanding of other PDE isoenzymes including PDE3 and 7 is essential if we are to improve the next generation of PDE inhibitors for the treatment of airways disease.

REFERENCES

1. Schmidt D, Dent G, Rabe KF. Selective phosphodiesterase inhibitors for the treatment of bronchial asthma and chronic obstructive pulmonary disease. *Clin Exp Allergy* 1999; 29(suppl 2):99–109.
2. Torphy TJ. Phosphodiesterase isozymes: molecular targets for novel antiasthma agents. *Am J Respir Crit Care Med* 1998; 157:351–370.
3. De RJ, Zwartkruis FJ, Verheijen MH, Cool RH, Nijman SM, Wittinghofer A, Bos JL. Epac is a Rap1 guanine-nucleotide-exchange factor directly activated by cyclic AMP. *Nature* 1998; 396:474–477.
4. Fimia GM, Sassone-Corsi P. Cyclic AMP signalling. *J Cell Sci* 2001; 114:1971–1972.
5. Colledge M, Scott JD. AKAPs: from structure to function. *Trends Cell Biol* 1999; 9:216–221.
6. Houslay MD, Adams DR. PDE4 cAMP phosphodiesterases: modular enzymes that orchestrate signalling cross-talk, desensitization and compartmentalization. *Biochem J* 2003; 370:1–18.
7. Houslay MD. PDE4 cAMP-specific phosphodiesterases. *Prog Nucleic Acid Res Mol Biol* 2001; 69:249–315.
8. Dent G, Giembycz MA. Phosphodiesterase inhibitors: Lily the Pink's medicinal compound for asthma? *Thorax* 1996; 51:647–649.
9. O'Connell JC, Mccallum JF, Mcphee I, Wakefield J, Houslay ES, Wishart W *et al.* The SH3 domain of Src tyrosyl protein kinase interacts with the N-terminal splice region of the PDE4A cAMP-specific phosphodiesterase RPDE-6 (RNPDE4A5). *Biochem J* 1996; 318:255–261.
10. Alvarez R, Sette C, Yang D, Eglen RM, Wilhelm R, Shelton ER, Conti M. Activation and selective inhibition of a cyclic AMP-specific phosphodiesterase, PDE-4D3. *Mol Pharmacol* 1995; 48:616–622.
11. Houslay MD, Baillie GS. The role of ERK2 docking and phosphorylation of PDE4 cAMP phosphodiesterase isoforms in mediating cross-talk between the cAMP and ERK signalling pathways. *Biochem Soc Trans* 2003; 31:1186–1190.
12. Muller T, Engels P, Fozard JR. Subtypes of the type 4 cAMP phosphodiesterases: structure, regulation and selective inhibition. *Trends Pharmacol Sci* 1996; 17:294–298.
13. Barber R, Baillie GS, Bergmann R, Shepherd MC, Sepper R, Houslay MD, Heeke GV. Differential expression of PDE4 cAMP phosphodiesterase isoforms in inflammatory cells of smokers with COPD, smokers without COPD, and nonsmokers. *Am J Physiol Lung Cell Mol Physiol* 2004; 287:L332–L343.
14. Jones NA, Leport M, Holand T, Vos T, Morgan M, Fink M *et al.* Phosphodiesterase 7 in inflammatory cells from patients with asthma and COPD. *Br J Pharmacol* 2005 (in press).
15. Barnes PJ, Shapiro SD, Pauwels RA. Chronic obstructive pulmonary disease: molecular and cellular mechanisms. *Eur Respir J* 2003; 22:672–688.
16. Wang P, Wu P, Ohleth KM, Egan RW, Billah MM. Phosphodiesterase 4B2 is the predominant phosphodiesterase species and undergoes differential regulation of gene expression in human monocytes and neutrophils. *Mol Pharmacol* 1999; 56:170–174.

17. Barnette MS, Christensen SB, Essayan DM, Grous M, Prabhakar U, Rush JA *et al*. SB 207499 (Ariflo), a potent and selective second-generation phosphodiesterase 4 inhibitor: *in vitro* anti-inflammatory actions. *J Pharmacol Exp Ther* 1998; 284:420–426.

18. Jones NA, Boswell-Smith V, Lever R, Page C. The effect of selective phosphodiesterase isoenzyme inhibition on neutrophil function *in vitro*. *Pulm Pharmacol* 2005; 18:93–101.

19. Nielson CP, Vestal RE, Sturm RJ, Heaslip R. Effects of selective phosphodiesterase inhibitors on the polymorphonuclear leukocyte respiratory burst. *J Allergy Clin Immunol* 1990; 86:801–808.

20. Schudt C, Winder S, Forderkunz S, Hatzelmann A, Ullrich V. Influence of selective phosphodiesterase inhibitors on human neutrophil functions and levels of cAMP and Cai. *Naunyn Schmiedebergs Arch Pharmacol* 1991; 344:682–690.

21. Yasui K, Agematsu K, Shinozaki K, Hokibara S, Nagumo H, Nakazawa T, Komiyama A. Theophylline induces neutrophil apoptosis through adenosine A2A receptor antagonism. *J Leukoc Biol* 2000; 67:529–535.

22. Cortijo J, Villagrasa V, Navarrete C, Sanz C, Berto L, Michel A *et al*. Effects of SCA40 on human isolated bronchus and human polymorphonuclear leukocytes: comparison with rolipram, SKF94120 and levcromakalim. *Br J Pharmacol* 1996; 119:99–106.

23. Au BT, Teixeira MM, Collins PD, Williams TJ. Effect of PDE4 inhibitors on zymosan-induced IL-8 release from human neutrophils: synergism with prostanoids and salbutamol. *Br J Pharmacol* 1998; 123:1260–1266.

24. Spond J, Chapman R, Fine J, Jones H, Kreutner W, Kung TT, Minnicozzi M. Comparison of PDE 4 inhibitors, rolipram and SB 207499 (ariflo), in a rat model of pulmonary neutrophilia. *Pulm Pharmacol Ther* 2001; 14:157–164.

25. Kuss H, Hoefgen N, Johanssen S, Kronbach T, Rundfeldt C. *In vivo* efficacy in airway disease models of N-(3,5-dichloropyrid-4-yl)-[1-(4-fluorobenzyl)-5-hydroxy-indole-3-yl]-glyo xylic acid amide (AWD 12–281), a selective phosphodiesterase 4 inhibitor for inhaled administration. *J Pharmacol Exp Ther* 2003; 307:373–385.

26. Sato Y, Sato S, Yamamoto T, Ishikawa S, Onizuka M, Sakakibira Y. Phosphodiesterase type 4 inhibitor reduces the retention of polymorphonuclear leukocytes in the lung. *Am J Physiol Lung Cell Mol Physiol* 2002; 282:L1376–L1381.

27. Sturton G, Fitzgerald M. Phosphodiesterase 4 inhibitors for the treatment of COPD. *Chest* 2002; 121:192S–196S.

28. Derian CK, Santulli RJ, Rao PE, Solomon HF, Barrett JA. Inhibition of chemotactic peptide-induced neutrophil adhesion to vascular endothelium by cAMP modulators. *J Immunol* 1995; 154:308–317.

29. Tenor H, Hatzelmann A, Kupferschmidt R, Stanciu L, Djukanovic R, Schudt C *et al*. Cyclic nucleotide phosphodiesterase isoenzyme activities in human alveolar macrophages. *Clin Exp Allergy* 1995; 25:625–633.

30. Manning CD, Burman M, Christensen SB, Cieslinski LB, Essayan DM, Grous M *et al*. Suppression of human inflammatory cell function by subtype-selective PDE4 inhibitors correlates with inhibition of PDE4A and PDE4B. *Br J Pharmacol* 1999; 128:1393–1398.

31. Smith SJ, Brookes-Fazakerley S, Donnelly LE, Barnes PJ, Barnette MS, Giembycz MA. Ubiquitous expression of phosphodiesterase 7A in human proinflammatory and immune cells. *Am J Physiol Lung Cell Mol Physiol* 2003; 284:L279–L289.

32. Hatzelmann A, Schudt C. Anti-inflammatory and immunomodulatory potential of the novel PDE4 inhibitor roflumilast *in vitro*. *J Pharmacol Exp Ther* 2001; 297:267–279.

33. Landells LJ, Spina D, Souness JE, O'Connor BJ, Page CP. A biochemical and functional assessment of monocyte phosphodiesterase activity in healthy and asthmatic subjects. *Pulm Pharmacol Ther* 2000; 13:231–239.

34. Griswold DE, Webb EF, Breton J, White JR, Marshall PJ, Torphy TJ. Effect of selective phosphodiesterase type IV inhibitor, rolipram, on fluid and cellular phases of inflammatory response. *Inflammation* 1993; 17:333–344.

35. Seldon PM, Giembycz MA. Suppression of granulocyte/macrophage colony-stimulating factor release from human monocytes by cyclic AMP-elevating drugs: role of interleukin-10. *Br J Pharmacol* 2001; 134:58–67.

36. Hichami A, Boichot E, Germain N, Coqueret O, Lagente V. Interactions between cAMP- and cGMP-dependent protein kinase inhibitors and phosphodiesterase IV inhibitors on arachidonate release from human monocytes. *Life Sci* 1996; 59:L255–L261.

37. Verghese MW, Mcconnell RT, Strickland AB, Gooding RC, Stimpson SA, Yarnall DP *et al*. Differential regulation of human monocyte-derived TNF alpha and IL-1 beta by type IV cAMP-phosphodiesterase (cAMP-PDE) inhibitors. *J Pharmacol Exp Ther* 1995; 272:1313–1320.

38. Molnar-Kimber K, Yonno L, Heaslip R, Weichman B. Modulation of TNF alpha and IL-1 beta from endotoxin-stimulated monocytes by selective PDE isozyme inhibitors. *Agents Actions* 1993; 39:C77–C79

39. Prabhakar U, Lipshutz D, Bartus JO, Slivjak MJ, Smith EF, III, Lee JC, Esser KM. Characterization of cAMP-dependent inhibition of LPS-induced TNF alpha production by rolipram, a specific phosphodiesterase IV (PDE IV) inhibitor. *Int J Immunopharmacol* 1994; 16:805–816.

40. Seldon PM, Barnes PJ, Giembycz MA. Interleukin-10 does not mediate the inhibitory effect of PDE-4 inhibitors and other cAMP-elevating drugs on lipopolysaccharide-induced tumor necrosis factor-alpha generation from human peripheral blood monocytes. *Cell Biochem Biophys* 1998; 29:179–201.

41. Smith SJ, Cieslinski LB, Newton R, Donnelly LE, Fenwick PS, Nicholson AG et al. Discovery of BRL 50481, a selective inhibitor of phosphodiesterase 7: *In vitro* studies in human monocytes, lung macrophages and CD8+ T-lymphocytes. *Mol Pharmacol* 2004; 66:1679–1689.

42. Beshay E, Croze F, Prud'homme GJ. The phosphodiesterase inhibitors pentoxifylline and rolipram suppress macrophage activation and nitric oxide production *in vitro* and *in vivo*. *Clin Immunol* 2001; 98:272–279.

43. Kambayashi T, Jacob CO, Zhou D, Mazurek N, Fong M, Strassmann G. Cyclic nucleotide phosphodiesterase type IV participates in the regulation of IL-10 and in the subsequent inhibition of TNF-alpha and IL-6 release by endotoxin-stimulated macrophages. *J Immunol* 1995; 155:4909–4916.

44. Tenor H, Staniciu L, Schudt C, Hatzelmann A, Wendel A, Djukanovic R et al. Cyclic nucleotide phosphodiesterases from purified human CD4+ and CD8+ T lymphocytes. *Clin Exp Allergy* 1995; 25:616–624.

45. Giembycz MA, Corrigan CJ, Seybold J, Newton R, Barnes PJ. Identification of cyclic AMP phosphodiesterases 3, 4 and 7 in human CD4+ and CD8+ T-lymphocytes: role in regulating proliferation and the biosynthesis of interleukin-2. *Br J Pharmacol* 1996; 118:1945–1958.

46. Schudt C, Tenor H, Hatzelmann A. PDE isoenzymes as targets for anti-asthma drugs. *Eur Respir J* 1995; 8:1179–1183.

47. Gamble E, Grootendorst DC, Brightling CE, Troy S, Qiu Y, Zhu J et al. Anti-inflammatory effects of the phosphodiesterase-4 inhibitor cilomilast (Ariflo) in chronic obstructive pulmonary disease. *Am J Respir Crit Care Med* 2003; 168:976–1014.

48. Di Stefano A, Caramori G, Ricciardolo FL, Capelli A, Adcock IM, Donner CF. Cellular and molecular mechanisms in chronic obstructive pulmonary disease: an overview. *Clin Exp Allergy* 2004; 34:1156–1167.

49. Fuke S, Betsuyaku T, Nasuhara Y, Morikawa T, Katoh H, Nishimura M. Chemokines in bronchiolar epithelium in the development of chronic obstructive pulmonary disease. *Am J Respir Cell Mol Biol* 2004; 31:405–412.

50. Fuhrmann M, Jahn HU, Seybold J, Neurohr C, Barnes PJ, Hippenstiel S et al. Identification and function of cyclic nucleotide phosphodiesterase isoenzymes in airway epithelial cells. *Am J Respir Cell Mol Biol* 1999; 20:292–302.

51. Dent G, White SR, Tenor H, Bodtke K, Schudt C, Leff AR et al. Cyclic nucleotide phosphodiesterase in human bronchial epithelial cells: characterization of isoenzymes and functional effects of PDE inhibitors. *Pulm Pharmacol Ther* 1998; 11:47–56.

52. Khairatkar-Joshi N, Deshpande S, Sonar S, Chile S. cAMP mediated anti-inflammatory effects of PDE4 inhibitors on airway epithelial cell functions. Immunology 2004. 12th International Congress of Immunology and 4th Annual Conference of FOCIS, July 18–23, 2004, Montreal; Proceedings, 499–504; Medimont Srl, Bologna; 499–504.

53. Dowling RB, Johnson M, Cole PJ, Wilson R. The effect of rolipram, a type IV phosphodiesterase inhibitor, on Pseudomonas aeruginosa infection of respiratory mucosa. *J Pharmacol Exp Ther* 1997; 282:1565–1571.

54. Kumar RK, Herbert C, Thomas PS, Wollin L, Beume R, Yang M et al. Inhibition of inflammation and remodeling by rofumilast and dexamethasone in murine chronic asthma. *J Pharmacol Exp Ther* 2003; 307:349–355.

55. Spina D. Theophylline and PDE4 inhibitors in asthma. *Curr Opin Pulm Med* 2003; 9:57–64.

56. Ellis JL, Undem BJ. Role of cysteinyl-leukotrienes and histamine in mediating intrinsic tone in isolated human bronchi. *Am J Respir Crit Care Med* 1994; 149:118–122.

57. Clayton RA, Mackenzie CA, Dick AJ, Hastings SF, Cooreman A, Anikin V. Phosphodiesterase expression and activity in human airways. *Eur Resp J* 2004 (Abstract).

58. Schmidt DT, Watson N, Dent G, Ruhlmann E, Branscheid D, Magnussen H, Rabe KF. The effect of selective and non-selective phosphodiesterase inhibitors on allergen- and leukotriene C(4)-induced contractions in passively sensitized human airways. *Br J Pharmacol* 2000; 131:1607–1618.

59. Nell H, Louw C, Leichtl S, Rathgeb F, Neuhauser M, Bardin P. Acute anti-inflammatory effect of the novel phosphodiesterase-4 inhibitor rofumilast on allergen challenge in asthmatics after a single dose. *Am J Respir Crit Care Med* 2000; 161 (Abstract).

60. Harbinson PL, MacLeod D, Hawksworth R, O'Toole S, Sullivan PJ, Heath P *et al*. The effect of a novel orally active selective PDE4 isoenzyme inhibitor (CDP840) on allergen-induced responses in asthmatic subjects. *Eur Respir J* 1997; 10:1008–1014.

61. Bundschuh DS, Eltze M, Barsig J, Wollin L, Hatzelmann A, Beume R. *In vivo* efficacy in airway disease models of rofumilast, a novel orally active PDE4 inhibitor. *J Pharmacol Exp Ther* 2001; 297:280–290.

62. Billah MM, Cooper N, Minnicozzi M, Warneck J, Wang P, Hey JA *et al*. Pharmacology of N-(3,5-dichloro-1-oxido-4-pyridinyl)-8-methoxy-2-(trifluoromethyl)-5-quinoline carboxamide (SCH 351591), a novel, orally active phosphodiesterase 4 inhibitor. *J Pharmacol Exp Ther* 2002; 302:127–137.

63. Spina D. The potential of PDE4 inhibitors in respiratory disease. *Curr Drug Targets Inflamm Allergy* 2004; 3:231–236.

64. Mehats C, Jin SL, Wahlstrom J, Law E, Umetsu DT, Conti M. PDE4D plays a critical role in the control of airway smooth muscle contraction. *FASEB J* 2003; 17:1831–1841.

65. Aubier M, Nagy GB, Sauer R, Schmid-Wirlitsch C, Albrecht A, Bredenbroker D. The novel selective PDE4 inhibitor rofumilast: early onset of efficacy in asthma. *Eur Respir J* 2003; 22 (Suppl 45), abstract.

66. Spina D, Harrison S, Page CP. Regulation by phosphodiesterase isoenzymes of non-adrenergic non-cholinergic contraction in guinea-pig isolated main bronchus. *Br J Pharmacol* 1995; 116:2334–2340.

67. Holbrook M, Gozzard N, James T, Higgs G, Hughes B. Inhibition of bronchospasm and ozone-induced airway hyperresponsiveness in the guinea-pig by CDP840, a novel phosphodiesterase type 4 inhibitor. *Br J Pharmacol* 1996; 118:1192–1200.

68. Ray DW, Hernandez C, Leff AR, Drazen JM, Solway J. Tachykinins mediate bronchoconstriction elicited by isocapnic hyperpnea in guinea-pigs. *J Appl Physiol* 1989; 66:1108–1112.

69. Underwood DC, Osborn RR, Kotzer CJ. Correlation of inhaled antigen or cysteinyl leukotriene-induced hypertussive activity with airway eosinophilia in guinea-pigs. *Am J Respir Crit Care Med* 2001; 163:A144–Ai44.

70. Lamontagne S, Meadows E, Luk P, Normandin D, Muise E, Boulet L *et al*. Localization of phosphodiesterase-4 isoforms in the medulla and nodose ganglion of the squirrel monkey. *Brain Res* 2001; 920:84–96.

71. Bredenbroker D, Syed J, Leichtl S, Rathgeb F, Wurst W. Roflumilast, a new orally active, selective phosphodiesterase 4 inhibitor, is effective in the treatment of chronic obstructive pulmonary disease. *Eur Respir J* 2002; 20:374s(Abstract).

72. Souness JE, Rao S. Proposal for pharmacologically distinct conformers of PDE4 cyclic AMP phosphodiesterases. *Cell Signal* 1997; 9:227–236.

73. Barnette MS, Grous M, Cieslinski LB, Burman M, Christensen SB, Torphy TJ. Inhibitors of phosphodiesterase IV (PDE IV) increase acid secretion in rabbit isolated gastric glands: correlation between function and interaction with a high-affinity rolipram binding site. *J Pharmacol Exp Ther* 1995; 273:1396–1402.

74. Duplantier AJ, Biggers MS, Chambers RJ, Cheng JB, Cooper K, Damon DB *et al*. Biarylcarboxylic acids and -amides: inhibition of phosphodiesterase type IV versus [3H]rolipram binding activity and their relationship to emetic behavior in the ferret. *J Med Chem* 1996; 39:120–125.

75. Barnette MS, Bartus JO, Burman M, Christensen SB, Cieslinski LB, Esser KM *et al*. Association of the anti-inflammatory activity of phosphodiesterase 4 (PDE4) inhibitors with either inhibition of PDE4 catalytic activity or competition for [3H]rolipram binding. *Biochem Pharmacol* 1996; 51:949–956.

76. Souness JE, Houghton C, Sardar N, Withnall MT. Evidence that cyclic AMP phosphodiesterase inhibitors suppress interleukin-2 release from murine splenocytes by interacting with a 'low-affinity' phosphodiesterase 4 conformer. *Br J Pharmacol* 1997; 121:743–750.

77. Torphy TJ, Barnette MS, Underwood DC, Griswold DE, Christensen SB, Murdoch RD *et al*. Ariflo (SB 207499), a second generation phosphodiesterase 4 inhibitor for the treatment of asthma and COPD: from concept to clinic. *Pulm Pharmacol Ther* 1999; 12:131–135.

78. Hughes B, Howat D, Lisle H, Holbrook M, James T, Gozzard N *et al*. The inhibition of antigen-induced eosinophilia and bronchoconstriction by CDP840, a novel stereo-selective inhibitor of phosphodiesterase type 4. *Br J Pharmacol* 1996; 118:1183–1191.

79. Robichaud A, Stamatiou PB, Jin SL, Lachance N, Macdonald D, Laliberte F *et al*. Deletion of phosphodiesterase 4D in mice shortens alpha(2)-adrenoceptor-mediated anesthesia, a behavioral correlate of emesis. *J Clin Invest* 2002; 110:1045–1052.

80. Takahashi M, Terwilliger R, Lane C, Mezes PS, Conti M, Duman RS. Chronic antidepressant administration increases the expression of cAMP-specific phosphodiesterase 4A and 4B isoforms. *J Neurosci* 1999; 19:610–618.

81. Jin SL, Conti M. Induction of the cyclic nucleotide phosphodiesterase PDE4B is essential for LPS-activated TNF-alpha responses. *Proc Natl Acad Sci USA* 2002; 99:7628–7633.

82. Trifilieff A, Wyss D, Walker C, Mazzoni L, Hersperger R. Pharmacological profile of a novel phosphodiesterase 4 inhibitor, 4-(8-benzo[1, 2, 5]oxadiazol-5-yl-[1, 7]naphthyridin-6-yl)-benzoic acid (NVP-ABE171), a 1,7-naphthyridine derivative, with anti-inflammatory activities. *J Pharmacol Exp Ther* 2002; 301:241–248.

83. Hersperger R, Bray-French K, Mazzoni L, Muller T. Palladium-catalyzed cross-coupling reactions for the synthesis of 6, 8-disubstituted 1,7-naphthyridines: a novel class of potent and selective phosphodiesterase type 4D inhibitors. *J Med Chem* 2000; 43:675–682.

84. Brunnee T, Engelstatter R, Steinijans VW, Kunkel G. Bronchodilatory effect of inhaled zardaverine, a phosphodiesterase III and IV inhibitor, in patients with asthma. *Eur Respir J* 1992; 5:982–985.

85. Boswell-Smith V, Spina D, Comer M, Page CP, Oxford AW, Jack D. The pharmacology and duration of action of novel trequinsin-like phosphodiesterase inhibitors. *Am J Respir Crit Care Med*; submitted ATS 2005, (Abstract).

86. Gantner F, Tenor H, Gekeler V, Schudt C, Wendel A, Hatzelmann A. Phosphodiesterase profiles of highly purified human peripheral blood leukocyte populations from normal and atopic individuals: a comparative study. *J Allergy Clin Immunol* 1997; 100:527–535.

87. Essayan DM, Kagey-Sobotka A, Lichtenstein LM, Huang SK. Differential regulation of human antigen-specific Th1 and Th2 lymphocyte responses by isozyme selective cyclic nucleotide phosphodiesterase inhibitors. *J Pharmacol Exp Ther* 1997; 282:505–512.

88. Ottonello L, Dapino P, Amelotti M, Barbera P, Arduino N, Bertolotto M, Dallegri F. Activation of neutrophil respiratory burst by cytokines and chemoattractants. Regulatory role of extracellular matrix glycoproteins. *Inflamm Res* 1998; 47:345–350.

89. Gantner F, Kupferschmid TR, Schudt C, Wendel A, Hatzelmann A. *In vitro* differentiation of human monocytes to macrophages: change of PDE profile and its relationship to suppression of tumour necrosis factor-alpha release by PDE inhibitors. *Br J Pharmacol* 1997; 121:221–231.

90. Compton CH, Gubb J, Nieman R, Edelson J, Amit O, Bakst A et al. Cilomilast, a selective phosphodiesterase-4 inhibitor for treatment of patients with chronic obstructive pulmonary disease: a randomised, dose-ranging study. *Lancet* 2001; 358:265–270.

91. Leichtl S, Syed J, Bredenbroker D. Efficacy of once-daily roflumilast, a new orally active, selective phosphodiesterase 4 inhibitor, in chronic obstructive pulmonary disease. *Am J Respir Crit Care Med* 2002; 165:A229.

92. Guay D, Hamel P, Blouin M, Brideau C, Chan CC, Chauret N et al. Discovery of L-791,943: a potent, selective, non emetic and orally active phosphodiesterase-4 inhibitor. *Bioorg Med Chem Lett* 2002; 12:1457–1461.

93. Draheim R, Egerland U, Rundfeldt C. Anti-inflammatory potential of the selective phosphodiesterase 4 inhibitor N-(3,5-dichloro-pyrid-4-yl)-[1-(4-fluorobenzyl)-5-hydroxy-indole-3-yl]-glyoxylic acid amide (AWD 12–281), in human cell preparations. *J Pharmacol Exp Ther* 2004; 308:555–563.

94. Vakkalanka SKVS, Balasubramaniam LA, Gharat LA, Joshi VD, Hussain N, Rao J, Page CP. (4 A.D.) The pharmacological and safety profile of a novel selective phosphodiesterase-4 (PDE4) inhibitor:- GRC-3886. *Eur Respir J* 2005 (Abstract), in press.

95. Grootendorst DC, Gauw SA, Benschop N, Sterk PJ, Hiemstra PS, Rabe KF. Efficacy of the novel phosphodiesterase-4 inhibitor BAY 19–8004 on lung function and airway inflammation in asthma and chronic obstructive pulmonary disease (COPD). *Pulm Pharmacol Ther* 2003; 16:341–347.

8

Phosphodiesterase 4 inhibitors: a new class of agents for the treatment of chronic obstructive pulmonary disease

K. F. Rabe

INTRODUCTION

Chronic inflammation is a hallmark of chronic obstructive pulmonary disease (COPD) and there is an unmet medical need for anti-inflammatory agents that target the inflammatory pathways underlying COPD. The degradation of 3',5'-cyclic adenosine monophosphate (cAMP) is modulated by phosphodiesterase (PDE) and has been identified as a putative target to reduce chronic inflammation in obstructive airway diseases. The PDE inhibitors, particularly inhibitors of the subtype PDE4, represent a new class of anti-inflammatory agents that have the potential to directly modulate the inflammatory pathophysiology underlying COPD, a limitation of current pharmacologic therapies. These agents modulate cAMP-mediated inflammation by targeting the cAMP-hydrolysing isozyme, PDE4, which is expressed in many immune effector cells implicated in the pathogenesis of COPD. Thus, targeted inhibition of PDE4 provides the rationale for the design of new drugs for the treatment of COPD.

The PDE4 inhibitors appear to impart significant anti-inflammatory effects in animal models of obstructive airway diseases and therapeutic efficacy in patients with COPD. The anti-inflammatory activity of PDE4 inhibitors may potentially alter or ameliorate disease progression, and may improve clinical symptoms. Thus, PDE4 inhibitors could overcome the limitations of current therapies.

This chapter provides a comprehensive review of the clinical progress of PDE inhibitors in COPD, focusing on PDE4 inhibitors in late-stage clinical development. A review of the rationale, mechanism of action, clinical profile, developmental status of the leading agents, and future perspectives for PDE4 inhibitors in the treatment of COPD are discussed.

RATIONALE FOR PDE INHIBITORS IN COPD

PHOSPHODIESTERASES

The chronic inflammation associated with COPD is characterised by an increase in the number and activity (i.e., mediator release, respiratory burst) of neutrophils,

Klaus F. Rabe, MD, PhD, Leiden University Medical Centre, Leiden, The Netherlands.

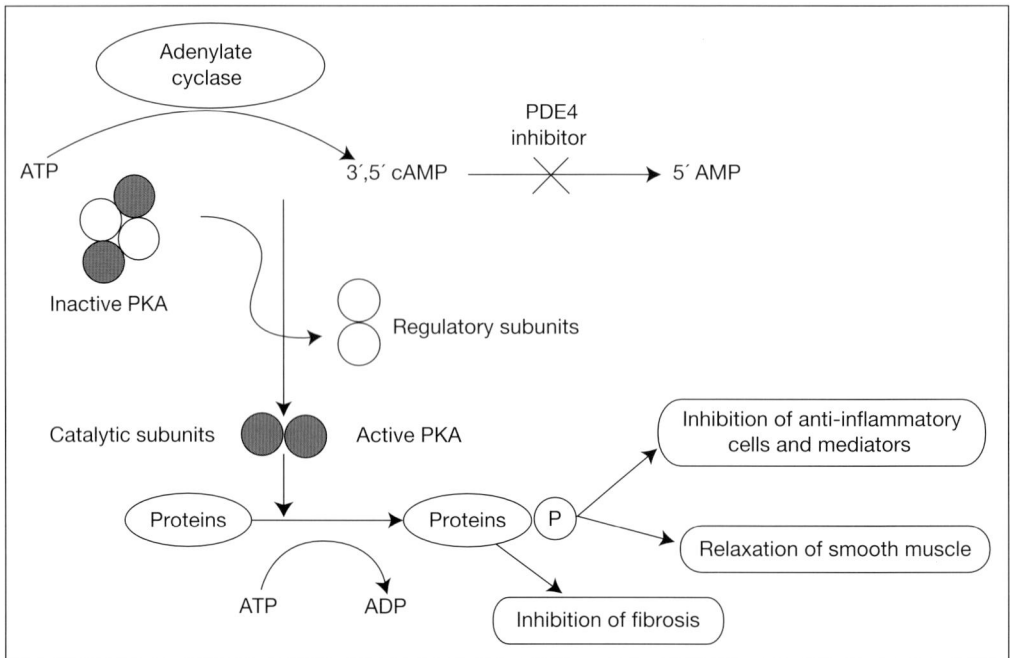

Figure 8.1 Increased levels of cyclic adenosine monophosphate (cAMP), *via* activation of adenylate cyclase or inhibition of cAMP metabolism, activate protein kinase A (PKA), which catalyses protein phosphorylation leading to inhibition of pro-inflammatory cells and mediators, relaxation of smooth muscle, and inhibition of fibrosis leading to airway remodelling [26]. ATP = Adenosine triphosphate; ADP = adenosine diphosphate; P = phosphate; T_H = T-helper cell; TNF-α = tumour necrosis factor-α. Adapted with permission from ALTANA Pharma AG [27].

CD8$^+$ T-lymphocytes, macrophages, and fibroblasts [1, 2]. The second messenger cAMP modulates the influx and activity of many of these pro-inflammatory cells. The intracellular level of cAMP is regulated via the activation of adenylate cyclase and the hydrolysis of cAMP to 5'-AMP by PDEs (Figure 8.1). At least 11 families of PDEs and more than 50 splice variants have been identified and characterised, based on substrate specificity and sensitivity to PDE inhibitors [3].

Phosphodiesterase 4 is a major regulator of cAMP metabolism in a variety of pro-inflammatory and immune cells associated with COPD [4–6], including neutrophils [7], macrophages, CD8$^+$ T cells [8], and eosinophils [7]. In animal and human *ex vivo* studies, PDE4 has also been localised to epithelial and endothelial cells, fibroblasts, and smooth muscle [1, 9–12]. Further, neutrophils, eosinophils, and monocytes contain PDE4 exclusively [13]. The localisation of the PDE isozymes, particularly PDE4, to inflammatory and immunocompetent cells [7, 8] has provided the impetus for development and clinical testing of PDE inhibitors that target these cells (Figure 8.2).

Within the PDE4 family, there are 4 PDE4 subtypes (PDE4A, B, C and D) that are the products of separate genes, along with a myriad of gene splice variants (e.g., PDE4A5) [14]. Inhibitors of PDE4 may display greater specificity for a particular subtype and different effector cells may exhibit differing sensitivities to PDE4 inhibitors [15]. Tissue-specific expression of splice variants affects how these gene products contribute to cellular responses to cAMP levels, and may account for the differential sensitivities of the various effector cells

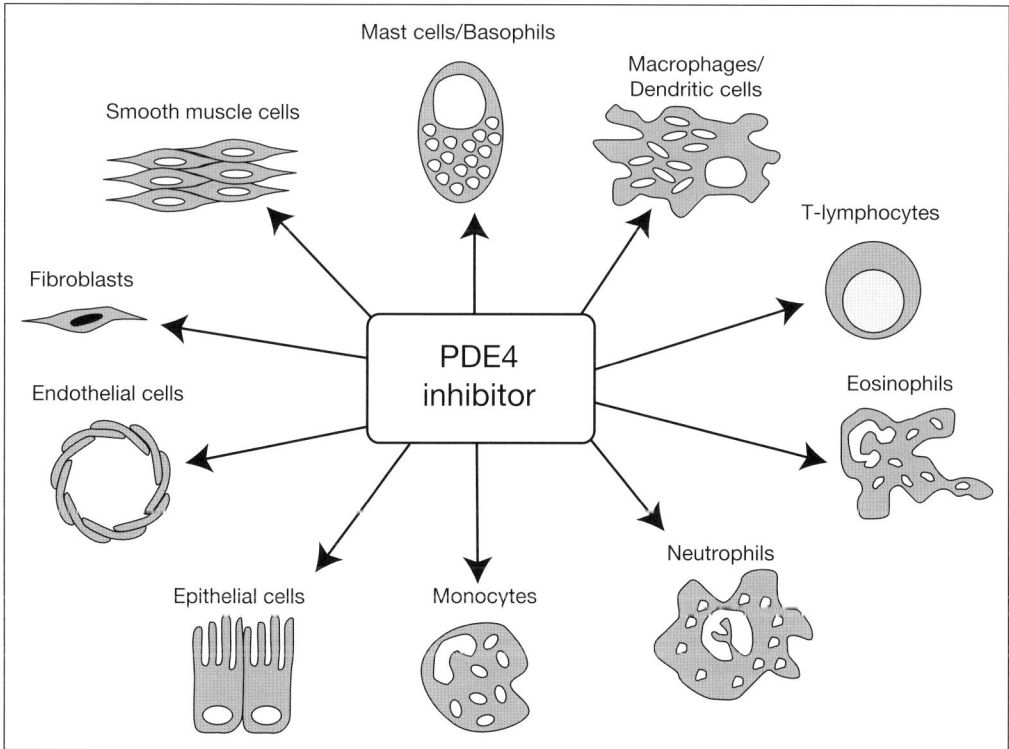

Figure 8.2 Phosphodiesterase (PDE) 4 inhibitors target multiple pro-inflammatory cells by maintaining increased levels of cAMP, leading to activation of protein kinase A and subsequent reduction in proliferation and infiltration of inflammatory cells as well as decreasing inflammatory cytokines and chemokines. Adapted with permission from ALTANA Pharma AG [27].

in response to PDE4 inhibitors. Investigation into the role of PDE4 splice variant diversity and cellular and subcellular localisation of these proteins is ongoing.

The PDE4 enzyme exists in at least two conformations [16]. Investigators have described these two conformations based on the selective binding affinity of rolipram, an archetypal PDE4 inhibitor, which is frequently used as a standard in preclinical testing of novel PDE4 inhibitors. The two conformations have been designated as the high-affinity rolipram-binding site (HARBS) and the low-affinity rolipram-binding site (LARBS) [17]. The high-affinity interaction with rolipram is thought to be related to the presence of metal cofactors (e.g., Mg^{2+}) located in the active site of PDE4 [18, 19]. Preferential binding to the HARBS has been suspected to be responsible for central nervous system (e.g., nausea and emesis) and cardiovascular effects, and would explain why rolipram has a poor safety profile and is unsuitable for clinical use.

Anti-Inflammatory Action of PDE4 Inhibitors

A large body of *in vitro*, *in vivo*, and *ex vivo* preclinical data supports the anti-inflammatory properties of PDE4 inhibitors. The anti-inflammatory action of PDE4 inhibitors can be broadly categorised as an inhibition of pro-inflammatory cell activities and pro-inflammatory cascades [1, 8, 20–25]. Additionally, the bronchodilatory activity associated with non-selective PDE4 inhibitors is mediated through increases in intracellular cAMP and subsequent relaxation of bronchiolar smooth muscle [26, 27]. However, acute bronchodilation in patients with COPD has not been observed with newer PDE4 inhibitors [28, 29]. Thus, the efficacy of PDE4 inhibitors in COPD may be related to their anti-inflammatory activity.

Inhibition of neutrophil chemotaxis and suppression of increased neutrophil activation, including production of reactive oxygen species, leukotriene B4, degranulation, and chemotaxis by PDE4 inhibitors has been well described [15, 21, 22, 30, 31]. The PDE4 inhibitors also reduce expression of tumour necrosis factor-α (TNF-α) [15, 30] and attenuate TNF-α-induced activation of cellular adhesion molecule expression [32].

There are also several reports of the effects of PDE4 inhibitors on airway epithelial cells, including inhibition of IL-1β-induced release of granulocyte/macrophage colony-stimulating factor (GM-CSF) in human cells *ex vivo* [33] and inhibition of mucus hypersecretion in an animal model *in vivo* [22]. The PDE4 inhibitors also suppress fibroblast chemotaxis and fibroblast-mediated collagen gel contraction [1], suggesting that these agents may inhibit fibroblast activity (i.e., fibrosis) and development of airway narrowing.

In summary, preclinical data suggest that PDE4 inhibitors potentially affect a multitude of pro-inflammatory effector cells and pathways involved in the pathogenesis of COPD. The anti-inflammatory action of PDE4 inhibitors is likely responsible, at least in part, for the clinical efficacy and therapeutic benefits of these agents in patients with COPD.

THERAPEUTIC USE OF PDE4 INHIBITORS

PDE INHIBITORS IN CLINICAL USE

Theophylline
Theophylline (3,7-dihydro-1,3-dimethyl-1H-purine-2,6-dione) is a methylxanthine, non-selective PDE inhibitor that has been used as a bronchodilator in patients with COPD for several decades (Figure 8.3) [34, 35]. Theophylline acts non-selectively through inhibition of all major PDE isozymes and adenosine receptor antagonism [36]. Theophylline also exhibits anti-inflammatory activity *in vitro* [37]. However, the concentration of theophylline that would be required to provide clinically effective anti-inflammatory therapy is greater than could reasonably be achieved in patients [37]. Thus, the anti-inflammatory contribution of theophylline in the clinic is still under debate.

Theophylline has demonstrated variable efficacy in improving exercise tolerance and clinical symptoms [38, 39], and is currently recommended as third-line therapy for COPD [34, 40]. Further, because of its non-selective mechanism of action, theophylline is associated with a high incidence of side-effects (e.g., cardiac arrhythmia, seizure, gastrointestinal disorder) [34, 41]. Taken together, the combination of the therapeutically limited anti-inflammatory activity of theophylline and the less than favourable safety profile in patients with COPD have led researchers to focus on improved PDE inhibitors, primarily those that inhibit PDE4, that have the potential for increased therapeutic ratios and more favourable safety profiles. Currently, there are only two PDE inhibitors, cilomilast and roflumilast, in late-stage clinical development for the treatment of COPD.

PDE INHIBITORS UNDER CLINICAL INVESTIGATION

Cilomilast
Cilomilast (SB 207499; *cis*-4-cyano-4-[3-(cyclopentyloxy)-4-methoxy-phenyl] cyclohexanecarboxylic acid) is a PDE4 inhibitor in phase III clinical development for the treatment of patients with COPD (Figure 8.3). Cilomilast is selective for PDE4 and does not appreciably bind to PDE1, 2, 3, or 5 at concentrations $\leq 10\,\mu$M [42]. Cilomilast is ~10-fold more selective for PDE4D than the other 3 isoforms in the PDE4 family (i.e., PDE4A, B, and C) [43], and has

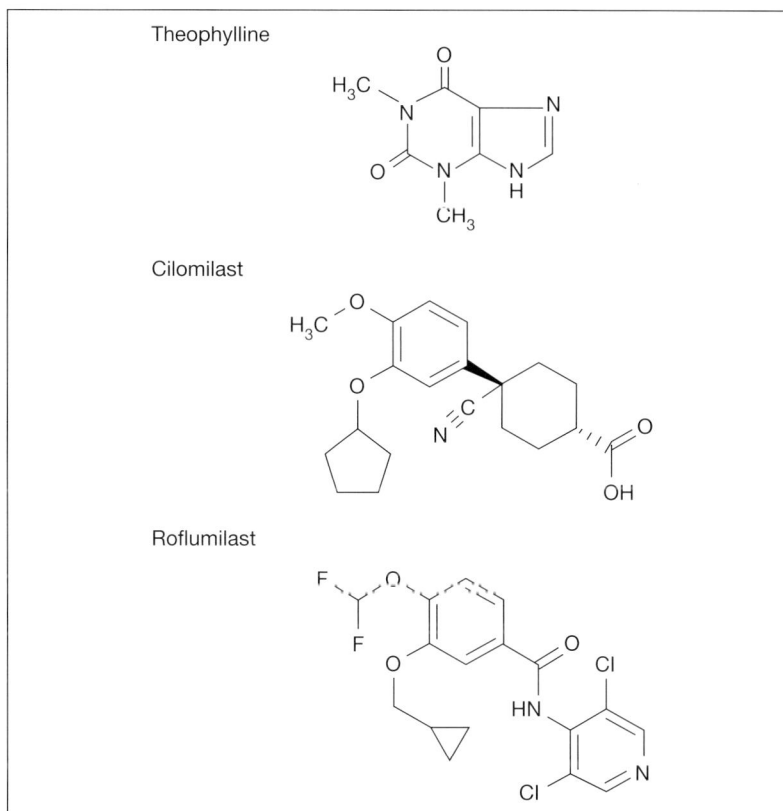

Figure 8.3 Chemical structures of the non-selective inhibitor theophylline and the PDE4 inhibitors cilomilast and roflumilast.

approximately equal affinity for the two conformations of PDE4: LARBS and HARBS [42]. This selectivity for the preferred PDE4 conformation, LARBS, provides an improved therapeutic ratio compared with less selective PDE4 inhibitors such as rolipram. In addition to numerous preclinical trials that have evaluated the anti-inflammatory potential of cilomilast [15, 30], the pharmacokinetic profile has also been examined. Further, the safety and efficacy of cilomilast have also been investigated in several clinical studies.

The pharmacokinetics of intravenous and oral cilomilast was evaluated in 16 healthy men [44]. In two separate experiments, volunteers received intravenous cilomilast 4 mg over 1 h or a single oral dose of cilomilast 15 mg [44]. Similar pharmacokinetic profiles were obtained with the two modes of administration. Cilomilast exhibited dose-dependent pharmacokinetics and a low clearance rate with a half-life of ~8 h, suggesting that bid cilomilast dosing might be an appropriate dosing regimen. The dose linearity of oral cilomilast ≤15 mg bid was confirmed in a randomised, placebo-controlled, dose-ranging study [45]. Oral cilomilast 15 mg was also shown to have a high oral bioavailability, with a mean absolute bioavailability of 103% [95% confidence interval (CI) = 98%, 109%].

The effects of food, administration timing, and coadministration with other medications on the pharmacokinetics of cilomilast and on the concomitant medications were also determined [44]. The effect of food absorption on cilomilast bioavailability was evaluated in 28 healthy volunteers who received two doses of oral cilomilast 15 mg. Patients were administered one dose after a 10-hour overnight fast and one dose 5 min after a high-fat breakfast. Overall, co-administration of cilomilast with food did not appear to affect cilomilast bioavailability. Additionally, neither co-administration of an antacid nor administration timing (morning or evening) appreciably affected the pharmacokinetics of cilomilast. Co-administration studies in healthy volunteers indicated a lack of significant pharmacody-namic interaction between cilomilast and digoxin, erythromycin, salbutamol, theophylline, or warfarin [46–50].

In patients with renal impairment, the half-life and area under the curve (AUC) of unbound cilomilast increased with increasing renal impairment as unbound cilomilast clear-ance and plasma protein binding decreased [49, 51]. The renal clearance of the active metabolite of cilomilast decreased with increasing renal impairment, with the AUC ratio of the unbound metabolite to cilomilast in severe renal impairment twice that observed in healthy volunteers (creatinine clearance <30 ml/min). These data led to the recommenda-tion that cilomilast not be administered to patients with severe renal impairment.

Efficacy and Safety in COPD

In a 12-week study designed to determine the ability of cilomilast to mitigate inflammatory pathways in the lung, patients (n = 59) with moderate COPD were randomised to receive cilomilast 15 mg twice daily or placebo [24]. Cilomilast reduced CD8$^+$ T-lymphocyte subsets by 48% (p < 0.01) and CD68$^+$ macrophages by 47% (p = 0.001) compared with placebo. Cilomilast did not effect forced expiratory volume in 1 s (FEV$_1$), although the study was not powered to show changes in pulmonary function. Overall, these data provided the rationale for further clinical studies of cilomilast. The acute bronchodilation effects of cilomilast were examined in patients with COPD (n = 21) who were administered a single dose of cilomi-last with or without concomitant administration of inhaled salbutamol and/or ipratropium bromide [28]. The mean maximum improvement in FEV$_1$ was ~140 ml with cilomilast versus ~152 ml with placebo, which is less than observed with bronchodilators such as salbutamol. Further, combined treatment with salbutamol or ipratropium bromide further increased FEV$_1$, suggesting that a single dose of cilomilast does not produce acute bronchodilation in patients with COPD.

The efficacy of cilomilast in COPD has been investigated in a number of clinical studies. The efficacy of cilomilast in patients with poorly reversible COPD (≤15% or ≤200 ml post-albuterol) was examined in four randomised, double-blind, placebo-controlled, parallel-group studies [52, 53]. Patients (n = 647–825) were treated with cilomilast 15 mg bid or placebo for 6 months after a 4-week run-in period. Only two studies demonstrated a signif-icant change from baseline in trough FEV$_1$ at study end point versus placebo, and only three studies showed a 30- to 40-ml improvement from baseline in FEV$_1$ for patients treated with cilomilast (Figure 8.4) [52–54]. These data indicate a maintenance of lung function rather than an improvement in lung function. Based on these data, the Pulmonary-Allergy Drugs Advisory Committee of the US Food and Drug Administration has recommended that long-term studies (e.g., 1 year) be conducted before approval of cilomilast for the maintenance of lung function (FEV$_1$). A 12-month, double-blind, placebo-controlled extension study exam-ined efficacy and safety in patients (n = 211) who received placebo for 12 months or cilomi-last 10 mg bid for 2 months followed by cilomilast 15 mg bid for the remaining 10 months [55]. Cilomilast improved FEV$_1$ by 210 ml versus 100 ml for placebo over 12 months, but this 110 ml improvement versus placebo was not significant (p = 0.094).

In a 3-month randomised, double-blind, parallel-group study in patients (n = 264) with both reversible and non-reversible COPD, cilomilast significantly improved FEV$_1$ versus placebo in patients with reversible disease, but not patients with non-reversible dis-ease [56]. In one of the 6-month studies, forced vital capacity (FVC; p = 0.001) and trough 25–75% forced expiratory flow (FEF$_{25-75}$; p = 0.003) significantly improved in cilomilast-treated patients versus patients treated with placebo [57, 58]. Further, in the 12-month,

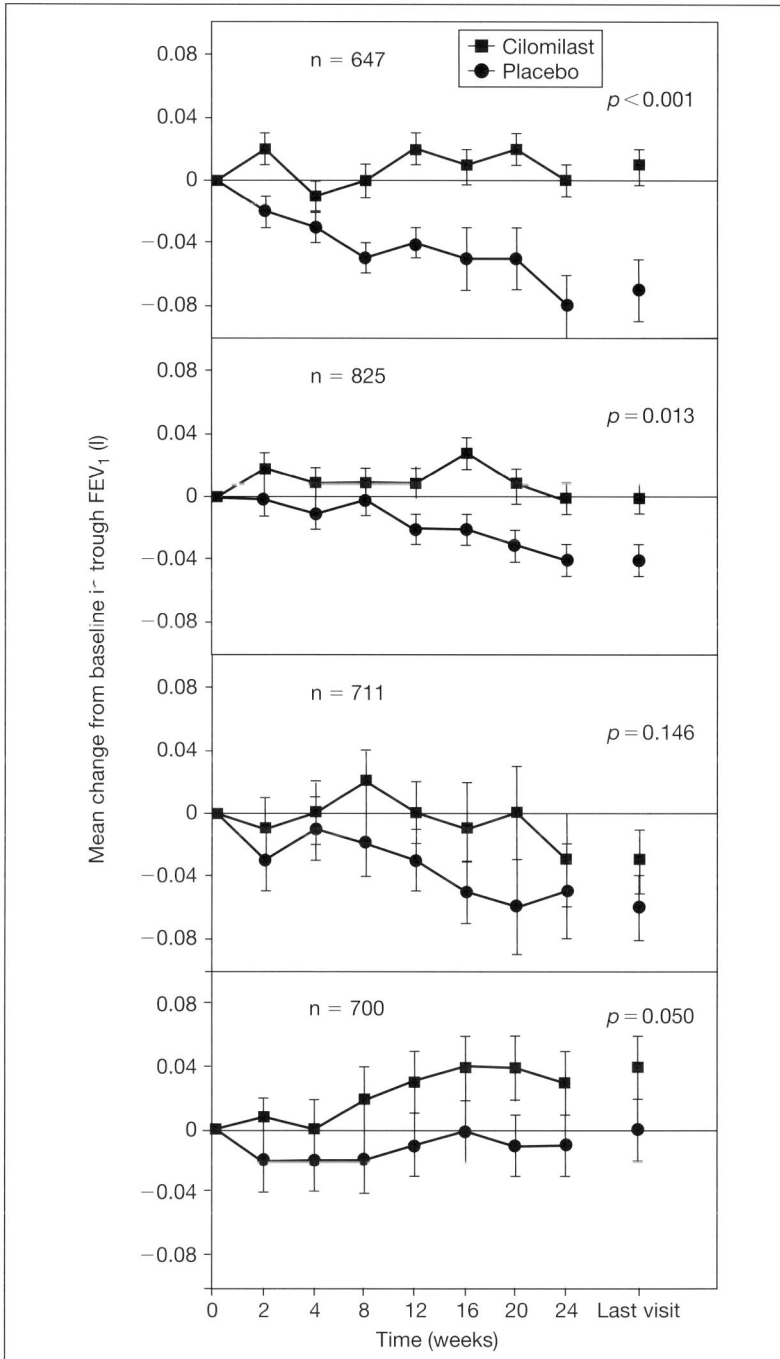

Figure 8.4   Change from baseline in trough FEV_1 in patients treated with cilomilast 15 mg bid versus placebo in four randomised, double-blind, phase III, 6-month trials. Data are mean ± standard errors. Adapted from US Food and Drug Administration [52]. EP = Endpoint; FEV_1 = forced expiratory volume in 1 second.

double-blind, placebo-controlled extension study, cilomilast-treated patients experienced improved FVC (p = 0.018) and peak expiratory flow (PEF; p = 0.01) compared with placebo [55].

Cilomilast also decreased the risk of a patient experiencing ≥1 COPD exacerbation by 44% (p = 0.0001) [59]. A total of 74% of patients treated with cilomilast were exacerbation-free during the 6-month study versus 62% of patients treated with placebo (p = 0.008). Additionally, a combined analysis of two of the 6-month studies examining the rate of prospectively defined COPD exacerbations reported a significant reduction (26%) in the frequency of moderate-to-severe exacerbations with cilomilast versus placebo [54].

In an open-label extension of one of the 6-month studies, health status was examined in patients who received cilomilast 15 mg bid from week 24 to week 120 [60]. Borker *et al* [60] reported that patients who received placebo in the initial 24-week study experienced a further improvement in health status or at least improvements achieved during the 6-month study were maintained. No lung function data from the open extension study have been reported. In addition, one of the 6-month studies demonstrated a significant improvement in quality of life as measured by St. George's Respiratory Questionnaire (SGRQ) total score [53]. Significant improvements in Short Form-36 scores for physical function (p = 0.017) and general health perceptions (p = 0.02) compared with placebo treatment were also noted [57].

Cilomilast was generally well tolerated. In a dose-ranging study, the most common drug-related adverse event was nausea, reported in 1% of patients in the placebo group, 12% of patients in the 10-mg dose group, and 11% of patients in the 15-mg dose group [61]. The most common serious adverse event was COPD exacerbation. Overall, there was no cilomilast dose-related trend or significant difference in incidence versus placebo for any serious adverse event. In a pooled analysis of the 6-month studies, gastrointestinal adverse events—including nausea, diarrhoea, abdominal pain, dyspepsia, and vomiting—were the most common and were reported more frequently in cilomilast-treated patients compared with placebo [62]. Gastrointestinal adverse events were generally mild to moderate in intensity and self-limited; however, they did account for the most discontinuations because of adverse events [53].

Roflumilast

Roflumilast (3-cyclopropylmethoxy-4-difluoromethoxy-N-[3,5-dichloropyridyl-4-yl]-benzamide) [30] is a PDE4 inhibitor in phase III clinical development in the treatment of COPD and asthma (Figure 8.3) [40]. Roflumilast is >100 times more potent in inhibiting PDE4 (IC_{50} = 0.8 nM) versus cilomilast (IC_{50} = 120 nM) [15]. *In vivo*, roflumilast is metabolised to a pharmacologically active metabolite, roflumilast N-oxide, which also has a high potency (IC_{50} = 2 nM), and may substantially contribute to the clinical efficacy of roflumilast.

The pharmacokinetics of a single oral dose of roflumilast 500 μg and intravenous roflumilast 150 μg infused over 15 min were evaluated in 12 healthy male volunteers. Pharmacokinetic analysis of a single dose of roflumilast indicated that roflumilast has a long elimination half-life [63, 64] and a high absolute oral bioavailability of 79% [63]. In a double-blind, parallel-group, dose-ranging study in 18 healthy volunteers who received escalating doses of oral roflumilast (250–1,000 μg) once daily for seven days, roflumilast exhibited linear pharmacokinetics in the dose range of 500–1,000 μg [63, 64]. The half-life of roflumilast and roflumilast N-oxide was ~15 h and 20 h, respectively, providing a rationale for a once-daily dosing regimen in clinical trials.

The pharmacokinetic implications of administration timing and food intake were also evaluated [65, 66]. The C_{max} of roflumilast was marginally lower with evening dosing and the time to C_{max} was slightly longer with evening dosing, but the AUC did not differ between the times of administration, indicating that exposure to roflumilast and roflumilast N-oxide was unaffected. Overall, administration timing did not significantly affect the pharmacokinetic profile of roflumilast or roflumilast N-oxide [65]. As with cilomilast [44], a high-fat meal reduced the absorption of roflumilast. The C_{max} was reduced for roflumilast, but not for roflumilast N-oxide; however, the AUC values for roflumilast and the active metabolite were not affected by food intake. Therefore, food intake did not appreciably affect the bioavailability of roflumilast or roflumilast N-oxide [66].

The effects of concomitant drug administration were investigated to determine potential interaction between roflumilast and erythromycin, budesonide, salbutamol, or warfarin; however, no significant effect of concomitant administration was observed with any of these medications [67–72]. Additionally, renal clearance rates suggest that roflumilast may be used in patients with renal impairment [73].

Efficacy and Safety in COPD
A phase II/III double-blind, dose-ranging, parallel-group study investigated the efficacy and safety of roflumilast in patients with moderate-to-severe COPD [74, 75]. Patients were administered oral roflumilast 250 µg (n = 175) or 500 µg (n = 169), or placebo (n = 172) once daily for 26 weeks. Roflumilast treatment significantly improved FEV_1, morning PEF, and FVC [43, 74, 75].

In a phase III, multicentre, double-blind, randomised, placebo-controlled study, 1,411 patients with COPD received oral roflumilast 250 µg (n = 576) or 500 µg (n = 555), or placebo (n = 280) once daily for 24 weeks [76, 77] Lung function, health-related quality of life (SGRQ), and COPD exacerbations were assessed. Roflumilast 250 and 500 µg significantly improved post-bronchodilator FEV_1 throughout the 24-week treatment period compared with placebo (p < 0.03). At the end of treatment, roflumilast 250 µg and roflumilast 500 µg improved mean FEV_1 by 74 ml and 97 ml, respectively (Figure 8.5; p < 0.0001 vs.

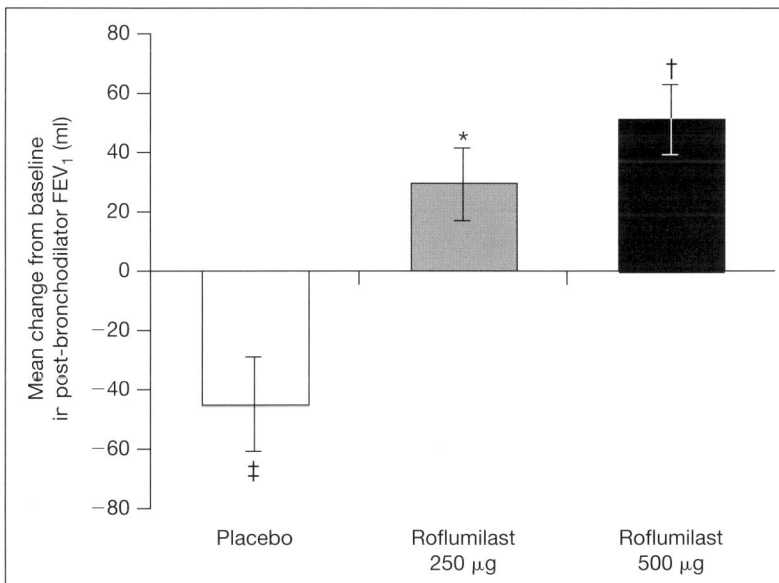

Figure 8.5 Change from baseline in post-bronchodilator FEV_1 at last visit for 1,411 patients administered roflumilast 250 µg, roflumilast 500 µg, or placebo in a randomised, double-blind, 6-month trial. Improvement was significant for roflumilast 250 and 500 µg versus baseline at last visit (*p < 0.05, ‡p < 0.01, †p < 0.001 vs. baseline). Improvement in FEV_1 was significantly greater for roflumilast 250 µg and 500 µg versus placebo (p < 0.0001 for both). Data are least squares mean ± standard error. Data from Rabe *et al.* [77].

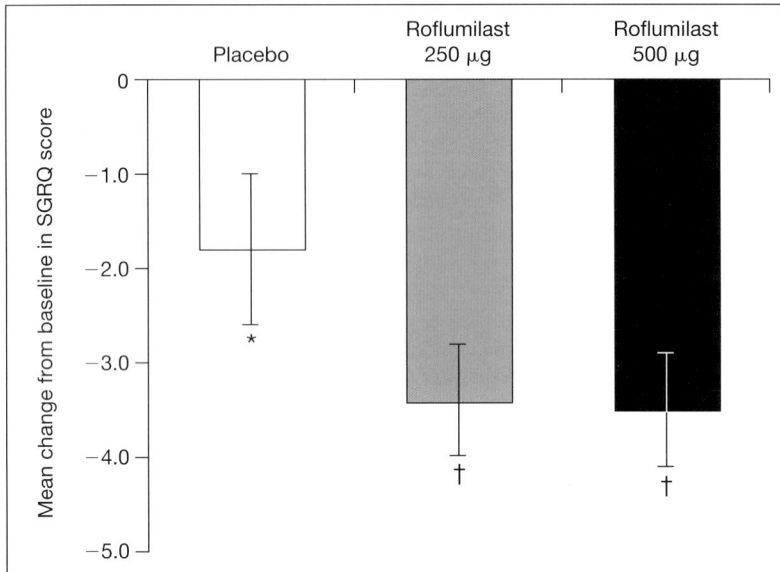

Figure 8.6   Change from baseline in St. George's Respiratory Questionnaire total score at last visit for 1,411 patients administered roflumilast 250 μg, roflumilast 500 μg, or placebo in a randomised, double-blind, 6-month trial. Roflumilast 250 and 500 μg improved SGRQ total score compared with placebo. Data are least squares mean ± standard errors. p values are relative to baseline at last visit (*p < 0.05, †p < 0.001 vs. baseline). Data from O'Donnell *et al* [78].

placebo for both). A similar pattern was seen for the secondary lung function parameters: post-bronchodilator FVC, FEV_6 and FEF_{25-75} improved in the roflumilast treatment groups versus placebo throughout the treatment period. For example, post-bronchodilator FVC improved by 71 ± 31 ml (p = 0.0193) and 114 ± 31 ml (p = 0.0002) for roflumilast 250 and 500 μg, respectively, compared with placebo.

Roflumilast 250 and 500 μg improved SGRQ total score (−3.4 and −3.5 units, respectively) compared with placebo (−1.8 units; Figure 8.6). Scores in the subcomponents activity, impacts, and symptoms also improved with roflumilast treatment compared with baseline (data not shown; p < 0.01 vs. baseline for both). Additionally, the percentage of patients who experienced a COPD exacerbation was lower in the roflumilast 500-μg group (28%) than in the roflumilast 250-μg (36%) or placebo group (35%). Roflumilast also reduced the overall number of exacerbations per patient compared with placebo with a 34% decrease in the rate of total exacerbations in the roflumilast 500-μg group compared with placebo.

Roflumilast was well tolerated at both dose levels tested. The most common adverse events during the study were exacerbations of COPD and nasopharyngitis [78]. Most adverse events (>90%) occurred across all treatment groups, were mild to moderate in intensity, and resolved during the course of the study. Discontinuations because of adverse events were slightly higher in the roflumilast 500-μg group (15% of patients) compared with the roflumilast 250-μg (10%) or placebo groups (8%). The most common reason for discontinuation was COPD exacerbation, with a similar incidence rate (3–4% of patients) reported in each group. Diarrhoea occurred more often in the roflumilast treatment groups, usually within the first 4 weeks of treatment, and was generally mild to moderate in intensity.

In another phase III, multicentre, double-blind, randomised, placebo-controlled study, 581 patients with COPD were randomised to roflumilast 500 μg (n = 200) for 24 weeks, placebo (n = 186) for 24 weeks, or roflumilast 500 μg for 12 weeks, followed by placebo for 12 weeks (n = 195) [79]. Over 24 weeks, roflumilast improved post-bronchodilator FEV_1 (p < 0.0001) from baseline. In patients withdrawn from active treatment after 12 weeks, post-bronchodilator FEV_1 deteriorated following withdrawal of roflumilast (p = 0.0047), but remained higher than with placebo. The improvement that persisted after roflumilast withdrawal raises the intriguing possibility that roflumilast administered over a longer time period may ameliorate disease pathophysiology. Roflumilast was also well tolerated in this study, and no adverse events were associated with withdrawal from roflumilast. Most adverse events were mild to moderate in severity and not related to the study drug.

The PDE4 inhibitors cilomilast and roflumilast share similar pharmacokinetic characteristics (e.g., bioavailability, oral administration), but clinical data suggest that roflumilast may offer a higher therapeutic index for patients with COPD. For example, the once-daily dosing of roflumilast versus bid dosing for cilomilast and the improved gastrointestinal side-effect profile in patients with COPD [62] compared with cilomilast provide a higher benefit-to-risk ratio in favour of roflumilast. The demonstrated efficacy of roflumilast in patients with COPD in early trials coupled with a favourable safety profile provide the rationale for the long-term studies of roflumilast in larger populations, which are currently underway.

PDE INHIBITORS UNDER PRECLINICAL INVESTIGATION

There are a number of experimental PDE inhibitors in various stages of preclinical investigation and pharmacokinetic analysis. Only a few have been reported to be in phase I or II clinical trials. GRC 3886 is an oral PDE4 inhibitor under investigation in inflammatory airway diseases. In animal models *in vitro* and *in vivo*, GRC 3886 inhibited pulmonary cell infiltration, including eosinophilia and neutrophilia [80]. The compound also demonstrated a favourable tolerability profile in animals. Currently, GRC 3886 is in phase I clinical trials. A second PDE4 inhibitor, AWD 12–281 inhibits pro-inflammatory cytokines and TNF-α release in human cells and whole blood *ex vivo* [81]. AWD 12–281 is currently in phase II clinical studies for inflammatory airway diseases, including COPD. The anti-inflammatory potential of the novel PDE4 inhibitor ONO-6126 has been tested in healthy subjects [82], and it is believed to be in phase II trials. Lastly, tofimilast (CP 325366) is a PDE4 inhibitor currently in phase II trials for COPD and asthma.

CONCLUSIONS

To date, there is no disease-modifying therapy available that effectively addresses the underlying chronic inflammation of COPD or effectively attenuates lung function decline. Current pharmacologic therapies (e.g., anticholinergics and long-acting β-agonists) are administered to treat or control the symptoms of the disease. However, the anti-inflammatory activities associated with PDE4 inhibitors may provide an opportunity to target the pathophysiology of COPD, leading to amelioration of the disease rather than solely treating the clinical symptoms. Significant improvements in lung function, reduction in COPD exacerbation rates, and improvement in quality of life have been demonstrated with PDE4 inhibitors in multiple clinical trials. Taken together, these data suggest that oral PDE4 inhibitors might be useful in the treatment and management of COPD. Further studies are needed to elucidate the long-term effects of PDE4 inhibitors on the pathophysiology of COPD and their affect on COPD progression. Long-term safety studies in patients treated with PDE4 inhibitors are also anticipated. The anti-inflammatory activity and disease-modifying potential of PDE4 inhibitors in patients with COPD will continue to provide a basis for further research. Further examination of the pathophysiological modifying potential may further validate PDE4 inhibitors for effective treatment of COPD. The more favourable safety profiles (e.g., gastrointestinal side-effects) observed with newer generation PDE4 inhibitors (e.g., roflumilast) suggest an improved therapeutic ratio. Further, efficacy data support improved lung function, reduction in COPD exacerbations, improved quality of life, and suggest the possibility of disease modification with long-term therapy.

REFERENCES

1. Kohyama T, Liu X, Wen FQ et al. PDE4 inhibitors attenuate fibroblast chemotaxis and contraction of native collagen gels. Am J Respir Cell Mol Biol 2002; 26:694–701.
2. Saetta M, Turato G, Facchini FM et al. Inflammatory cells in the bronchial glands of smokers with chronic bronchitis. Am J Respir Crit Care Med 1997; 156:1633–1639.
3. Houslay MD, Sullivan M, Bolger GB. The multienzyme PDE4 cyclic adenosine monophosphate-specific phosphodiesterase family: intracellular targeting, regulation, and selective inhibition by compounds exerting anti-inflammatory and antidepressant actions. Adv Pharmacol 1998; 44:225–342.
4. Dent G, Giembycz MA, Evans PM, Rabe KF, Barnes PJ. Suppression of human eosinophil respiratory burst and cyclic AMP hydrolysis by inhibitors of type IV phosphodiesterase: interaction with the beta adrenoceptor agonist albuterol. J Pharmacol Exp Ther 1994; 271:1167–1174.
5. Giembycz MA. Could isoenzyme-selective phosphodiesterase inhibitors render bronchodilator therapy redundant in the treatment of bronchial asthma? Biochem Pharmacol 1992; 43:2041–2051.
6. Torphy TJ, Undem BJ. Phosphodiesterase inhibitors: new opportunities for the treatment of asthma. Thorax 1991; 46:512–523.
7. Pryzwansky KB, Madden VJ. Type 4A cAMP-specific phosphodiesterase is stored in granules of human neutrophils and eosinophils. Cell Tissue Res 2003; 312:301–311.
8. Giembycz MA, Corrigan CJ, Seybold J, Newton R, Barnes PJ. Identification of cyclic AMP phosphodiesterases 3, 4 and 7 in human CD4$^+$ and CD8$^+$ T-lymphocytes: role in regulating proliferation and the biosynthesis of interleukin-2. Br J Pharmacol 1996; 118:1945–1958.
9. Dent G, White SR, Tenor H et al. Cyclic nucleotide phosphodiesterase in human bronchial epithelial cells: characterization of isoenzymes and functional effects of PDE inhibitors. Pulm Pharmacol Ther 1998; 11:47–56.
10. Le Jeune IR, Shepherd M, Van Heeke G, Houslay MD, Hall IP. Cyclic AMP-dependent transcriptional up-regulation of phosphodiesterase 4D5 in human airway smooth muscle cells. Identification and characterization of a novel PDE4D5 promoter. J Biol Chem 2002; 277:35980–35989.
11. Campos-Toimil M, Lugnier C, Droy-Lefaix MT, Takeda K. Inhibition of type 4 phosphodiesterase by rolipram and Ginkgo biloba extract (EGb 761) decreases agonist-induced rises in internal calcium in human endothelial cells. Arterioscler Thromb Vasc Biol 2000; 20:E34-E40.
12. Thompson WJ, Ashikaga T, Kelly JJ et al. Regulation of cyclic AMP in rat pulmonary microvascular endothelial cells by rolipram-sensitive cyclic AMP phosphodiesterase (PDE4). Biochem Pharmacol 2002; 63:797–807.
13. Schudt C, Tenor H, Hatzelmann A. PDE isoenzymes as targets for anti-asthma drugs. Eur Respir J 1995; 8:1179–1183.
14. Obernolte R, Ratzliff J, Baecker PA et al. Multiple splice variants of phosphodiesterase PDE4C cloned from human lung and testis. Biochim Biophys Acta 1997; 1353:287–297.
15. Hatzelmann A, Schudt C. Anti-inflammatory and immunomodulatory potential of the novel PDE4 inhibitor roflumilast in vitro. J Pharmacol Exp Ther 2001; 297:267–279.
16. Souness JE, Rao S. Proposal for pharmacologically distinct conformers of PDE4 cyclic AMP phosphodiesterases. Cell Signal 1997; 9:227–236.
17. Schneider HH, Schmiechen R, Brezinski M, Seidler J. Stereospecific binding of the antidepressant rolipram to brain protein structures. Eur J Pharmacol 1986; 127:105–115.
18. Liu S, Laliberte F, Bobechko B et al. Dissecting the cofactor-dependent and independent bindings of PDE4 inhibitors. Biochemistry (Mosc) 2001; 40:10179–10186.
19. Laliberte F, Han Y, Govindarajan A et al. Conformational difference between PDE4 apoenzyme and holoenzyme. Biochemistry (Mosc) 2000; 39:6449–6458.
20. Burnett D, Chamba A, Hill SL, Stockley RA. Neutrophils from subjects with chronic obstructive lung disease show enhanced chemotaxis and extracellular proteolysis. Lancet 1987; 2:1043–1046.
21. Langen RC, Korn SH, Wouters EF. ROS in the local and systemic pathogenesis of COPD. Free Radic Biol Med 2003; 35:226–235.

22. Fitzgerald MF, Spicer J, Clark E, Bowyer N. Efficacy of the selective phosphodiesterase (PDE) 4 inhibitor, BAY 19–8004, in a rat model of neutrophilic lung inflammation [poster abstract online]. Available at: https://www.ersnetsecure.org/public/prg_congres.abstract?ww_i_presentation=775. Accessed October 14, 2003.

23. Jin SLC, Conti M. Induction of the cyclic nucleotide phosphodiesterase PDE4B is essential for LPS-activated TNF-α responses. *Proc Natl Acad Sci USA* 2002; 99:7628–7633.

24. Gamble E, Grootendorst DC, Brightling CE *et al*. Anti-inflammatory effects of the phosphodiesterase-4 inhibitor cilomilast (Ariflo) in chronic obstructive pulmonary disease. *Am J Respir Crit Care Med* 2003; 168;976–982.

25. Trifilieff A, Wyss D, Walker C, Mazzoni L, Hersperger R . Pharmacological profile of a novel phosphodiesterase 4 inhibitor, 4-(8-benzo[1,2,5]oxadiazol-5-yl-[1,7]naphthyridin-6-yl)-benzoic acid (NVP-ABE171), a 1,7-naphthyridine derivative, with anti-inflammatory activities. *J Pharmacol Exp Ther* 2002; 301:241–248.

26. Giembycz MA, Raeburn D. Putative substrates for cyclic nucleotide-dependent protein kinases and the control of airway smooth muscle tone. *J Auton Pharmacol* 1991; 11:365–398.

27. Data on file. Konstanz, Germany; Altana Pharma AG, 2003.

28. Grootendorst DC, Gauw SA, Baan R *et al*. Does a single dose of the phosphodiesterase 4 inhibitor, cilomilast (15 mg), induce bronchodilation in patients with chronic obstructive pulmonary disease? *Pulm Pharmacol Ther* 2003; 16:115–120.

29. Clayton RA, Mackenzie A, Dick CAJ *et al*. Phosphodiesterase expression and activity in human airways. *Eur Respir J* 2004; 24:21s (Abstract 266).

30. Bundschuh DS, Eltze M, Barsig J, Wollin L, Hatzelmann A, Beume R. *In vivo* efficacy in airway disease models of roflumilast, a novel orally active PDE4 inhibitor. *J Pharmacol Exp Ther* 2001; 297:280–290.

31. Noguera A, Batle S, Miralles C *et al*. Enhanced neutrophil response in chronic obstructive pulmonary disease. *Thorax* 2001; 56:432–437.

32. Blease K, Burke-Gaffney A, Hellewell PG. Modulation of cell adhesion molecule expression and function on human lung microvascular endothelial cells by inhibition of phosphodiesterases 3 and 4. *Br J Pharmacol* 1998; 124:229–237.

33. Wright LC, Seybold J, Robichaud A, Adcock IM, Barnes PJ. Phosphodiesterase expression in human epithelial cells. *Am J Physiol* 1998; 275:L694–L700.

34. Uniphyl® Tablets. [package insert]. Stamford, Conn; The Purdue Fredrick Company, 2002.

35. Barnes PJ. Theophylline: new perspectives for an old drug. *Am J Respir Crit Care Med* 2003; 167:813–818.

36. Rabe KF, Magnussen H, Dent G. Theophylline and selective PDE inhibitors as bronchodilators and smooth muscle relaxants. *Eur Respir J* 1995; 8:637–642.

37. Torphy TJ. Phosphodiesterase isozymes: molecular targets for novel antiasthma agents. *Am J Respir Crit Care Med* 1998; 157:351–370.

38. Ram FS, Jones PW, Castro AA *et al*. Oral theophylline for chronic obstructive pulmonary disease. *Cochrane Database Syst Rev* 2002:CD003902.

39. Mahler DA. The role of theophylline in the treatment of dyspnea in COPD. *Chest* 1987; 92:2S–6S.

40. Martin TJ. PDE4 inhibitors—a review of the recent patent literature. *IDrugs* 2001; 4:312–338.

41. Tsiu SJ, Self TH, Burns R. Theophylline toxicity: update. *Ann Allergy* 1990; 64:241–257.

42. Christensen SB, Guider A, Forster CJ *et al*. 1,4-Cyclohexanecarboxylates: potent and selective inhibitors of phosphodiesterase 4 for the treatment of asthma. *J Med Chem* 1998; 41:821–835.

43. Giembycz MA. Development status of second generation PDE4 inhibitors for asthma and COPD: the story so far. *Monaldi Arch Chest Dis* 2002; 57:48–64.

44. Zussman BD, Davie CC, Kelly J *et al*. Bioavailability of the oral selective phosphodiesterase 4 inhibitor cilomilast. *Pharmacotherapy* 2001; 21:653–660.

45. Murdoch RD, Cowley H, Upward J *et al*. The safety and tolerability of Ariflo™ (SB 207499), a novel selective phosphodiesterase 4 inhibitor, in healthy male volunteers. *Am J Respir Crit Care Med* 1998; 157(suppl) (Abstract A409).

46. Kelly J, Murdoch RD, Clark DJ, Webber DM, Fuder H. Warfarin pharmacodynamics unaffected by cilomilast. *Ann Pharmacother* 2001; 35:1535–1539.

47. Murdoch RD, Cowley H, Kelly J, Higgins R, Webber D. Cilomilast (Ariflo) does not potentiate the cardiovascular effects of inhaled salbutamol. *Pulm Pharmacol Ther* 2002; 15:521–527.

48. Zussman BD, Kelly J, Murdoch RD *et al*. Cilomilast: pharmacokinetic and pharmacodynamic interactions with digoxin. *Clin Ther* 2001; 23:921–931.

49. Kelly J, Walls C, Murdoch R *et al*. No interaction when erythromycin is co-administered with cilomilast at steady state. *Am J Respir Crit Care Med* 2002; 165(suppl):A536 (Abstract).

50. Murdoch RD, Zussman B, Schofield JP, Webber DM. Lack of pharmacokinetic interactions between cilomilast and theophylline or smoking in healthy volunteers. *J Clin Pharmacol* 2004; 44:1046–1053.

51. Zussman B, Kelly J, Rost K *et al*. The effect of renal impairment on the disposition of cilomilast, a novel and selective oral PDE4 inhibitor. *Am J Respir Crit Care Med* 2002; 165(suppl):A596 (Abstract).

52. US Food and Drug Administration. NDA 21–573, Ariflo™ tablets 15 mg, by GlaxoSmithKline, for use in chronic obstructive pulmonary disease (COPD). Available at: http://www.fda.gov/ohrms/dockets/ac/03/slides/3976s1.htm. Accessed October 15, 2003.

53. US Food and Drug Administration. Ariflo™ [PADAC briefing document]. Available at: http://www.fda.gov/ohrms/dockets/ac/03/briefing/3976b1.htm. Accessed October 14, 2003.

54. Lim S, Zhu J, Lake P. Cilomilast decreases exacerbations and maintains lung function in patients with poorly reversible COPD. Presented at the European Respiratory Society's annual meeting. September 4–9, 2004; Glasgow, Scotland (Abstract P648).

55. Compton C, Duggan M, Cedar E *et al*. Ariflo efficacy in a 12-month study of patients with asthma. Presented at the American Thoracic Society's International Conferences. May 17–23, 2002; Atlanta, GA (Abstract C12).

56. Knobil K, Morris A, Zhu J, Fischer T, Reisner C. Cilomilast is efficacious in chronic obstructive pulmonary disease (COPD). Presented at the 99th Annual International Conference of the American Thoracic Society. May 16–21, 2003. Seattle, WA (Abstract A035).

57. Edelson JD, Compton C, Nieman R *et al*. Cilomilast (Ariflo®) improves health status in patients with COPD: results of a 6-month trial. *Am J Respir Crit Care Med* 2001; 163(suppl):A277 (Abstract).

58. Edelson JD, Compton C, Nieman R *et al*. Cilomilast (Ariflo®), a potent, selective inhibitor of phosphodiesterase 4, improves lung function in COPD patients: results of a 6-month trial. *Am J Respir Crit Care Med* 2001; 163(suppl):A277 (Abstract).

59. Kelsen SG, Rennard SI, Chodosh S, Schryver B, Vleisides C, Zhu J. COPD exacerbation in a 6-month trial of cilomilast (Ariflo®), a potent, selective phosphodiesterase 4 inhibitor. *Am J Respir Crit Care Med* 2002; 165(suppl):A271 (Abstract).

60. Borker R, Zhu J, Lake P, Knobil K, Sam L. Long-term health status in patients with poorly reversible chronic obstructive pulmonary disease (COPD) treated with cilomilast. Presented at the European Respiratory Society's annual meeting. September 4–9, 2004; Glasgow, Scotland (Abstract P3350).

61. Compton CH, Gubb J, Nieman R *et al*. Cilomilast, a selective phosphodiesterase-4 inhibitor for treatment of patients with chronic obstructive pulmonary disease: a randomised, dose-ranging study. *Lancet* 2001; 358: 265–270.

62. Compton CH, Edelson JD, Cedar E *et al*. Cilomilast (Ariflo®) 15 mg BID safety in a 6-month clinical trial program. *Am J Respir Crit Care Med* 2001; 163(suppl):A909 (Abstract).

63. Zech K, David M, Seiberling M, Weimar C, Bethke T, Wurst W. High oral absolute bioavailability of roflumilast, a new, orally active, once daily PDE4 inhibitor. *Eur Respir J* 2001; 18(suppl 33):20s (Abstract 256).

64. Manegold A, Hauns B, David M, Zech K, Bethke TD, Wurst W. Pharmacokinetic characteristics of roflumilast administered in gradually increasing doses of 500 µg to 1,000 µg are dose-linear in healthy subjects. *Eur Respir J* 2002; 20(suppl 38):108s (Abstract P742).

65. Hauns B, Huennemeyer A, Seiberling M *et al*. Investigation of pharmacokinetics of roflumilast and roflumilast N-oxide after single morning or evening oral administration of 500 µg roflumilast in healthy subjects—an open, randomized, two-period crossover study. *Am J Respir Crit Care Med* 2003; 167(suppl):A92 (Abstract).

66. Drollmann A, Huennemayer A, Hartmann M *et al*. Pharmacokinetic characteristics of roflumilast and its active metabolite roflumilast-N-oxide are not affected by food intake. *Eur Respir J* 2002; 20(suppl 38):109s (Abstract P747).

67. Manegold A, Hauns B, Huennemeyer A, Koch M, Zech K, Bethke D. Pharmacokinetics of roflumilast and its active metabolite roflumilast N-oxide are not influenced by erythromycin. *Eur Respir J* 2004; 24:128s (Abstract P867).

68. Hünnemeyer A, Hauns B, Drollmann A *et al*. Pharmacokinetics of roflumilast and its active metabolite, roflumilast-N-oxide, is not influenced by smoking. *Am J Respir Crit Care Med* 2002; 165:A594 (Abstract).

69. Hünnemeyer A, Bethke T, David M, Westphal K, Siegmund W, Wurst W. No interaction of roflumilast and its active metabolite, roflumilast-N-oxide, with inhaled budesonide. *Am J Respir Crit Care Med* 2002; 165(suppl):A595.
70. Bethke T, Hartmann M, Zech K, David M, Weimar C, Wurst W. No dose adjustment of roflumilast in patients with severe renal impairment. *Am J Respir Crit Care Med* 2002; 165(suppl):A594 (Abstract).
71. Weimar C, Bethke T, Westphal K, Zech K, Siegmund W, Wurst W. Roflumilast and its active metabolite, roflumilast-N-oxide, do not interact with inhaled salbutamol. *Am J Respir Crit Care Med* 2002; 165(suppl):A594 (Abstract).
72. Hauns B, Huennemeyer A, Duursema L *et al.* Roflumilast and its active metabolite roflumilast N-oxide do not interact with R- and S-warfarin. *Eur Respir J* 2003; 22(suppl 45):103s (Abstract P717).
73. Drollmann A, Hartmann M, Zech K, David M, Weimer C, Bethke TD. Patients with severe renal impairment do not require dose adjustments of roflumilast. *Eur Respir J* 2002; 20(suppl 38):108s (Abstract P743).
74. Leichtl S, Syed J, Bredenbröker D, Rathgeb F, Wurst W. Efficacy of once-daily roflumilast, a new, orally active, selective phosphodiesterase 4 inhibitor, in chronic obstructive pulmonary disease. *Am J Respir Crit Care Med* 2002; 165(suppl) (Abstract A229).
75. Bredenbröker D, Syed J, Leichtl S, Rathgeb F, Wurst W. Safety of once-daily roflumilast, a new, orally active, selective phosphodiesterase 4 inhibitor, in patients with COPD. *Am J Respir Crit Care Med* 2002; 165(suppl):A595.
76. Rabe KF, Chapman KR, Joubert J, Vetter N, Witte S, Bredenbroeker D. Roflumilast, a novel, selective phosphodiesterase 4 inhibitor, improves lung function in patients with moderate to severe COPD. *Am J Respir Crit Care Med* 2004; 169:A518 (Abstract).
77. Rabe KF, O'Donnell D, Muir JF *et al.* Roflumilast, an oral, once-daily PDE4 inhibitor, improves lung function and reduces exacerbation rates in patients with COPD. *Eur Respir J* 2004; 24:21s (Abstract).
78. O'Donnell D, Muir JF, Jenkins C *et al.* Roflumilast, a novel, selective phosphodiesterase 4 inhibitor, improves quality of life and lowers exacerbation rate in patients with moderate to severe COPD. *Am J Respir Crit Care Med* 2004; 167:A602 (Abstract).
79. Fabbri LM, Calverley PMA, Kraft M, Welte T. Simplifying the complexities of obstructive lung disease: exploring a new therapeutic target. Presented in conjunction with the European Respiratory Society's annual meeting. September 6, 2004; Glasgow, Scotland.
80. Vakkalanka SKVS, Balasubramaniam G, Charat LA *et al.* The pharmacological and safety profile of a novel selective phosphodiesterase-4(PDE4) inhibitor:- GRC- 3886. *Eur Respir J* 2004; 24:220s (Abstract P1391).
81. Draheim R, Egerland U, Rundfeldt C. Anti-inflammatory potential of the selective phosphodiesterase 4 inhibitor N-(3,5-dichloro-pyrid-4-yl)-[1-(4-fluorobenzyl)-5-hydroxy-indole-3-yl]-gly oxylic acid amide (AWD 12–281), in human cell preparations. *J Pharmacol Exp Ther* 2004; 308:555–563.
82. Furuie H, Nakagawa S, Kawashima M, Murakami M, Irie S. Suppressive effect of novel phosphodiesterase4 (PDE4) inhibitor ONO-6126 on TNF-α release was increased after repeated oral administration in healthy Japanese subjects. Presented at the 13th Annual European Respiratory Society's Annual Congress. September 27, 2003; Vienna, Austria (Abstract 2557).

9

Combination therapy with bronchodilators

S. I. Rennard

INTRODUCTION

Bronchodilators are first-line therapy for symptomatic relief in the management of stable patients with chronic obstructive pulmonary disease (COPD) [1, 2]. Three classes of bronchodilators are available and are reviewed in detail in other chapters in this volume: β-adrenoceptor agonists (Chapters 3, 4), anticholinergics (Chapters 5, 6) and phosphodiesterase inhibitors/theophylline (Chapters 7, 8). There are several theoretical and practical reasons to combine bronchodilators in the routine management of COPD patients. The use of combinations, however, raises a number of practical issues with which the clinician must deal. Oftentimes the available clinical data upon which the clinician must base therapeutic decisions are limited. Nevertheless, available information suggests that combination therapy can be of significant benefit to patients with COPD.

RATIONALE FOR COMBINATION THERAPY

AIRFLOW LIMITATION

Airflow limitation in COPD results from several distinct histophysiologic processes that are present in varying degrees of severity in COPD patients [3]. Fixed airflow limitation results primarily from two distinct lesions. Loss of alveolar wall, the characteristic and defining lesion in emphysema, leads to loss of lung elastic recoil and destruction of alveolar insertions in small airways. As a result, there is decreased pressure in the distal airways and small airway collapse with forced exhalation, both of which decrease expiratory airflow. In addition, small airways are characteristically fibrotic [4] and, like all fibrotic tissues, undergo contraction. The narrowing of the airways that results limits airflow [5]. In addition to these lesions, airflow may be limited by airway oedema, inflammation and the accumulation of secretions within the airway lumen [4].

AIRWAY SMOOTH MUSCLE

All airways have some degree of resting smooth muscle tone that slightly narrows airways. Bronchodilators, therefore, improve airflow modestly, about 3–5% in normal individuals [6]. While not clinically meaningful in normal subjects, even modest improvement in airflow may be of benefit in the COPD patient. Should increased resting tone be present, the benefit of bronchodilators will be even greater. Currently available bronchodilator drugs, moreover, also have biological effects in addition to causing smooth muscle relaxation [7–12]. It is possible that these 'non-bronchodilator effects' may also be beneficial in COPD patients (see below).

Stephen I. Rennard, MD, Larson Professor of Medicine, University of Nebraska Medical Center, Omaha, Nebraska, USA.

MAXIMAL BRONCHODILATATION

Early discussions of combined bronchodilator use were heavily influenced by the concept of 'maximal bronchodilatation' [13]. The concept proposed was that a single bronchodilator, if given in sufficient amount, should be able to result in the maximally attainable bronchodilatation. This led to a series of studies with a similar design: a given bronchodilator would be administered in sequentially increasing doses until a maximal response had been obtained. After this, a second bronchodilator would be administered to determine if more bronchodilatation could be achieved. Several studies performed with sequential administration of bronchodilators failed to show added benefits of a second bronchodilator [14–18]. In addition, dose-ranging studies have suggested that the conventionally used clinical dose of ipratropium [19] and β-adrenoceptor agonist [20] are less than maximally effective. Results of these studies, therefore, supported the concept that maximal bronchodilatation could be achieved by appropriately increasing the dose of a single agent. Such an approach suggested the use of combination bronchodilators would be unnecessarily complicated and the use of fixed-dose combinations unnecessarily constraining.

Attitudes towards combination bronchodilators in general, and to fixed-dose combinations specifically, have changed dramatically for a number of reasons. First, bronchodilator response to both β-adrenoceptor agonists [20, 21] and anticholinergic [21, 22] bronchodilators in an individual with COPD is variable on a day-to-day basis. Thus, maximally achieved bronchodilatation is not a fixed concept, but a variable one. This variability, of course, greatly confounds the assessment of dose response in an individual COPD patient and may have contributed to the methodologic constraints that led to the conclusions of no benefit from combinations. In addition, the majority of studies that showed no benefit of multiple bronchodilators enrolled relatively small numbers of subjects. This raises the possibility of a type II statistical error. In fact, larger studies consistently support the therapeutic benefit of bronchodilators in combination (see reference [23] for a review of these studies). Finally, inhaled bronchodilators are relatively safe, but are not entirely free of side-effects that are dose related (see Chapters 3–6). Since different classes of bronchodilators have distinctly different side-effects, combinations have the possibility of being better tolerated by minimising dose-related adverse effects.

POPULATION VERSUS INDIVIDUAL RESPONSE

Most of the studies available to date that show a benefit of combination bronchodilators have used a parallel group design. In these studies, a group treated with the combination is compared to groups treated with either agent alone and sometimes with a placebo. Benefit in such a study could result from either an improved number of subjects who achieved bronchodilation or improved bronchodilation in individual subjects receiving the combination. Consistent with the first possibility, two clinical trials characterised COPD patients for reversibility to salmeterol and ipratropium [24, 25]. About 70–80% of subjects responded to albuterol and 60–70% to ipratropium, using 12% and 200 ml improvement in reversibility as the definition of response. However, some subjects responded to only one of the bronchodilators, thus the number of responders would be expected to be increased using a combination. Consistently, a retrospective analysis of 1067 subjects in two parallel group studies that compared ipratropium combined with albuterol to either agent alone was performed by Dorinsky *et al.* [26]. Using either a 12 or 15% improvement in FEV_1 as a definition of response, significantly more subjects treated with the combination reversed than those treated with ipratropium or albuterol alone.

In order to determine if maximal bronchodilation is improved within a given subject with a combination, a crossover design is preferable. While data are limited, several studies using such a design, most commonly with subjects assessed on separate days and the combination bronchodilators being given at the same time, have demonstrated improved bronchodilatation with combination therapy. Several of these studies used only a single dose of each component of bronchodilator. Thus, whether the combination resulted in increased 'maximal' bronchodilatation may not have been assessed. A smaller number of studies are available that have performed dose-ranging crossover comparisons within subjects, but several of these have also demonstrated a benefit for combination [14, 17, 18, 27–32]. Thus, while the available data have limitations, evidence supports the concept that combination bronchodilators are superior to individual drugs. This will be true both because a larger number of COPD patients will respond to the combination and because a greater degree of bronchodilation will be achieved.

LONG- AND SHORT-ACTING BRONCHODILATORS

Both long-acting and short-acting agents are available for both the anticholinergic and β-adrenoceptor classes of bronchodilators. The long-acting bronchodilators in these classes achieve their long duration of action by interacting with the cell surface and/or the receptor differently than do the short-acting bronchodilators (see Chapters 3–6). Long-acting theophylline preparations are also available, but they achieve their long duration of action through slow release of the drug rather than a distinct pharmacologic mechanism. Despite the pharmacologic differences, available evidence to date suggests that any β-adrenoceptor agonist, whether short or long acting, can be combined effectively with any anticholinergic (Table 9.1). Similarly, theophylline can likely be added to any inhaled β-adrenoceptor agonist or anticholinergic bronchodilator or bronchodilator combination. Whether long-acting bronchodilators can be combined with short-acting bronchodilators within a class is a separate question, but is much more relevant for the treatment of acute exacerbations than for chronic stable COPD (see below).

MECHANISMS AND CLINICAL IMPLICATIONS

There are several theoretical reasons that could explain increased maximal bronchodilation with combined bronchodilators within an individual COPD patient, and these considerations

Table 9.1 Selected studies showing a benefit of combinations of β-agonist and anticholinergic bronchodilators

β-Agonist	Anticholinergic		
	Ipratropium	Oxitropium	Tiotropium
Isoprenaline	[74]		
Isoetharine	[75]		
Metaproterenol	[76]		
Terbutaline	[77]		
Albuterol	[17, 26, 68, 78–88]		
Fenoterol	[28, 29, 89–95]	[96]	
Formoterol	[30]		[97]
Salmeterol	[98, 99]	[31]	[100]

Studies demonstrating a significant benefit for at least one outcome are included. Studies showing trends or no significant effect are not listed. Additional combinations are under investigation; reports presented only as abstracts have not been included.

may help guide clinical care. First, smooth muscle tone maintains some degree of airway narrowing from the proximal to the distal airways. However, the distribution of cholinergic and adrenergic receptors is not uniform along the axis of the airways. Autoradiographic studies demonstrate that the proximal airways are relatively more richly endowed with cholinergic receptors [33] while the more distal airways are relatively enriched with β-receptors [34]. Concordantly, a study using intrabronchial catheters has demonstrated a greater proximal effect of anticholinergic bronchodilators and a relatively greater distal effect of β-agonist bronchodilators [35]. Thus, greater bronchodilator effect is possible within an individual using a combination, as different sites within the airway may be responding to different bronchodilators.

Whether true mechanistic synergy occurs within a cell responding to two distinct bronchodilators remains to be determined. It is possible that a β-adrenoceptor agonist that increased cAMP would synergise with a PDE inhibitor that prevented cAMP breakdown. Consistent with this, patients have been reported to prefer a combination of β-adrenoceptor agonist with theophylline [36], and increased bronchodilator effect has been observed in many clinical trials [36–45].

The three classes of bronchodilators cause smooth muscle relaxation by different mechanisms (Figure 9.1). There are, however, a number of mechanistic interactions between cholinergic and β-adrenergic signalling that could theoretically lead to synergistic interactions. In addition, at least one clinical trial provides supportive evidence for a synergistic interaction. Specifically, van Noord et al. administered placebo, salmeterol or salmeterol together with ipratropium [46]. The maximal bronchodilator response was greatest with the combination of salmeterol and ipratropium, consistent with improved 'maximal' bronchodilation within an individual. This peak bronchodilator effect occurred at approximately 2h, the time expected from the known pharmacokinetics of the two drugs. Interestingly, 10–12h after administration of the two drugs, the effect of the combination was still greater than that of salmeterol alone. At such a time point, the effect of ipratropium alone would be expected to have abated. While not a direct proof of the hypothesis, this study provides evidence consistent with a potential synergy between anticholinergic and β-agonist bronchodilators.

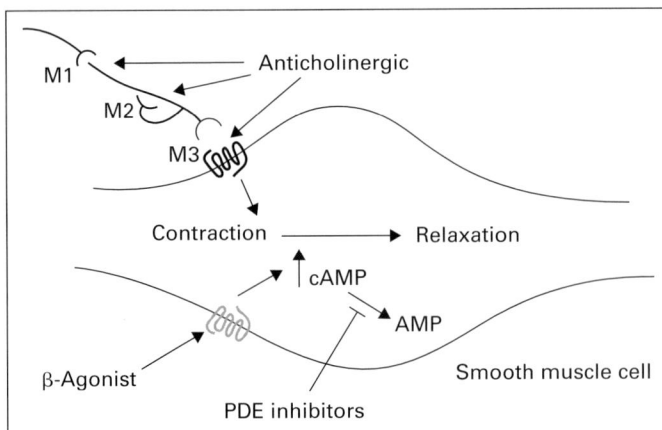

Figure 9.1 Mechanisms of action of bronchodilators. Currently available bronchodilators improve airflow primarily by relaxing airway smooth muscle. Anticholinergic agents accomplish this by blocking the M3 muscarinic stimulus that provides for 'resting' tone. β-Adrenoceptor agonists achieve bronchodilation by increasing intracellular cAMP resulting in relaxation of contracted smooth muscle. Phosphodiesterase inhibitors act similarly by preventing the breakdown of cAMP to AMP.

DISEASE INHOMOGENEITY

COPD is not homogeneous anatomically. This may create a particularly important advantage for combination bronchodilator therapy. In this context, it is now clear that a major factor in causing dyspnoea in COPD patients, particularly dyspnoea with exertion, is dynamic hyperinflation [47].

DYNAMIC HYPERINFLATION AND VARIABLE TIME CONSTANTS

The lungs are characteristically hyperinflated in patients with COPD. This occurs for at least two reasons (Figure 9.2). First, functional residual capacity (FRC) represents the balance point between lung elastic recoil and the elastic force generated by the chest wall, which causes the lung to expand. Loss of lung elastic recoil, which is characteristic of emphysema, results in an increase in FRC and thus in hyperinflation. Second, limitation of expiratory airflow can sufficiently delay emptying of the lungs after inhalation such that subsequent inhalations begin before FRC is reached. Hyperinflation resulting from expiratory airflow limitation is related to expiratory time and, therefore, to respiratory rate and is termed dynamic hyperinflation. With increasing respiratory rate, dynamic hyperinflation increases. The work of breathing increases with hyperinflation, and dyspnoea is thought to be related to the inspiratory effort required to maintain the increased work of breath. Dynamic hyperinflation, therefore, is believed to be a major cause of dyspnoea in patients with COPD, particularly dyspnoea on exertion where respiratory rates increase [48, 49].

Because the anatomic lesions in COPD are heterogeneously distributed throughout the lung, it is likely that dynamic hyperinflation is as well. Thus, areas of the lung with more severe expiratory airflow limitation will become more severely hyperinflated than adjoining lung regions with better-preserved airflow. Because the total lung capacity is limited, if hyperinflation becomes severe enough, the residual lung may become functionally restricted [47]. Dynamic hyperinflation, therefore, can result in compression of relatively

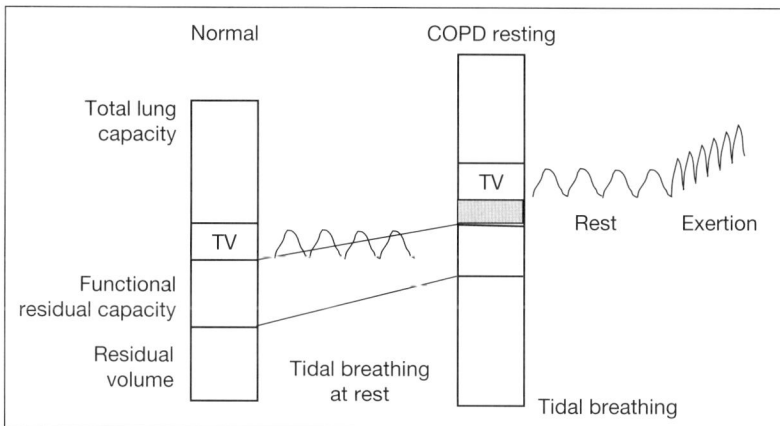

Figure 9.2 Dynamic hyperinflation. In the normal lung (left) tidal volume (TV) begins at functional residual capacity (FRC) with each breath. In COPD (right), there is hyperinflation at rest (centre). This is due to loss of lung elastic recoil and total lung capacity. FRC and residual volume are all increased. Because of the prolonged expiratory time required for tidal breathing to return to FRC, there may be further hyperinflation (shaded region), even at rest. With exertion, or any other cause of increased respiratory rate, there is less time for the lungs to empty and each breath causes further hyperinflation until a new equilibrium is met.

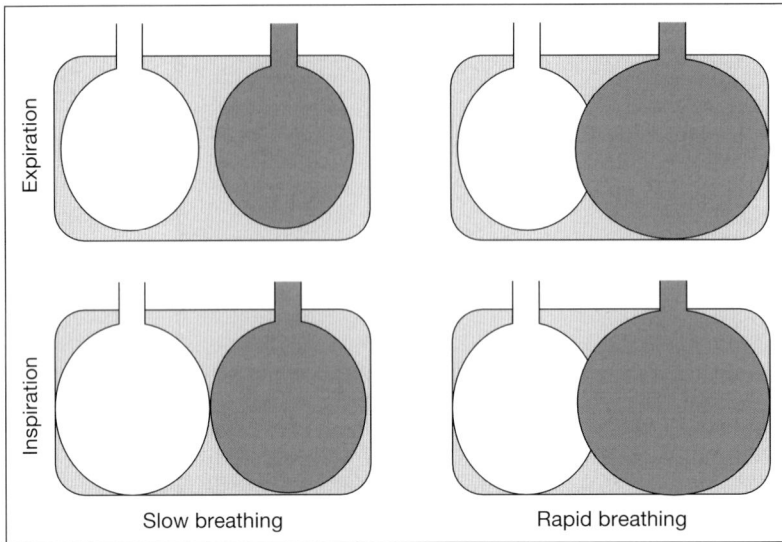

Figure 9.3 Heterogeneity of dynamic hyperinflation. Airflow limitation is characteristically heterogeneous. Nevertheless, with slow breathing, there may be sufficient time for all segments to empty and dynamic hyperinflation will be minimal (left). With increasing respiratory rate, the most obstructed segments (shaded) will hyperinflate (right). This not only prevents those segments from supporting ventilation, but can compress the relatively more normal lung compromising the function of those regions also. The more heterogeneously distributed the airflow limitation, the more important this effect will be. As different bronchodilators may affect different regions of the lung differently, combinations of bronchodilators may be more effective in reducing inhomogeneities than single agents.

normal lung compromising its function (Figure 9.3). Compression of intrapulmonary airways has also been suggested to further worsen airflow limitation [50].

It is currently believed that 'deflation' of the lungs is one major physiological benefit of bronchodilators. In this context, all classes of bronchodilators have been demonstrated to result in a decrease in both resting and dynamic hyperinflation [48, 49, 51, 52]. The reduction in hyperinflation, moreover, is better correlated with the reduction in dyspnoea and improvement in exercise capacity than is the effect on airflow. Because different classes of bronchodilators can affect airways at different sites within the lung, combination bronchodilators have the possibility of improving airflow more diffusely within the lung. As a result, combination bronchodilators may be more beneficial at reducing dynamic hyperinflation than would individual bronchodilators. Such benefits of combination bronchodilator therapy may be important clinically even in the absence of dramatic effects of the combination on resting airflow. While such a mechanism is appealing conceptually, it remains to be tested directly.

Theophylline can be added effectively to either β-adrenoceptor bronchodilators [36–45] or to anticholinergic bronchodilators [53]. While the available data are limited, combination of all three bronchodilators can result in further improvement in airflows [54, 55]. Because theophylline is administered orally, there may be a special advantage to its use in combination. Specifically, inhaled bronchodilators may not effectively reach areas within the lung that are severely airflow limited. Theophylline, because it reaches the lung through the circulation, may have the potential for bronchodilating such regions. Such an effect could improve airflow directly, could improve the distribution of inhaled bronchodilators and could reduce dynamic hyperinflation by reducing inhomogeneities in airflow distribution.

COMBINATION OF BRONCHODILATORS WITHIN A CLASS

Combinations of bronchodilators within a class are of more than theoretical interest. Specifically, the addition of a short-acting (and presumably rapid-acting) bronchodilator for the acute management of respiratory distress in a patient chronically treated with a long-acting bronchodilator is important in both the management of acute exacerbations and for 'rescue' therapy. There are several reasons for concern about the potential effectiveness of short-acting agents when added to the management of patients chronically taking long-acting bronchodilators. The long-acting agents theoretically could either induce tachyphylaxis or could serve as blockers of the short-acting agents. Although not specifically studied in COPD patients, the issue is highly relevant for patients with asthma who are chronically treated with long-acting β-agonist bronchodilators. The addition of albuterol to long-acting β-adrenoceptor bronchodilators can result in further bronchodilation, although the effectiveness may be partially diminished [56, 57]. Consistent with this, in clinical trials of patients with asthma treated with long-acting bronchodilators who had exacerbations, the addition of albuterol resulted in improved airflow [57, 58].

Less is known about the anticholinergics. Tiotropium interacts irreversibly with the M3 muscarinic receptor. Whether the addition of ipratropium results in further bronchodilation in the presence of tiotropium has not been specifically studied in patients with COPD exacerbations. It is likely, however, that the addition of ipratropium to patients treated with tiotropium has minimal adverse side-effects.

In contrast to the theoretical potential for problems noted above, there is also theoretical potential for combinations of bronchodilators within a class to have advantages. It is now recognised, for example, that receptors such as the β-adrenergic receptor can adopt a number of distinct confirmations [59]. It is likely that these various combinations have differing signalling mechanisms and biological effects. It is also likely, moreover, that different β-agonist agents interact with the various receptor confirmations differently. This raises the possibility that combinations of β-agonists may have effects distinct from either agent alone. Whether such effects can be exploited for medical benefit remains to be determined.

ACUTE EXACERBATIONS

Current recommendations for the management of acute exacerbations of COPD recommend the use of short-acting β-adrenoceptor bronchodilators and/or short-acting anticholinergic bronchodilators [1, 2, 60, 61]. These agents should be used even if the patient had been chronically managed with a long-acting bronchodilator. Since the long-acting bronchodilator will likely persist, this will result in some interval of overlapping therapy. If a patient had been treated with a single long-acting bronchodilator agent, it would be rational to treat with a short-acting bronchodilator of a different class, although clinical data assessing the outcome of such a strategy in COPD exacerbations are not available.

Aminophylline can be used for the treatment of acute exacerbations, although it has generally been found to have relatively little benefit. Its addition to a therapeutic regimen, however, can be considered in selected patients where additional bronchodilation is needed.

NON-BRONCHODILATOR EFFECTS

All classes of bronchodilators have non-bronchodilator effects. β-Adrenergic receptors are located on most cells, and β-adrenoceptor agonists have numerous effects in addition to bronchodilation (see reference [7] for review). These include a variety of anti-inflammatory effects, which may be of benefit in patients with COPD. β-Adrenoceptor agonists may also modulate mucociliary clearance and have a cytoprotective effect on airway epithelial cells. Similarly, muscarinic cholinergic receptors are also widely distributed [62]. As these receptors are believed to contribute to a variety of pro-inflammatory effects, it is plausible that anti-cholinergics could also have an anti-inflammatory effect. Finally, theophylline has many pharmacologic effects that may also have important non-bronchodilator actions of relevance to COPD [10–12]. Moreover, activation of histone deacetylase by theophylline has been suggested to provide an important anti-inflammatory mechanism in COPD patients [63, 64]. Other phosphodiesterase inhibitors, particularly inhibitors of PDE4, may have their primary actions through down-regulation of inflammatory responses [65].

The importance of the various non-bronchodilator effects of these agents in the therapy of COPD remains to be determined. There is, however, great potential for these agents to interact and to have synergistic beneficial actions. Evaluation of these effects and their clinical significance in COPD patients will be important lines of future research.

ACCEPTABLE COMBINATIONS

To date, a limited number of combinations have been approved for registration (Table 9.2). Uniformly, these are fixed combinations of a short-acting β-agonist bronchodilator combined with a short-acting anticholinergic bronchodilator. They are administered as a combined formulation through either a metered-dose inhaler [66], a soft mist inhaler [67] or as a nebulised solution [68]. There is considerably more experience with these fixed-dose combinations than with other bronchodilator combinations for at least two reasons. First, the clinical trials required for registration of these products required adequately sized, well-controlled and well-executed clinical studies, the results of which are available. In addition, the availability of fixed combinations is extremely popular, both with patients and physicians [69, 70]. As a result, after their introduction, considerable clinical experience has been gained with these products. While data are limited, a variety of other combinations have been assessed (Table 9.1) and, as noted above, any combination of a bronchodilator from one class with a bronchodilator of another class is reasonable.

Whether it is better to prescribe two bronchodilators has been evaluated in several contexts. One is cost. Hilleman *et al.* [71] demonstrated that the combination of ipratropium and albuterol reduces total costs of care compared to either agent alone, primarily because of reduced hospitalisation and their associated costs. As exacerbations and hospitalisations were more common with more severe disease, this effect was more prominent in patients with worse lung function. Long-acting bronchodilators have a greater effect on exacerbations and may be expected to have a similar beneficial effect on total costs. Such cost estimates, of course, will depend on the cost structure of individual health care systems.

A separate issue is the value of combination of bronchodilators administered through a fixed-combination device versus individual components. Benayoun *et al.* [72] evaluated this question in a retrospective analysis of 641 individuals treated with a fixed combination

Table 9.2 Fixed combination bronchodilators

Agent	Formulation	Components (dose)
Combivent	Metered dose inhaler (CFC)	Per actuation: ipratropium (21 ug); Albuterol (120 ug); usual dose 2 puffs
DuoNeb	Nebuliser solution	Per vial: ipratropium (0.5 mg); albuterol sulphate (3.0 mg)
Berodual*	Metered dose inhaler (CFC)	Per actuation: ipratropium (20 ug); fenoterol (50 ug); usual dose 2 puffs
Berodual*	Respimat (soft mist inhaler)	Per actuation: ipratropium (20 ug); fenoterol (50 ug); usual dose one actuation

*Not available in United States.

compared to 411 subjects treated with ipratropium bromide and inhaled β_2-agonists administered separately. There was increased usage of bronchodilator when administered with a single device, and this was associated with significantly lower overall health care costs, presumably as a result of better overall management of the subject's COPD. Similarly, Chrischilles *et al.* [73] compared 428 patients who received a fixed-combination bronchodilator with 658 patients who received separate inhaler therapy. These investigators also observed improved compliance with a single inhaler which was associated with decreased respiratory morbidity and an overall reduction in respiratory-related health care costs. Thus, available data support the concept that combination bronchodilator therapy can reduce costs and that administration of bronchodilators in a single fixed-dose combination device can result in further benefits.

Fixed-dose combinations prevent the clinician from adjusting the dose of one of the components. This can, of course, be achieved by adding an additional inhaler. Since the conventional clinical formulation of short-acting bronchodilators, particularly ipratropium, is often submaximal [19], increasing the dosage is not unreasonable. Such a strategy is supported by the observation that increased bronchodilatation is observed across the dose range for oxitropium when added to salmeterol [31]. Thus, while data are limited, individualising dosing regimens for bronchodilator combinations can be considered by the clinician who feels comfortable with such an approach.

SUMMARY

Bronchodilators are currently first-line treatment for patients with COPD. The several classes of bronchodilators act by different mechanisms and affect different sites within the lung. Their use in combination is therefore rational and benefits are supported by clinical data. Combination bronchodilators, moreover, by minimising the dose of individual components, may reduce the risk for side-effects. The use of fixed-dose combinations has proved effective in practice settings.

REFERENCES

1. Global Strategy for the Diagnosis, Management, and Prevention of Chronic Obstructive Pulmonary Disease, 2003.
2. Standards for the Diagnosis and Management of Patients with COPD, 2004, ATS/ERS.
3. Niewoehner DE, Sobonya RE. Structure-function correlations in chronic airflow obstruction. In: Baum GL, Wolinsky E (eds) Textbook of Pulmonary Diseases. Lippincott Williams & Wilkins, 1989, pp 913–932.
4. Hogg JC *et al*. The nature of small-airway obstruction in chronic obstructive pulmonary disease. *N Engl J Med* 2004; 350:2645–2653.
5. Kuwano K *et al*. Small airways dimensions in asthma and in chronic obstructive pulmonary disease. *Am Rev Respir Dis* 1993; 148:1220–1225.
6. Taylor RG, Maclagan J, Cook DG. Bronchodilator action of inhaled fenoterol and ipratropium in normal subjects: a teaching exercise for medical students. *Br J Clin Pharmacol* 1989; 28:709–713.
7. Johnson M, Rennard S. Alternative mechanisms for long-acting beta(2)-adrenergic agonists in COPD. *Chest* 2001; 120:258–270.
8. Sato E *et al*. Acetylcholine stimulates alveolar macrophages to release inflammatory cell chemotactic activity. *Am J Physiol* 1998; 274(6 Pt 1):L970–L979.
9. Koyama S, Rennard SI, Robbins RA. Acetylcholine stimulates bronchial epithelial cells to release neutrophil and monocyte chemotactic activity. *Am J Physiol* 1992; 262:L466–L471.
10. Aubier M. Effect of theophylline on diaphragmatic muscle function. *Chest* 1987; 92:S27–S31.

11. Wanner A. Effects of methylxanthines on airway mucociliary function. *Am J Med* 1985; 79:16–21.
12. Pasteline G *et al*. The search for a digitalis substitute II milrinone (Win 47203). Its action on the heart-lung preparation of the dog. *Life Sci* 1983; 33:1787–1796.
13. Levy SF. Bronchodilators in COPD. *Chest* 1991; 99:793–794.
14. Newnham DM *et al*. Bronchodilator reversibility to low and high doses of terbutaline and ipratropium bromide in patients with chronic obstructive pulmonary disease. *Thorax* 1995; 48:1151–1155.
15. Lloberes P *et al*. Effect of three different bronchodilators during an exacerbation of chronic obstructive pulmonary disease. *Eur Respir J* 1988; 1:536–539.
16. LeDoux EJ *et al*. Standard and double dose ipratropium bromide and combined ipratropium bromide and inhaled metaproterenol in COPD. *Chest* 1989; 95:1013–1016.
17. Easton PA *et al*. A comparison of the bronchodilating effects of a beta-2 adrenergic agent (albuterol) and an anti-cholinergic agent (ipratropium bromide), given by aerosol alone or in sequence. *N Engl J Med* 1986; 315:735–739.
18. Ikeda A *et al*. Comparative dose-response study of three anti-cholinergic agents and fenoterol using a metered dose inhaler in patients with chronic obstructive pulmonary disease. *Thorax* 1995; 50:62–66.
19. Gross NJ *et al*. Dose response to ipratropium as a nebulized solution in patients with chronic obstructive pulmonary disease. *Am Rev Respir Dis* 1989; 139:1188–1191.
20. Jaeschke R *et al*. The effect of increasing doses of β-agonists on airflow in patients with chronic airflow limitation. *Respir Med* 1993; 87:433–438.
21. Anthonisen NR, Wright E. Bronchodilator response in chronic obstructive pulmonary disease. *Am Rev Respir Dis* 1986; 133:814–819.
22. Nisar M *et al*. Acute bronchodilator trials in chronic obstructive pulmonary disease. *Am Rev Respir Dis* 1992; 146:555–559.
23. Rennard SI. Anti-cholinergics in combination bronchodilator therapy in COPD. In: Spector SL (ed.) Anti-cholinergic Agents in the Upper and Lower Airways. Marcel Dekker, Inc., New York, 1999; pp 119–136.
24. Mahler DA *et al*. Efficacy of salmeterol xinafoate in the treatment of COPD. *Chest* 1999; 115:957–965.
25. Rennard SI *et al*. Use of a long-acting inhaled beta(2)-adrenergic agonist, salmeterol xinafoate, in patients with chronic obstructive pulmonary disease. *Am J Respir Crit Care Med* 2001; 163:1087–1092.
26. Dorinsky PM *et al*. The combination of ipratropium and albuterol optimizes pulmonary function reversibility testing in patients with COPD. *Chest* 1999; 115:966–971.
27. Gutersohn J, Joos H, Herzog H. The effect of R_{aw} on Sch 1000 MDI or fenoterol MDI and the combined administration of subthreshold dosages of both compounds. *Postgrad Med J* 1975; 51:113–114.
28. Serra C, Giacopelli A, Luciani G. Acute controlled study of the dose-response relationship of fenoterol, ipratropium bromide and their combination. *Respiration* 1986; 50:144–147.
29. Wesseling G, Mostert R, Wouters EFM. A comparison of the effects of anti-cholinergic and beta-2 agonist and combination therapy on respiratory impedance in COPD. *Chest* 1992; 101:166–173.
30. Sichletidis L *et al*. Bronchodilatory responses to formoterol, ipratropium, and their combination in patients with stable COPD. *Int J Clin Pract* 1999; 53:185–188.
31. Cazzola M *et al*. Acute effect of pretreatment with single conventional dose of salmeterol on dose-response curve to oxitropium bromide in chronic obstructive pulmonary disease. *Thorax* 1999; 54:1083–1086.
32. Kassner F, Hodder R, Bateman ED. A review of ipratropium bromide/fenoterol hydrobromide (Berodual) delivered *via* Respimat Soft Mist Inhaler in patients with asthma and chronic obstructive pulmonary disease. *Drugs* 2004; 64:1671–1682.
33. Barnes PJ, Basbaum CB, Nadel JA. Autoradiographic localization of autonomic receptors in airway smooth muscle. Marked differences between large and small airways. *Am Rev Respir Dis* 1983; 127:758–762.
34. Hoffman EA, Chiplunkar R, Casale TB. CT scanning confirms beta receptor distribution is greater for smaller vs. larger airways. *Am J Respir Crit Care Med* 1997; 155:A855.
35. Ohrui T, Yanai M, Sekizawa K *et al*. Effective site of bronchodilation by beta-adrenergic and anti-cholinergic agents in patients with chronic obstructive pulmonary disease: Direct measurement of intrabronchial pressure with a new catheter. *Am Rev Respir Dis* 1992; 146:88–91.
36. Taylor DR *et al*. The efficacy of orally administered theophylline, inhaled salbutamol, and a combination of the two as chronic therapy in the management of chronic bronchitis with reversible air-flow obstruction. *Am Rev Respir Dis* 1985; 131:747–751.
37. Kirsten DK *et al*. Effects of theophylline withdrawal in severe chronic obstructive pulmonary disease. *Chest* 1993; 104:1101–1107.

38. Thomas P, Pugsley JA, Stewart JH. Theophylline and salbutamol improve pulmonary function in patients with irreversible chronic obstructive pulmonary disease. *Chest* 1992; 101:160–165.

39. Dullinger D, Kronenberg R, Niewoehner DE. Efficacy of inhaled metaproterenol and orally-administered theophylline in patients with chronic airflow obstruction. *Chest* 1986; 89:171–173.

40. Jenne JW. Theophylline as a bronchodilator in COPD and its combination with inhaled β-adrenergic drugs. *Chest* 1987; 92:S7–S14.

41. Tandon MK, Kailis SG. Bronchodilator treatment for partially reversible chronic obstructive airways disease. *Thorax* 1991; 46:248–251.

42. Mahler DA. Sustained-released theophylline reduces dyspnea in nonreversible obstructive airway disease. *Am Rev Respir Dis* 1985; 131:22–25.

43. Filuk RB, Easton PA, Anthonisen NR. Responses to large doses of salbutamol and theophylline in patients with chronic obstructive pulmonary disease. *Am Rev Respir Dis* 1985; 132:871–874.

44. Lamont H *et al*. The combined effect of theophylline and terbutaline in patients with chronic obstructive airway diseases. *Eur J Respir Dis* 1982; 63:13–22.

45. ZuWallach RL *et al*. Salmeterol plus theophylline combination therapy in the treatment of COPD. *Chest* 2001; 119:1661–1670.

46. Van Noord JA *et al*. A randomised controlled comparison of tiotropium and ipratropium in the treatment of chronic obstructive pulmonary disease. The Dutch Tiotropium Study Group. *Thorax* 2000; 55:289–294.

47. O'Donnell DE, Revill SM, Webb KA. Dynamic hyperinflation and exercise intolerance in chronic obstructive pulmonary disease. *Am J Respir Crit Care Med* 2001; 164:770–777.

48. Belman MJ, Botnick WC, Shin JW. Inhaled bronchodilators reduce dynamic hyperinflation during exercise in patients with chronic obstructive pulmonary disease. *Am J Respir Crit Care Med* 1996; 153:967–975.

49. O'Donnell DE, Lam M, Webb KA. Measurement of symptoms, lung hyperinflation, and endurance during exercise in chronic obstructive pulmonary disease. *Am J Respir Crit Care Med* 1998; 158(5 Pt 1):1557–1565.

50. Pellegrino R, Brusasco V. Lung hyperinflation and flow limitation in chronic airway obstruction. *Eur Respir J* 1997; 10:543–549.

51. O'Donnell DE. Assessment of bronchodilator efficacy in symptomatic COPD: is spirometry useful? *Chest* 2000; 117(2 suppl):S42–S47.

52. O'Donnell DE *et al*. Effects of tiotropium on lung hyperinflation, dyspnoea and exercise tolerance in COPD. *Eur Respir J* 2004; 23:832–840.

53. Bleecker ER, Britt EJ. Acute bronchodilating effects of ipratropium bromide and theophylline in chronic obstructive pulmonary disease. *Am J Med* 1991; 91:S24–S27.

54. Nishimura K *et al*. Is oral theophylline effective in combination with both inhaled anti-cholinergic agent and inhaled beta2-agonist in the treatment of stable COPD? *Chest* 1993; 104:179–184.

55. Nishimura K *et al*. The additive effect of theophylline on a high-dose combination of inhaled salbutamol and ipratropium bromide in stable COPD. *Chest* 1995; 107:718–723.

56. Aziz I, Lipworth BJ. *In vivo* effect of albuterol on methacholine-contracted bronchi in conjunction with salmeterol and formoterol. *J Allergy Clin Immunol* 1999; 103(5 Pt 1):816–822.

57. FitzGerald JM *et al*. Sustained bronchoprotection, bronchodilatation, and symptom control during regular formoterol use in asthma of moderate or greater severity. The Canadian FO/OD1 Study Group. *J Allergy Clin Immunol* 1999; 103(3 Pt 1):427–435.

58. Taylor D.R *et al*. Asthma control during long-term treatment with regular inhaled salbutamol and salmeterol. *Thorax* 1998; 53:744–752.

59. Liggett SB. Update on current concepts of the molecular basis of beta2-adrenergic receptor signaling. *J Allergy Clin Immunol* 2002; 110(6 suppl):S223–S228.

60. McCrory DC *et al*. Management of acute exacerbations of COPD. *Chest* 2001; 119:1190–1209.

61. Soto FJ, Varkey B. Evidence-based approach to acute exacerbations of COPD. *Curr Opin Pulm Med* 2003; 9:117–124.

62. Wessler I *et al*. The non-neuronal cholinergic system in humans: expression, function and pathophysiology. *Life Sci* 2003; 72:2055–2061.

63. Ito K *et al*. A molecular mechanism of action of theophylline: induction of histone deacetylase activity to decrease inflammatory gene expression. *Proc Natl Acad Sci USA* 2002; 99:8921–8926.

64. Cosio BG *et al*. Theophylline restores histone deacetylase activity and steroid responses in COPD macrophages. *J Exp Med* 2004; 200:689–695.

65. Gamble E et al. Antiinflammatory effects of the phosphodiesterase 4 inhibitor cilomilast (Ariflo) in COPD. Am J Resp Crit Care Med 2003; 168:976–982.

66. Levin DC et al. Ipratropium bromide inhalant solution delivered by small volume nebulizer persistently augments the extent and duration of FEV1 and FVC increases achieved by albuterol alone when compared over an 85-day period. Submitted.

67. Kilfeather SA et al. Improved delivery of ipratropium bromide/fenoterol from Respimat Soft Mist Inhaler in patients with COPD. Respir Med 2004; 98:387–397.

68. Gross N et al. Inhalation by nebulization of albuterol-ipratropium combination (Dey combination) is superior to either agent alone in the treatment of chronic obstructive pulmonary disease. Dey Combination Solution Study Group. Respiration 1998; 65:354–362.

69. Rammeloo RHU et al. Therapeutic equivalence of a fenoterol-ipratropium bromide combination (Berodual) inhaled as a dry powder and by metered dose inhaler in chronic obstructive airway disease. Respiration 1992; 59:322–326.

70. Morton O. Response to duovent of chronic reversible airways obstruction – a controlled trial in general practice. Postgrad Med J 1984; 60:32–35.

71. Hilleman DE et al. Pharmacoeconomic evaluation of COPD. Chest 2000; 118:1278–1285.

72. Benayoun S, Ernst P, Suissa S. The impact of combined inhaled bronchodilator therapy in the treatment of COPD. Chest 2001; 119:85–92.

73. Chrischilles E et al. Delivery of ipratropium and albuterol combination therapy for chronic obstructive pulmonary disease: effectiveness of a two-in-one inhaler versus separate inhalers. Am J Manag Care 2002; 8:902–911.

74. Poppius H et al. Exercise asthma and disodium cromoglycate. Br Med J 1970; 4:337–339.

75. Shrestha M et al. Decreased duration of emergency department treatment of chronic obstructive pulmonary disease exacerbations with the addition of ipratropium bromide to beta-agonist therapy. Ann Emerg Med 1991; 20:1206–1209.

76. Tashkin DP et al. Results of a multicenter study of nebulized inhalant bronchodilator solution. Am J Med 1996; 100:S62–S69.

77. Krivoy N et al. Combination therapy of ipratropium bromide, terbutaline and slow release theophylline in asthma and chronic airways obstruction. Postgrad Med J 1987; 63:21a.

78. Barros MJ, Rees PJ. Bronchodilator responses to salbutamol followed by ipratropium bromide in partially reversible airflow obstruction. Respir Med 1990; 84:371–375.

79. Brown IG et al. Assessment of the clinical usefulness of nebulised ipratropium bromide in patients with chronic airflow limitation. Thorax 1984; 39:272–276.

80. Group CIAS. In chronic obstructive pulmonary disease, a combination of ipratropium and albuterol is more effective than either agent alone. Chest 1994; 105:1411–1419.

81. Ikeda A et al. Bronchodilating effects of combined therapy with clinical dosages of ipratropium bromide and salbutamol for stable COPD: comparison with ipratropium bromide alone. Chest 1995; 107:401–405.

82. Lees AW Allan GW, Smith J. Nebulised ipratropium bromide and salbutamol in chronic bronchitis. Br J Clin Pract 1980; 34:340–342.

83. Levin DC et al. Addition of anti-cholinergic solution prolongs bronchodilator effect of beta 2 agonists in patients with chronic obstructive pulmonary disease. Am J Med 1996; 100:S40–S48.

84. Lightbody IM et al. Ipratropium bromide, salbutamol and prednisolone in bronchial asthma and chronic bronchitis. Br J Dis Chest 1978; 72:181–186.

85. Petrie GR, Palmer KNV. Comparison of aerosol ipratropium bromide and salbutamol in chronic bronchitis and asthma. Br Med J 1975; 1:430–432.

86. Ullah MI, Newman GB, Saunders KB. Influence of age on response to ipratropium and salbutamol in asthma. Thorax 1981; 36:523–529.

87. Sansores R et al. Effect of the combination of two bronchodilators on breathlessness in patients with chronic obstructive pulmonary disease. A crossover clinical trial. Arch Med Res 2003; 34:292–297.

88. Karpel JP et al. A comparison of inhaled ipratropium, oral theophylline plus inhaled beta-agonist, and the combination of all three in patients with COPD. Chest 1994; 105:1089–1094.

89. Dubois PEP et al. Bronchodilating and density dependence effects of fenoterol, ipratropium bromide and duovent in reversible chronic obstructive pulmonary disease. Respiration 1986; 50:280–284.

90. Huhti E, Poukkula A. Comparison of fenoterol, ipratropium bromide and their combination in patients with asthma or chronic airflow obstruction. Respiration 1986; 50:298–301.

91. Kaik G. The effect on total airways resistance (R_t) of adding Sch 1000 MDI to beta-adrenergics, and vice versa, in patients with chronic bronchitis and emphysema. Postgrad Med J 1975; 51:114–115.

92. Marlin GE, Berend N, Harrison AC. Combined cholinergic antagonist and beta2-adrenoceptor agonist bronchodilator therapy by inhalation. *Aust NZJ Med* 1979; 9:511–514.
93. Molkenboer JFWM, Cornelissen PJG. A double-blind randomized crossover study assessing the efficacy of Berodual in comparison to its components ipratropium bromide and fenoterol in chronic bronchitis. *Postgrad Med J* 1987; 63:19a.
94. Nossen GD *et al.* Berodual versus its single components fenoterol and ipratropium bromide. A placebo controlled trial in chronic bronchitis. *Postgrad Med J* 1987; 63:19a.
95. Tang OT, Flatley M. A comparison of effects on inhaling a combined preparation of fenoterol with ipratropium bromide (Duovent) with those of fenoterol and salbutamol. *Postgrad Med J* 1984; 60:24–27.
96. Frith PA, Jenner B, Atkinson J. Effects of inhaled oxitropium and fenoterol, alone and in combination, in chronic airflow obstruction. *Respiration* 1986; 50:294–297.
97. Cazzola M *et al.* The pharmacodynamic effects of single inhaled doses of formoterol, tiotropium and their combination in patients with COPD. *Pulm Pharmacol Ther* 2004; 17:35–39.
98. Chapman KR *et al.* The addition of salmeterol 50 microg bid to anti-cholinergic treatment in patients with COPD: a randomized, placebo controlled trial. Chronic obstructive pulmonary disease. *Can Respir J* 2002; 9:178–185.
99. van Noord JA *et al.* Long-term treatment of chronic obstructive pulmonary disease with salmeterol and the additive effect of ipratropium. *Eur Respir J* 2000; 15:878–885.
100. Cazzola M *et al.* The functional impact of adding salmeterol and tiotropium in patients with stable COPD. *Respir Med* 2004; 98:1214–1221.

10

Corticosteroids: basic pharmacology

G. Caramori, I. M. Adcock

INTRODUCTION

Chronic obstructive pulmonary disease (COPD) is amongst the commonest diseases in the world, with an alarming increase in global prevalence [1]. Cigarette smoking is the major risk factor for the development of COPD and cigarette smokers constitute over 90% of COPD patients in developed countries. The incidence of COPD is rising worldwide and there is a need to develop new treatments to prevent the progression of the disease, which results in a large consumption of health care resources [2]. COPD involves fixed airflow limitation and chronic inflammation of the lower airways and is characterised by the expression of multiple inflammatory proteins, including cytokines, chemokines, adhesion molecules, enzymes producing inflammatory mediators and inflammatory mediator receptors [2, 3]. Most of these proteins are regulated at the transcriptional level, suggesting that in both diseases transcription factors may play an important role [4, 5]. Nuclear factor-kappaB (NF-κB) regulates many of the genes that are abnormally expressed in COPD and is activated in the lower airways of patients with COPD [6]. One clear difference between COPD and other chronic inflammatory diseases of the lower airways such as asthma is the clinical responsiveness to corticosteroids.

Even high doses of inhaled or oral corticosteroids are virtually ineffective in patients with COPD compared to the marked responses seen in asthma, suggesting that the inflammation in COPD is essentially steroid resistant [2]. In COPD, there is a marked increase in oxidative stress which may contribute to corticosteroid-insensitivity [7, 8]. Understanding the molecular mechanisms involved may lead to the development of an effective therapeutic strategy for COPD [9, 10].

COPD IS A CHRONIC INFLAMMATORY DISEASE OF THE LOWER AIRWAYS

COPD can be defined as 'a disease state characterised by airflow limitation that is not fully reversible. The airflow limitation is usually both progressive and associated with an abnormal inflammatory response of the lungs to noxious particles or gases' [11]. This chronic inflammatory process within the lower airways is enhanced during exacerbations [2]. The pathological hallmarks of COPD are destruction of the lung parenchyma (pulmonary emphysema), inflammation, mucus plugging and fibrosis of the peripheral airways (obstructive respiratory bronchiolitis) [12] and inflammation of the central airways [13]. Pathological studies show

Ian Michael Adcock, PhD, Professor of Respiratory Cell and Molecular Biology, Airways Disease Section, National Heart & Lung Institute, Imperial College, London, UK.

Gaetano Caramori, MD, PhD, Centro di Ricerca su Asma e BPCO, Università di Ferrara, Ferrara, Italy.

that inflammation in COPD occurs in the central and peripheral airways (bronchioles) and lung parenchyma [13]. Most patients with COPD have all three pathological conditions (chronic obstructive bronchitis/bronchiolitis, emphysema and mucus plugging), but the relative extent of emphysema and obstructive bronchitis within individual patients can vary widely [14]. There is a marked increase in macrophages and neutrophils in bronchoalveolar lavage (BAL) and induced sputum [13]. Patients with COPD have infiltration of T cells (with an increased ratio between CD8+ and CD4+ T cells), macrophages and an increased number of neutrophils within the bronchial mucosa and lung parenchyma [13]. The bronchioles are obstructed by fibrosis and mucus plugging and infiltrated predominantly by macrophages and T-lymphocytes. In contrast to the situation with asthma, eosinophils are not prominent except in patients with concomitant asthma or in some patients during exacerbations [13].

In COPD there is a marked increase in local and systemic oxidative stress [7, 8, 15], particularly during exacerbations [16]. Most striking are the increases in reactive oxygen and nitrogen species such as 4-hydroxynonenal, acrolein, nitro-tyrosine, hydrogen peroxide and 8-isoprostane that have been reported in sputum, BAL, exhaled breath condensate and urine [17–20]. Oxidative stress is increased because of the high concentration of oxidants in cigarette smoke, the production of oxidants by activated inflammatory cells and a reduction in endogenous antioxidant mechanisms.

Although the diagnosis, the assessment of severity, and the monitoring of COPD still rely on lung function tests, there is an increasing interest to characterise the type and intensity of airway inflammation, and to investigate whether they provide useful information for the management of this disease. For example, COPD patients with a significant reversibility after a course of glucocorticoids have the pathological characteristics of asthma [21].

CLINICAL PHARMACOLOGY OF CORTICOSTEROIDS IN COPD

The role of corticosteroids in the management of COPD remains controversial. The Global Initiative for Chronic Obstructive Lung Disease (GOLD) guidelines [11] state that regular treatment with inhaled corticosteroids (ICS), alone or in combination with inhaled long-acting β_2-agonists should be prescribed only to severe COPD patients with an FEV_1 <50% of predicted value, and repeated exacerbations requiring treatment with antibiotics and/or oral corticosteroids.

ICSs are commonly prescribed in high doses, and in some countries are used as frequently in patients with COPD as in those with asthma, but evidence for a beneficial effect in patients with pure COPD is weak. Long-term clinical trials with high doses of ICS in the treatment of stable COPD have been disappointing, as they do not appear to arrest the progressive decline in lung function even when treatment was started before the disease became symptomatic and have a small and inconsistent effect on symptoms, quality of life (QOL), or severity and number of exacerbations (Table 10.1). At the same time this treatment, particularly when prolonged for many years, can produce systemic adverse effects, including skin bruising, adrenal suppression, cataracts and loss of bone density [11, 22, 23]. However, not all studies report a significant change in bone density [24]. Responsiveness to ICS may be severity-dependent [22, 25]. Thus, treatment of patients with stage 3 COPD with ICS results in improved exacerbation rates [25] and quality-adjusted life expectancy seemingly without additional cost compared to other therapies [26]. Although it is well known that corticosteroids are effective at suppressing airway inflammation in asthma, their effects on lower airways inflammation in COPD is still controversial.

CLINICAL EFFECTS OF CORTICOSTEROIDS IN COPD

The evidence for clinical effectiveness of oral or ICS in COPD is weak except in patients with some asthmatic/eosinophilic component [27].

Table 10.1   Effects of inhaled and systemic corticosteroids in COPD

Study	Lung function[1]	QOL	Exacerbations	Side-effects	Ref
ICS in stable COPD					
Placebo-controlled – 1 year or longer					
ISOLDE	No effect	↑	↓		[22]
EUROSCOP	No effect				[34]
Copenhagen City Lung Study	No effect		No effect		[28]
Lung Health Study	No effect	↑	↓	↑	[35]
TRISTAN	↑	↑	↓	↑[2]	[112]
Calverley et al., 2003	No effect	↑	No effect	No effect	[113]
Szafranski et al., 2003	↑	No effect	↓	No effect	[114]
Placebo-controlled – less than 1 year					
Gizycki et al., 2002					[69]
Hanania et al., 2003	↑	↑	No effect	↑[2]	[120]
Hattotuwa et al., 2002					[71]
Mahler et al., 2002	↑	No effect	No effect	↑[2]	[121]
Paggiaro et al., 1998			↓		[39]
Thompson et al., 2002	↑				[38]
Withdrawal studies					
COPE	↑	↑	↓		[43]
O'Brien et al., 2001	↑	↑	↓		[42]
Systemic corticosteroids Stable COPD					
Rice et al., 2000	No effect	No effect	No effect	↑[3]	[122]
Exacerbations					
Aaron et al., 2003	↑	No effect	↓	↑	[123]
Davies et al.,	↑		↓		[46]
Niewoehner 2002	↑		↓	↑	[49]

[1]Rate of decline in FEV_1
[2]Oropharyngeal candidiasis
[3]Body mass index

DIFFERENTIAL DIAGNOSIS BETWEEN ASTHMA AND COPD

In the past a short (1–2 weeks) trial with high doses of systemic glucocorticoids has often been used in the differential diagnosis between asthma and COPD [28]. In fact a clinical trial has shown that COPD patients with high BAL eosinophil counts and a thickened basement membrane improved their forced expiratory volume in one second (FEV_1) by >12% after 2 weeks prednisolone [21]. Similar FEV_1 responsiveness and improvements in QOL scores have also been reported and found to correlate with reductions in sputum eosinophilia but not with changes in neutrophils or neutrophil proteases [29]. Patients without sputum eosinophilia did not show clinical benefit from short-term prednisone therapy [29]. Furthermore, in a trial of high-dose inhaled beclomethasone dipropionate (3,000 μg per day for 4 weeks) only those subjects with an asthma component showed any improvement in FEV_1 [30].

However, evidence from the ISOLDE study suggests that prednisolone testing is an unreliable predictor of the benefit from inhaled fluticasone propionate in individual patients and that patients with COPD cannot be separated into discrete groups of corticosteroid responders and non-responders according to a short-term prednisolone trial [31]. Future research should examine the mechanisms underlying this difference in responsiveness and any clinical biomarkers that may be associated with this. It can be argued therefore, that as recommended in the GOLD guidelines, all patients with COPD should undergo a formal trial (3 months) of ICS to determine whether or not they respond to prednisolone [32, 33].

EFFECTS ON STABLE COPD PATIENTS

When asthmatic patients were rigorously excluded from patients with COPD, four large studies in Europe and the USA all failed to show any clinically relevant effect on the rate of decline in FEV_1 [22, 28, 34, 35]. In addition, a small, possibly, underpowered population-based study [36] reported no effect on mortality and morbidity of ICS treatment following hospitalisation for COPD and no reduction in the risk of an exacerbation [37].

However, recent findings suggest that corticosteroids may be effective in more severe disease. Thus, treatment with an ICS for >3 months improved pre-bronchodilator airflow limitation and oxygenation while decreasing dyspnoea in patients with moderate-to-severe COPD [38]. In addition, the severity of exacerbations was reduced in patients with moderate-to-severe COPD who were treated for 6 months with high doses of inhaled fluticasone [39]. Furthermore, subgroup analysis of the ISOLDE study reported that 3 years of regular treatment with high doses of inhaled fluticasone resulted in fewer exacerbations, a reduced rate of decline in health status, and higher FEV_1 values in patients with moderate-to-severe disease [22]. Overall, there appears to be a significant improvement in exacerbation rates [40] and survival in patients with ICS [41].

Importantly, withdrawal of ICS therapy has been shown to lead to deterioration in ventilatory function, increased exercise-induced dyspnoea, increased severity and rate of exacerbations and a decrease in QOL in patients with severe irreversible airway limitation [42]. Interestingly, 40% of the subjects in the COPE study experienced no untoward effect from the withdrawal of ICSs, suggesting a large subgroup of responders and non-responders, although this needs to be confirmed in other studies. For this reason the recently published ATS/ERS guidelines on COPD suggest that when therapy with inhaled glucocorticoids is thought to be ineffective, a trial with the withdrawal of treatment is reasonable. Some patients will exacerbate when this occurs, which is a reason for re-instituting this therapy [44]. In contrast, discontinuation of chronic systemic glucocorticoid treatment in glucocorticoid-dependent COPD patients does not cause a significant increase in COPD exacerbations, but did result in reduced body weight [45].

In view of the well-known side-effects of long-term treatment with oral glucocorticoids, it is not surprising that no prospective studies have been performed on the long-term effects of these drugs in COPD [11]. Therefore, based on the lack of evidence of benefit, and the large body of evidence of side-effects, long-term treatment with oral glucocorticoids is not recommended in COPD [11]. The results of the forthcoming large randomised trials (e.g., TORCH) with mortality as an outcome will help clarify the role of inhaled glucocorticoids in stable COPD.

EFFECTS ON COPD EXACERBATIONS

Results from recent clinical trials indicate that systemic corticosteroids have a significant though modest effect in shortening the duration of severe exacerbations of COPD [46, 47]. Thus, systemic corticosteroids administered intravenously or orally to hospitalised patients with exacerbations of COPD reduced the absolute treatment failure rate by about 10%, increased the FEV_1 by about 100 ml, and shortened the hospital stay by 1–2 days. Furthermore, oral corticosteroids probably give similar results in the treating of moderately severe COPD exacerbations in an out-patient setting. It is unclear what the optimal starting dose should be and the treatment should not be given for longer than 2 weeks since maximal benefit appears to occur within the first 72 h of treatment [48]. Not unsurprisingly, adverse events occur with hyperglycemia being the most common adverse event, but secondary infections (pneumonia), psychosis, and myopathies may also occur [48, 49].

EFFECTS OF ICS ON INFLAMMATION IN ASTHMA

ICSs clearly reverse the chronic inflammation seen in the airways of asthmatic patients [50–53]. This results in a marked reduction in the number of mast cells, macrophages, T-lymphocytes and eosinophils in the sputum, BAL and bronchial wall [54, 55]. Furthermore, at higher concentrations, ICSs reverse the epithelial shedding, goblet-cell hyperplasia and basement membrane thickening characteristic of asthmatic biopsies [52, 56]. The inflammatory component of asthmatic airways most responsive to glucocorticoid treatment seems to be eosinophilic inflammation. In *in vitro* experiments, corticosteroids decrease cytokine-mediated survival of eosinophils by stimulating apoptosis [57]. This process may explain the reduction in the number of eosinophils in the circulation and airways of patients during ICS therapy [54, 58]. In general, corticosteroids substantially reduce the mast cell/eosinophil/lymphocyte-driven processes, while leaving behind or even augmenting a neutrophil-mediated process [59]. In addition to their suppressive effects on inflammatory cells, corticosteroids may also inhibit plasma exudation [60, 61] and mucus secretion [62, 63] in inflamed airways. Not all of these parameters have been investigated in COPD.

EFFECTS OF ICS ON INFLAMMATION IN COPD

Whilst some studies suggest that ICS may be clinically effective and have changes in inflammatory parameters in COPD, many other studies have reported little or no effect on inflammatory cells and mediators in the sputum or biopsies of patients with stable COPD [27] (Table 10.2).

In vitro, corticosteroids attenuate neutrophil recruitment and activation [64], and reduce neutrophil chemotaxis [65] whilst *in vivo*, they attenuate sputum chemotactic activity, increase neutrophil elastase inhibitory capacity [66], and in non-placebo-controlled clinical trials decrease neutrophil and total cell counts in induced sputum [67, 68]. However, a placebo-controlled clinical trial has reported that ICS therapy results in an increase in neutrophil numbers [69]. Dexamethasone, *in vitro*, can also reduce fibronectin digestion by neutrophils from COPD patients in a concentration-dependent manner [70]. Moreover, inhaled fluticasone (500 µg bid, 12 weeks) reduced in bronchial biopsies the numbers of mucosal and subepithelial mast cells in mild-to-moderate COPD patients without affecting mononuclear cell numbers [69]. Fluticasone was also reported to reduce in bronchial mucosa the epithelial CD8/CD4 ratio [71], again without significantly affecting macrophage numbers, although an effect on macrophage numbers in bronchial mucosa has been reported in another study [72]. In non-placebo-controlled clinical trials, ICSs have been reported to induce significant reductions in BAL IL-8 and myeloperoxidase levels, as well as reductions in cell numbers, the proportion of neutrophils, symptom score and bronchitis index [73]. Furthermore, beclamethasone has shown to significantly reduce exhaled NO levels in a small group of COPD patients without affecting hydrogen peroxide levels in their breath condensate [74].

The findings reported above (and Table 10.2) would seem to support the use of ICSs in treating COPD, although long-term treatment with ICSs must be associated with a high risk of adverse systemic effects [75]. However, other placebo-controlled clinical trials examining the effects of ICS in COPD and *in vitro* data have reported conflicting results [75, 76]. ICSs, often even in high doses, have been reported not to reduce inflammatory cells [77], mediators or proteases in induced sputum or bronchial biopsies of patients with COPD [71, 77–79]. It is clear, however, that recommended doses of ICS do not affect fracture risk in COPD patients [80] or bone mineral density [81], although some effects on bruising and wound healing are seen [81]. The risk of fracture in patients on high dose ICS is currently unclear.

Table 10.2 Effects of ICS on inflammation in COPD

	Ref
Positive studies with ICS in COPD	
In vitro	
Reduce neutrophil recruitment, chemotaxis and activation	[64, 65]
Reduce fibronectin degradation by neutrophils	[70]
Reduce neutrophil elastase activity and sputum chemotaxis	[66]
Non-placebo-controlled clinical trials	
Reduce neutrophil and total cell counts	[67, 68]
Reduce BAL IL-8 and myeloperoxidase levels	[73]
Placebo-controlled clinical trials	
In bronchial biopsies reduce mast cell number	[69]
In bronchial biopsies reduce CD8/CD4 ratio	[71]
In bronchial biopsies reduce macrophage number	[72]
Reduce exhaled NO levels	[74]
Negative studies with ICS in COPD	
In vitro	
No suppression of IL-8 and TNF-α	[85]
No suppression of MMP9 or elastin expression	[83–85]
No effect on ROS production	[86]
Placebo-controlled clinical trials	
In bronchial biopsies, increase neutrophil numbers and no reduction in macrophages, CD3, CD4, CD8, mast cells, eosinophils, CD1a+ and CD15+ cells	[69, 71, 72, 77]
No effect on sputum cell numbers	[79]
No effect on hydrogen peroxide levels in exhaled breath condensate	[74]
No effect on inflammatory mediators including sputum NOS2, IL-8, TNF-α, EPO, MPO, NHL, ECP , MMP1, MMP9, TIMP-1 or SLPI	[77–79]

It has recently been demonstrated that there is a resistance to corticosteroids at the level of single cells in patients with COPD. Alveolar macrophages, activated by endotoxin and cigarette smoke-conditioned medium (CSM), release TNF-α, IL-8 and MMP9. There is a greater release of these inflammatory proteins from alveolar macrophages from cigarette smokers with normal lung function (normal smokers) than from macrophages derived from non-smoking normal individuals, whereas there is an even greater spontaneous and stimulated release from macrophages derived from patients with COPD [82–84]. The release of these inflammatory proteins is suppressed by corticosteroids in normal macrophages, is reduced in normal smokers, but in patients with COPD, corticosteroids are much less effective [85]. This suggests that there may be an active molecular mechanism of steroid resistance in alveolar macrophages from patients with COPD. In addition, fluticasone had no effect on oxidant production from BAL macrophages from smoking COPD patients after 6 months treatment [86]. The reasons for these differences are currently unclear.

Systemic inflammation is also present in COPD and has been linked to cardiovascular morbidity and mortality. Withdrawal of ICS in 41 patients with mild-to-moderate COPD increased baseline C-reactive protein (CRP) levels significantly, whereas restoration of increasing doses of fluticasone was associated with reduced CRP levels. Thus, inhaled and oral corticosteroids are effective in reducing serum CRP levels in patients with COPD and suggest a potential use for improving cardiovascular outcomes in COPD [87].

MOLECULAR MECHANISM OF ACTION OF CORTICOSTEROIDS

Corticosteroids are 21-carbon steroid hormones (Figure 10.1) composed of four rings [88, 89]. Modern topical corticosteroids are based on the cortisol structure with modification to enhance the anti-inflammatory effects such as insertion of a C=C double bond at C1, C2 or by the introduction of 6α-fluoro, 6α-methyl, 9α-fluoro and/or further substitutions with α-hydroxyl, α-methyl or β-methyl at the 16 position, for example in dexamethasone (Figure 10.1). Lipophilic substituents, for example, 16α-, 17α-acetals, 17α-esters or 21α-esters attached to the D ring were found to further enhance receptor affinity, prolong local topical deposition and enhance hepatic metabolism and are exemplified by the structures of budesonide and fluticasone (Figure 10.1). However, the exact structural and lipophilic requirements to optimise corticosteroid pharmacokinetics, tissue retention and longevity of action are still unclear and corticosteroids with improved clinical characteristics are likely to be synthesised as our knowledge in this area increases.

Classically corticosteroids exert their effects by binding to a single 777 amino acid receptor, glucocorticoid receptor (GR) that is localised to the cytoplasm of target cells. GRs are expressed in almost all cell types and their density varies from 200 to 30,000 per cell [90] with an affinity for cortisol of ~30 nM, which falls within the normal range for plasma concentrations of free hormone. GR has several functional domains (Figure 10.2). The corticosteroid ligand-binding domain (LBD) is at the carboxyl terminus of the molecule and is separated from the DNA-binding domain (DBD) by a hinge region. There is an N-terminal transactivation domain that is involved in activation of genes once binding to DNA has occurred. This region may also be involved in binding to other transcription factors. The inactive GR is part of a large protein complex (~300 kDa) that includes two subunits of the

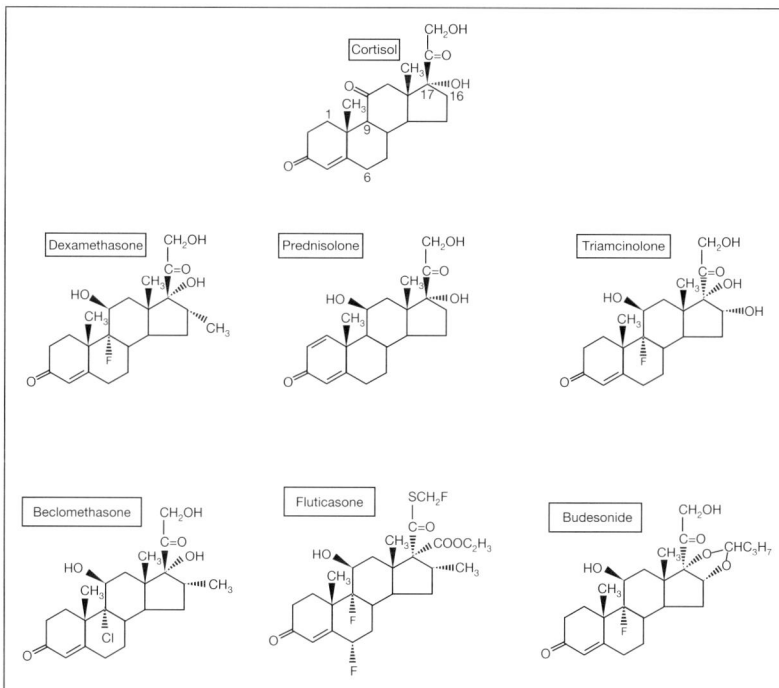

Figure 10.1 Structural modifications of cortisol that produce the clinically used corticosteroids dexamethasone, prednisolone, triamcinolone, beclomethasone, fluticasone and budesonide.

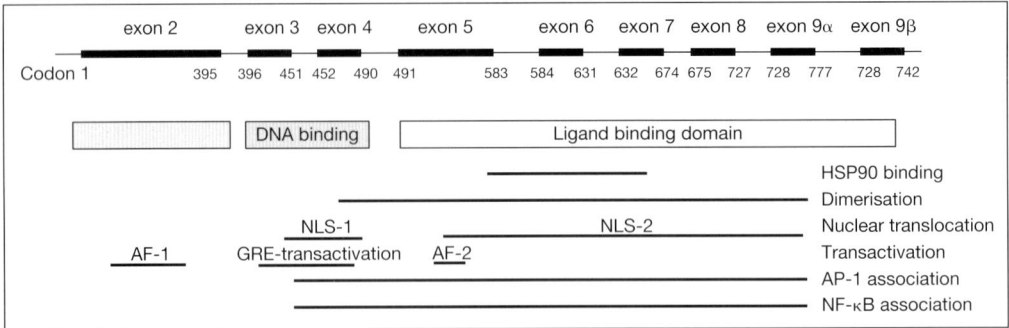

Figure 10.2 Modular structure of the corticosteroid receptor (glucocorticoid receptor, GR). The coding region of GR results from splicing together of exons 2–9 of the GR gene. The GRβ isoform of GR results from the use of the short 9β exon which removes the ligand-binding domain seen in GRα. The modular design of GR enables distinct regions of the protein to function in isolation as ligand-binding domains, dimerisation domains, nuclear localisation domains, transactivation and transrepression (AP-1 and NF-κB interacting) domains. NLS: nuclear localisation signal; AF-1/2: activating factor 1/2; GRE: glucocorticoid response element (composed of two palindromic half sites (AGAACA) separated by three nucleotides).

heat shock protein hsp90, which blocks the nuclear localisation of GR and one molecule of the immunophilin p59 [90].

Corticosteroids are thought to freely diffuse from the circulation into cells across the cell membrane and bind to cytoplasmic GR (Figure 10.3). Once the corticosteroid binds to GR, hsp90 dissociates allowing the nuclear localisation of the activated GR-cortisteroid complex and its binding to DNA [90]. GR combines with another GR to form a dimer at consensus DNA sites termed glucocorticoid response elements (GREs) in the regulating regions of corticosteroid-responsive genes. This interaction allows GR to associate with a complex of DNA-protein modifying and remodelling proteins including steroid receptor coactivator-1 (SRC-1) and CREB binding protein (CBP), which produce a DNA-protein structure that allows enhanced gene transcription [90]. The particular ligand and the number of GREs and their position relative to the transcriptional start site may be an important determinant of the magnitude of the transcriptional response to corticosteroids [90].

The GR complex can regulate gene products in at least four other ways. Firstly, GR acting as a monomer can bind directly, or indirectly, with the transcription factors activator protein-1 (AP-1) and NF-κB, which are up-regulated during inflammation, thereby inhibiting the pro-inflammatory effects of a variety of cytokines [90]. Secondly, the GR dimer can bind to a GRE which overlaps the DNA-binding site for a pro-inflammatory transcription factor or the start site of transcription thus blocking gene expression [90]. Thirdly, the GR dimer can induce the expression of the NF-κB inhibitor IκBα in certain cell types [91]. Lastly, corticosteroids can increase the levels of cell ribonucleases and mRNA destabilising proteins, thereby reducing the levels of mRNA [92] (Figure 10.3). However, it is becoming clear the context in which GR is seen by a specific gene promoter can have profound effects on GR function. For example, GR activated in the presence of TNF-α, with or without the presence of IFNγ, can markedly up-regulate Toll-like receptor (TLR)2 expression *via* a mechanism involving an interaction between GR, NF-κB and STAT protein [93, 94]. It is likely that the altered transcription of many different genes is involved in the anti-inflammatory action of corticosteroids, but the drugs' most important action may be to inhibit transcription of cytokine and chemokine genes implicated in inflammation [90]. Evidence for this has been described in a series of elegant experiments using mice expressing mutated GRs unable to dimerise and subsequently bind to DNA. Thus, Reichardt and colleagues [95, 96] have confirmed a role for GR

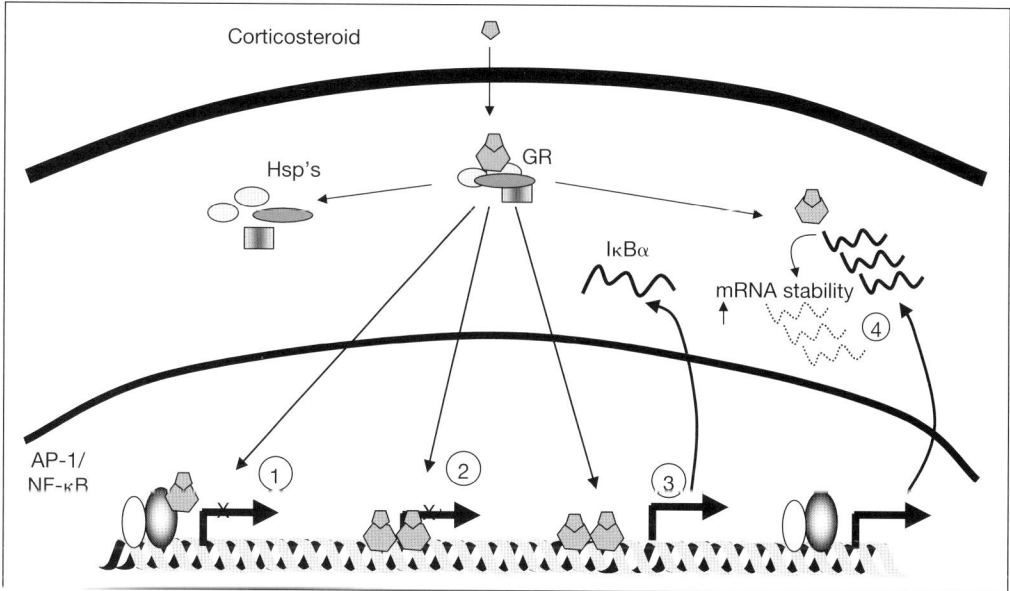

Figure 10.3 Mechanisms of gene repression by the corticosteroid receptor. The corticosteroid can freely migrate across the plasma membrane where it associates with the cytoplasmic corticosteroid receptor (glucocorticoid receptor, GR). This results in activation of the GR and dissociation from the heat shock protein (hsp90)-chaperone complex. Activated GR translocates to the nucleus where it can bind as a monomer either directly or indirectly with the transcription factors activator protein-1 (AP-1) and nuclear factor kappaB (NF-κB) preventing their ability to switch on inflammatory gene expression (1). Secondly, the GR dimer can bind to a GRE that overlaps the DNA binding site for a pro-inflammatory transcription factor or the start site of transcription to prevent inflammatory gene expression (2). Thirdly, the GR dimer can induce the expression of the NF-κB inhibitor IκBα (3) and fourthly, corticosteroids can increase the levels of cell ribonucleases and mRNA destabilising proteins, thereby reducing the levels of mRNA (4).

DNA binding as a dimer in the control of pro-opiomelanocortin (POMC) expression and T-cell apoptosis but not in that of inflammatory genes regulated by AP-1 or NF-κB.

EFFECTS OF OXIDATIVE STRESS ON GR FUNCTION

The relative lack of response to corticosteroids has been linked to oxidative stress. Cigarette smoking is the primary cause of COPD, and the smoke contains more than 10^{18} oxidant molecules per puff [18, 97]. This suggests that oxidative stress may be an important factor in inducing corticosteroid resistance in COPD. The resistance may be due to cigarette smoking itself, since corticosteroids are much less effective in reducing inflammatory cells in BAL and sputum from smoking asthmatic patients compared with non-smoking patients [98, 99]. The resistance to corticosteroid action is maintained even in subjects who are no longer smoking. This implies that either the oxidant stress is persistent or that the initial chronic insult permanently alters the expression of a component involved in corticosteroid action. There is good evidence for prolonged persistence of oxidative stress involving long-acting lipid peroxidation products such as 4-hydroxynonenal and isoprostanes and a reduction in the anti-oxidant protein gamma-glutamylcysteine synthetase [18, 97].

Okamoto et al. [100] have suggested that oxidative stress may influence corticosteroid function by inhibiting GR nuclear translocation. Indeed, we have recently reported that many patients with severe corticosteroid-insensitive asthma have a defect in GR nuclear translocation [101]. Of interest is the fact that respiratory viruses are important exacerbation triggers [102] and recent evidence has suggested that rhinoviral infection can reduce GR nuclear transloca-tion and reduced corticosteroid function [103]. In further experiments, we have reported that cigarette smoke can suppress GR-function without affecting nuclear translocation [104].

Other potential causes of reduced corticosteroid function involve nuclear events. Histone deacetylases (HDACs) are important for corticosteroid-mediated suppression of NF-κB activity and the expression and activity of HDAC2 is decreased in BAL macrophages and biopsy specimens from smokers and patients with COPD [105]. This decrease in HDAC2 activity correlates with increased inflammatory gene expression and reduced responsive-ness to corticosteroids [106] and can be mimicked by pre-treatment of macrophages with hydrogen peroxide [106]. This reduction in HDAC2 activity and expression by oxidative stress relates to nitration of tyrosine residues within the active site of HDAC2, possibly leading to an initial loss of activity prior to HDAC2 degradation in the proteosome [107]. The results suggest that oxidative stress, by repression of HDAC activity, can enhance the inflammatory response and modulate corticosteroid function in BAL macrophages.

IMPROVING CORTICOSTEROID RESPONSIVENESS IN COPD

Many new drugs are now in development for the treatment of COPD. There has been an intensive search for anti-inflammatory treatments that are as effective as glucocorticoids but with fewer side-effects [108]. Whereas one approach is to seek glucocorticoids with a greater therapeutic effect, other approaches involve developing different classes of anti-inflammatory drugs [108]. It would be expected that anti-oxidants should be anti-inflammatory and also improve steroid function in COPD but currently available drugs lack *in vivo* potency [109, 110]. Preliminary *in vitro* and *in vivo* data suggest that the combination of long-acting inhaled β$_2$-agonists and inhaled glucocorticoids may have a synergistic effect [111]. The results of the first large clinical trials of combination therapy in COPD have recently been published and it shows that combination therapy produces better control of symptoms and lung function, with no greater risk of side-effects than that with use of either component alone [111–114]. Further large scale, long-term clinical studies to evaluate the exacerbation rates and the decline of FEV$_1$ in COPD patients treated with the combination therapy are underway.

The elucidation of the molecular mechanisms of glucocorticoids raises the possibility that novel nonsteroidal anti-inflammatory treatments might be developed that mimic the actions of glucocorticoids on inflammatory gene regulation. Activation of HDACs may have thera-peutic potential, and theophylline has been shown to have this property, resulting in marked potentiation of the anti-inflammatory effects of glucocorticoids both *in vitro* and *in vivo* [115]. This action of theophylline is not mediated *via* phosphodiesterase inhibition or adeno-sine receptor antagonism and, therefore, appears to be a novel action of theophylline [115]. It may be possible to discover similar drugs that could form the basis of a new class of anti-inflammatory drugs without the side-effects that limit the use of theophylline [115].

Many of the anti-inflammatory effects of glucocorticoids appear to be mediated *via* inhi-bition of the transcriptional effects of NF-κB, and small-molecule inhibitors of IKK-2, which activate NF-κB, are in development. However, glucocorticoids have additional effects, so it is uncertain whether IKK-2 inhibitors will parallel the clinical effectiveness of glucocorti-coids. They may have side-effects, such as increased susceptibility to infections, however, as a corollary to this, if glucocorticoids were discovered today, they would be unlikely to be used in humans because of the low therapeutic ratio and their side-effect profile [116]. p38 mitogen-activated protein kinase (MAPK) inhibitors also have therapeutic potential as glucocorticoid-sparing agents [117–119].

There is a pressing need to develop drugs to prevent and treat the exacerbations and to prevent the progression of COPD [11]. Even if the several classes of new drugs currently in preclinical and clinical development prove effective, except for phosphodiesterase 4 inhibitors, no innovative treatment is likely to become available for use in COPD patients within the next 5 years. This should encourage future intensive research on the cellular and molecular pathogenesis of COPD, with the hope that a better understanding of the mechanisms of COPD will provide new targets for the development of drugs.

NEW DEVICES FOR THE ADMINISTRATION OF INHALED GLUCOCORTICOIDS

The principal site of airflow limitation in COPD is the small airways (<2 mm in diameter) [105]. The chronic airflow limitation present in patients with COPD is due to a combination of small airways disease, and loss of lung elasticity due to destruction of the lung parenchyma (emphysema) but the relative extent of obstructive bronchitis and emphysema within individual patients can vary [117]. Recently, the introduction of hydrofluoroalkanes (HFAs) as propellants in pressurised metered-dose inhalers (pMDIs) has allowed for the erogation of smaller particles of the drug and increased by 4- to 5-fold lung deposition and increased delivery of the drug to the small airways [118]. Treatment with ICS administered with HFAs-based pMDIs allows similar control of asthma symptoms with lower doses of the same drug as when administered through non-HFA pMDIs devices [118]. It is tempting to speculate that the long-term treatment of COPD with these new HFAs-based pMDIs could potentially improve ICS efficacy. However, the efficacy of these drugs administered to COPD patients through the new HFAs-based pMDIs has never been investigated in large, long-term, controlled clinical studies [119].

CONCLUSIONS

Apart from a few exceptions, COPD is caused by tobacco smoking, and smoking cessation is the only truly effective treatment of COPD. Once smoking has caused COPD, the disease is still largely irreversible and progressive. Current pharmacological treatment of COPD is unsatisfactory, as it does not significantly influence the severity of the disease or its natural course. Bronchodilators are the only pharmacological treatment that improve symptoms, QOL, and lung function in COPD patients, but they do not significantly influence the natural course of the disease. Apart from the treatment of exacerbations, systemic and inhaled glucocorticoids have not been shown to be consistently effective in COPD, either in reducing symptoms or for improving lung function and the course of the disease. Even if the new anti-inflammatory drugs for COPD that are in the pipeline prove fruitful, no really innovative treatment options are likely to be available in the next 5 years. This rather nihilistic conclusion should encourage further research on the pathogenesis of COPD, with the hope that a better understanding of the mechanisms of its development and evolution will provide valuable information for novel drug development.

ACKNOWLEDGEMENTS

Work in our groups is supported by Associazione per la Ricerca e la Cura dell'Asma (ARCA, Padua, Italy), Asthma UK, The British Lung Foundation, The Clinical Research Committee (Brompton Hospital), The National Institutes of Health (USA), AstraZeneca, Boehringer Ingelheim, GlaxoSmithKline (UK) and Mitsubishi (Japan).

REFERENCES

1. Lopez AD, Murray CC. The global burden of disease, 1990–2020. *Nat Med* 1998; 4:1241–1243.
2. Barnes PJ. Chronic obstructive pulmonary disease. *N Engl J Med* 2000; 343:269–280.
3. Caramori G, Adcock I. Pharmacology of airway inflammation in asthma and COPD. *Pulm Pharmacol Ther* 2003; 16:247–277.
4. Barnes PJ, Adcock IM. Transcription factors and asthma. *Eur Respir J* 1998; 12:221–234.
5. Barnes PJ. Mechanisms in COPD: differences from asthma. *Chest* 2000; 117:S10–S14.

6.   Di Stefano A, Caramori G, Oates T, Capelli A, Lusuardi M, Gnemmi I *et al*. Increased expression of nuclear factor-kB in bronchial biopsies from smokers and patients with COPD. *Eur Respir J* 2002; 20:556–563.
7.   Montuschi P, Collins JV, Ciabattoni G, Lazzeri N, Corradi M, Kharitonov SA, Barnes PJ. Exhaled 8-isoprostane as an *in vivo* biomarker of lung oxidative stress in patients with COPD and healthy smokers. *Am J Respir Crit Care Med* 2000; 162:1175–1177.
8.   Paredi P, Kharitonov SA, Leak D, Ward S, Cramer D, Barnes PJ. Exhaled ethane, a marker of lipid peroxidation, is elevated in chronic obstructive pulmonary disease. *Am J Respir Crit Care Med* 2000; 162:369–373.
9.   Barnes PJ. Genetics and pulmonary medicine. 9. Molecular genetics of chronic obstructive pulmonary disease. *Thorax* 1999; 54:245–252.
10. Barnes PJ. New treatments for chronic obstructive pulmonary disease. *Curr Opin Pharmacol* 2001; 1:217–222.
11. Pauwels RA, Buist AS, Ma P, Jenkins CR, Hurd SS. Global strategy for the diagnosis, management, and prevention of chronic obstructive pulmonary disease: National Heart, Lung, and Blood Institute and World Health Organization Global Initiative for Chronic Obstructive Lung Disease (GOLD): executive summary. *Respir Care* 2001; 46:798–825.
12. Hogg JC, Chu F, Utokaparch S, Woods R, Elliott WM, Buzatu L *et al*. The nature of small-airway obstruction in chronic obstructive pulmonary disease. *N Engl J Med* 2004; 350:2645–2653.
13. Saetta M, Turato G, Maestrelli P, Mapp CE, Fabbri LM. Cellular and structural bases of chronic obstructive pulmonary disease. *Am J Respir Crit Care Med* 2001; 163:1304–1309.
14. Boschetto P, Miniati M, Miotto D, Braccioni F, De Rosa E, Bononi I *et al*. Predominant emphysema phenotype in chronic obstructive pulmonary. *Eur Respir J* 2003; 21:450–454.
15. Macnee W. Oxidative stress and lung inflammation in airways disease. *Eur J Pharmacol* 2001; 429:195–207.
16. Biernacki WA, Kharitonov SA, Barnes PJ. Increased leukotriene B4 and 8-isoprostane in exhaled breath condensate of patients with exacerbations of COPD. *Thorax* 2003; 58:294–298.
17. Rahman I, van Schadewijk AA, Crowther AJ, Hiemstra PS, Stolk J, Macnee W, De Boer WI. 4-Hydroxy-2-nonenal, a specific lipid peroxidation product, is elevated in lungs of patients with chronic obstructive pulmonary disease. *Am J Respir Crit Care Med* 2002; 166:490–495.
18. Rahman I. Oxidative stress, transcription factors and chromatin remodelling in lung inflammation. *Biochem Pharmacol* 2002; 64:935–942.
19. Kostikas K, Papatheodorou G, Psathakis K, Panagou P, Loukides S. Oxidative stress in expired breath condensate of patients with COPD. *Chest* 2003; 124:1373–1380.
20. Sugiura H, Ichinose M, Yamagata S, Koarai A, Shirato K, Hattori T. Correlation between change in pulmonary function and suppression of reactive nitrogen species production following steroid treatment in COPD. *Thorax* 2003; 58:299–305.
21. Chanez P, Vignola AM, O'Shaugnessy T, Enander I, Li D, Jeffery PK, Bousquet J. Corticosteroid reversibility in COPD is related to features of asthma. *Am J Respir Crit Care Med* 1997; 155:1529–1534.
22. Burge PS, Calverley PM, Jones PW, Spencer S, Anderson JA, Maslen TK. Randomised, double blind, placebo controlled study of fluticasone propionate in patients with moderate to severe chronic obstructive pulmonary disease: the ISOLDE trial. *Br Med J* 2000; 320:1297–1303.
23. Israel E, Banerjee TR, Fitzmaurice GM, Kotlov TV, LaHive K, LeBoff MS. Effects of inhaled glucocorticoids on bone density in premenopausal women. *N Engl J Med* 2001; 345:941–947.
24. Halpern MT, Schmier JK, Van Kerkhove MD, Watkins M, Kalberg CJ. Impact of long-term inhaled corticosteroid therapy on bone mineral density: results of a meta-analysis. *Ann Allergy Asthma Immunol* 2004; 92:201–207.
25. Jones PW, Willits LR, Burge PS, Calverley PM. Disease severity and the effect of fluticasone propionate on chronic obstructive pulmonary disease exacerbations. *Eur Respir J* 2003; 21:68–73.
26. Sin DD, Golmohammadi K, Jacobs P. Cost-effectiveness of inhaled corticosteroids for chronic obstructive pulmonary disease according to disease severity. *Am J Med* 2004; 116:325–331.
27. Cazzola M, Dahl R. Inhaled combination therapy with long-acting β2-agonists and corticosteroids in stable COPD. *Chest* 2004; 126:220–237.
28. Vestbo J, Sorensen T, Lange P, Brix A, Torre P, Viskum K. Long-term effect of inhaled budesonide in mild and moderate chronic obstructive pulmonary disease: a randomised controlled trial. *Lancet* 1999; 353:1819–1823.
29. Pizzichini E, Pizzichini MM, Gibson P, Parameswaran K, Gleich GJ, Berman L *et al*. Sputum eosinophilia predicts benefit from prednisone in smokers with chronic obstructive bronchitis. *Am J Respir Crit Care Med* 1998; 158:1511–1517.

30. Nishimura K, Koyama H, Ikeda A, Tsukino M, Hajiro T, Mishima M, Izumi T. The effect of high-dose inhaled beclomethasone dipropionate in patients with stable COPD. *Chest* 1999; 115:31–37.
31. Burge PS, Calverley PM, Jones PW, Spencer S, Anderson JA. Prednisolone response in patients with chronic obstructive pulmonary disease: results from the ISOLDE study. *Thorax* 2003; 58:654–658.
32. O'Brien A, Ward NS. Steroid therapy in chronic obstructive pulmonary disease. *Med Health R I* 2002; 85:52–55.
33. Senderovitz T, Vestbo J, Frandsen J, Maltbaek N, Norgaard M, Nielsen C, Kampmann JP. Steroid reversibility test followed by inhaled budesonide or placebo in outpatients with stable chronic obstructive pulmonary disease. The Danish Society of Respiratory Medicine. *Respir Med* 1999; 93:715–718.
34. Pauwels RA, Lofdahl CG, Laitinen LA, Schouten JP, Postma DS, Pride NB, Ohlsson SV. Long-term treatment with inhaled budesonide in persons with mild chronic obstructive pulmonary disease who continue smoking. European Respiratory Society Study on Chronic Obstructive Pulmonary Disease. *N Engl J Med* 1999; 340:1948–1953.
35. Lung Health Study Research Group. Effect of inhaled triamcinolone on the decline in pulmonary function in chronic obstructive pulmonary disease. *N Engl J Med* 2000; 343:1902–1909.
36. Suissa S. Effectiveness of inhaled corticosteroids in chronic obstructive pulmonary disease: immortal time bias in observational studies. *Am J Respir Crit Care Med* 2003; 168:49–53.
37. de Melo MN, Ernst P, Suissa S. Inhaled corticosteroids and the risk of a first exacerbation in COPD patients. *Eur Respir J* 2004; 23:692–697.
38. Thompson WH, Carvalho P, Souza JP, Charan NB. Controlled trial of inhaled fluticasone propionate in moderate to severe COPD. *Lung* 2002; 180:191–201.
39. Paggiaro PL, Dahle R, Bakran I, Frith L, Hollingworth K, Efthimiou J. Multicentre randomised placebo-controlled trial of inhaled fluticasone propionate in patients with chronic obstructive pulmonary disease. International COPD Study Group. *Lancet* 1998; 351:773–780.
40. Alsaeedi A, Sin DD, McAlister FA. The effects of inhaled corticosteroids in chronic obstructive pulmonary disease: a systematic review of randomized placebo-controlled trials. *Am J Med* 2002; 113:59–65.
41. Sin DD, Tu JV. Inhaled corticosteroids and the risk of mortality and readmission in elderly patients with chronic obstructive pulmonary disease. *Am J Respir Crit Care Med* 2001; 164:580–584.
42. O'Brien A, Russo-Magno P, Karki A, Hiranniramol S, Hardin M, Kaszuba M *et al*. Effects of withdrawal of inhaled steroids in men with severe irreversible airflow obstruction. *Am J Respir Crit Care Med* 2001; 164:365–371.
43. Van der Valk P, Monninkhof E, van der Palen J, Zielhuis G, van Herwaarden C. Effect of discontinuation of inhaled corticosteroids in patients with chronic obstructive pulmonary disease: the COPE study. *Am J Respir Crit Care Med* 2002; 166:1358–1363.
44. Celli BR, Macnee W. Standards for the diagnosis and treatment of patients with COPD: a summary of the ATS/ERS position paper. *Eur Respir J* 2004; 23:932–946.
45. Berry JK, Baum CL. Malnutrition in chronic obstructive pulmonary disease: adding insult to injury. *AACN Clin Issues* 2001; 12:210–219.
46. Davies L, Angus RM, Calverley PM. Oral corticosteroids in patients admitted to hospital with exacerbations of chronic obstructive pulmonary disease: a prospective randomised controlled trial. *Lancet* 1999; 354:456–460.
47. Calverley PM. Modern treatment of chronic obstructive pulmonary disease. *Eur Respir J Suppl* 2001; 34:S60–S66.
48. Wood-Baker R, Walters EH, Gibson P. Oral corticosteroids for acute exacerbations of chronic obstructive pulmonary disease. *Cochrane Database Syst Rev* 2001; CD001288.
49. Niewoehner DE. The role of systemic corticosteroids in acute exacerbation of chronic obstructive pulmonary disease. *Am J Respir Med* 2002; 1:243–248.
50. Jeffery PK, Godfrey RW, Adelroth E, Nelson F, Rogers A, Johansson SA. Effects of treatment on airway inflammation and thickening of basement membrane reticular collagen in asthma. A quantitative light and electron microscopic study. *Am Rev Respir Dis* 1992; 145:890–899.
51. Adelroth E, Rosenhall L, Johansson SA, Linden M, Venge P. Inflammatory cells and eosinophilic activity in asthmatics investigated by bronchoalveolar lavage. The effects of antiasthmatic treatment with budesonide or terbutaline. *Am Rev Respir Dis* 1990; 142:91–99.
52. Laitinen, LA, Laitinen, A, Haahtela, T. A comparative study of the effects of an inhaled corticosteroid, budesonide, and a beta2-agonist, terbutaline, on airway inflammation in newly diagnosed asthma: a randomized, double-blind, parallel-group controlled trial. *J Allergy Clin Immunol* 1992; 90:32–42.

53. Laursen LC, Taudorf E, Borgeskov S, Kobayasi T, Jensen H, Weeke B. Fiberoptic bronchoscopy and bronchial mucosal biopsies in asthmatics undergoing long-term high-dose budesonide aerosol treatment. *Allergy* 1988; 43:284–288.

54. Barnes PJ. Inhaled glucocorticoids for asthma. *N Engl J Med* 1995; 332:868–875.

55. van Rensen EL, Straathof KC, Veselic-Charvat MA, Zwinderman AH, Bel EH, Sterk PJ. Effect of inhaled steroids on airway hyperresponsiveness, sputum eosinophils, and exhaled nitric oxide levels in patients with asthma. *Thorax* 1999; 54:403–408.

56. Olivieri D, Chetta A, Del Donno M, Bertorelli G, Casalini A, Pesci A *et al*. Effect of short-term treatment with low-dose inhaled fluticasone propionate on airway inflammation and remodeling in mild asthma: a placebo-controlled study. *Am J Respir Crit Care Med* 1997; 155:1864–1871.

57. Schleimer RP, Bochner BS. The effects of glucocorticoids on human eosinophils. *J Allergy Clin Immunol* 1994; 94:1202–1213.

58. Laitinen LA, Laitinen A, Haahtela T. A comparative study of the effects of an inhaled corticosteroid, budesonide, and a beta2-agonist, terbutaline, on airway inflammation in newly diagnosed asthma: a randomized, double-blind, parallel-group controlled trial. *J Allergy Clin Immunol* 1992; 90:32–42.

59. Wenzel SE, Szefler SJ, Leung DY, Sloan SI, Rex MD, Martin RJ. Bronchoscopic evaluation of severe asthma. Persistent inflammation associated with high dose glucocorticoids. *Am J Respir Crit Care Med* 1997; 156:737–743.

60. Boschetto P, Rogers DF, Fabbri LM, Barnes PJ. Corticosteroid inhibition of airway microvascular leakage. *Am Rev Respir Dis* 1991; 143:605–609.

61. Van de Graaf EA, Out TA, Roos CM, Jansen HM. Respiratory membrane permeability and bronchial hyperreactivity in patients with stable asthma. Effects of therapy with inhaled steroids. *Am Rev Respir Dis* 1991; 143:362–368.

62. Shimura S, Sasaki T, Ikeda K, Yamauchi K, Sasaki H, Takishima T. Direct inhibitory action of glucocorticoid on glycoconjugate secretion from airway submucosal glands. *Am Rev Respir Dis* 1990; 141:1044–1049.

63. Lundgren JD, Kaliner MA, Shelhamer JH. Mechanisms by which glucocorticosteroids inhibit secretion of mucus in asthmatic airways. *Am Rev Respir Dis* 1990; 141:52–58.

64. Lomas DA, Ip M, Chamba A, Stockley RA. The effect of *in vitro* and *in vivo* dexamethasone on human neutrophil function. *Agents Actions* 1991; 33:279–285.

65. Llewellyn-Jones CG, Hill SL, Stockley RA. Effect of fluticasone propionate on neutrophil chemotaxis, superoxide generation, and extracellular proteolytic activity *in vitro*. *Thorax* 1994; 49:207–212.

66. Llewellyn-Jones CG, Harris TA, Stockley RA. Effect of fluticasone propionate on sputum of patients with chronic bronchitis and emphysema. *Am J Respir Crit Care Med* 1996; 153:616–621.

67. Confalonieri M, Mainardi E, Della PR, Bernorio S, Gandola L, Beghe B, Spanevello A. Inhaled corticosteroids reduce neutrophilic bronchial inflammation in patients with chronic obstructive pulmonary disease. *Thorax* 1998; 53:583–585.

68. Yildiz F, Kaur AC, Ilgazli A, Celikoglu M, Kacar OS, Paksoy N, Ozkarakas O. Inhaled corticosteroids may reduce neutrophilic inflammation in patients with stable chronic obstructive pulmonary disease. *Respiration* 2000; 67:71–76.

69. Gizycki MJ, Hattotuwa KL, Barnes N, Jeffery PK. Effects of fluticasone propionate on inflammatory cells in COPD: an ultrastructural examination of endobronchial biopsy tissue. *Thorax* 2002; 57:799–803.

70. Burnett D, Chamba A, Hill SL, Stockley RA. Effects of plasma, tumour necrosis factor, endotoxin and dexamethasone on extracellular proteolysis by neutrophils from healthy subjects and patients with emphysema. *Clin Sci (Lond)* 1989; 77:35–41.

71. Hattotuwa KL, Gizycki MJ, Ansari TW, Jeffery PK, Barnes NC. The effects of inhaled fluticasone on airway inflammation in chronic obstructive pulmonary disease: a double-blind, placebo-controlled biopsy study. *Am J Respir Crit Care Med* 2002; 165:1592–1596.

72. Verhoeven GT, Hegmans JP, Mulder PG, Bogaard JM, Hoogsteden HC, Prins JB. Effects of fluticasone propionate in COPD patients with bronchial hyperresponsiveness. *Thorax* 2002; 57:694–700.

73. Balbi B, Majori M, Bertacco S, Convertino G, Cuomo A, Donner CF, Pesci A. Inhaled corticosteroids in stable COPD patients: do they have effects on cells and molecular mediators of airway inflammation? *Chest* 2000; 117:1633–1637.

74. Ferreira IM, Hazari MS, Gutierrez C, Zamel N, Chapman KR. Exhaled nitric oxide and hydrogen peroxide in patients with chronic obstructive pulmonary disease: effects of inhaled beclomethasone. *Am J Respir Crit Care Med* 2001; 164:1012–1015.

75. Barnes PJ. Inhaled corticosteroids are not beneficial in chronic obstructive pulmonary disease. *Am J Respir Crit Care Med* 2000; 161:342–344.

76. Calverley PM. Inhaled corticosteroids are beneficial in chronic obstructive pulmonary disease. *Am J Respir Crit Care Med* 2000; 161:341–342.

77. Loppow D, Schleiss MB, Kanniess F, Taube C, Jorres RA, Magnussen H. In patients with chronic bronchitis a four week trial with inhaled steroids does not attenuate airway inflammation. *Respir Med* 2001; 95:115–121.

78. Keatings VM, Jatakanon A, Worsdell YM, Barnes PJ. Effects of inhaled and oral glucocorticoids on inflammatory indices in asthma and COPD. *Am J Respir Crit Care Med* 1997; 155:542–548.

79. Culpitt SV, Maziak W, Loukidis S, Nightingale JA, Matthews JL, Barnes PJ. Effect of high dose inhaled steroid on cells, cytokines, and proteases in induced sputum in chronic obstructive pulmonary disease. *Am J Respir Crit Care Med* 1999; 160:1635–1639.

80. Johannes CB, Schneider GA, Dube TJ, Alfredson TD, Davis KJ, Walker AM. The risk of nonvertebral fracture related to inhaled corticosteroid exposure among adults with chronic respiratory disease. *Chest* 2005; 127(1):89–97.

81. Tashkin DP, Murray HE, Skeans M, Murray RP. Skin manifestations of inhaled corticosteroids in COPD patients: results from Lung Health Study II. *Chest* 2004; 126(4):1123–1133.

82. Lim S, Roche N, Oliver BG, Mattos W, Barnes PJ, Fan CK. Balance of matrix metalloprotease-9 and tissue inhibitor of metalloprotease-1 from alveolar macrophages in cigarette smokers. Regulation by interleukin-10. *Am J Respir Crit Care Med* 2000; 162:1355–1360.

83. Russell RE, Thorley A, Culpitt S, Donnelly LE, Mattos CD, Wiggins J *et al*. Elastin degradation is increased in alveolar macrophages and BAL in COPD. *Am J Physiol Lung Cell Mol Physiol* 2002; 283.867–873.

84. Russell RE, Culpitt SV, DeMatos C, Donnelly L, Smith M, Wiggins J, Barnes PJ. Release and activity of matrix metalloproteinase-9 and tissue inhibitor of metalloproteinase-1 by alveolar macrophages from patients with chronic obstructive pulmonary disease. *Am J Respir Cell Mol Biol* 2002; 26:602–609.

85. Culpitt SV, Rogers DF, Shah P, De Matos C, Russell RE, Donnelly LE, Barnes PJ. Impaired inhibition by dexamethasone of cytokine release by alveolar macrophages from patients with chronic obstructive pulmonary disease. *Am J Respir Crit Care Med* 2003; 167:24–31.

86. Verhoeven GT, Wijkhuijs AJ, Hooijkaas H, Hoogsteden HC, Sluiter W. Effect of an inhaled glucocorticoid on reactive oxygen species production by bronchoalveolar lavage cells from smoking COPD patients. *Mediators Inflamm* 2000; 9:109–113.

87. Sin DD, Lacy P, York E, Man SF. Effects of Fluticasone on systemic markers of inflammation in chronic obstructive pulmonary disease. *Am J Respir Crit Care Med* 2004; June 30[Epub ahead of print].

88. Johnson M. Pharmacodynamics and pharmacokinetics of inhaled glucocorticoids. *J Allergy Clin Immunol* 1996; 97:169–176.

89. Brattsand R, Thalen A, Roempke K, Kallstrom L, Gruvstad E. Influence of 16 alpha, 17 alpha-acetal substitution and steroid nucleus fluorination on the topical to systemic activity ratio of glucocorticoids. *J Steroid Biochem* 1982; 16:779–786.

90. Adcock IM. Glucocorticoids: new mechanisms and future agents. *Curr Allergy Asthma Rep* 2003; 3:249–257.

91. Auphan N, Didonato JA, Rosette C, Helmberg A, Karin M. Immunosuppression by glucocorticoids: inhibition of NF-kappa B activity through induction of I kappa B synthesis. *Science* 1995; 270:286–290.

92. Shim J, Karin M. The control of mRNA stability in response to extracellular stimuli. *Mol Cells* 2002; 14:323–331.

93. Hermoso MA, Matsuguchi T, Smoak K, Cidlowski JA. Glucocorticoids and tumor necrosis factor alpha cooperatively regulate toll-like receptor 2 gene expression. *Mol Cell Biol* 2004; 24(11): 4743–4756.

94. Homma T, Kato A, Hashimoto N, Batchelor J, Yoshikawa M, Imai S *et al*. Corticosteroid and cytokines synergistically enhance toll-like receptor 2 expression in respiratory epithelial cells. *Am J Respir Cell Mol Biol* 2004; 31(4):463–469.

95. Reichardt HM, Tuckermann JP, Gottlicher M, Vujic M, Weih F, Angel P *et al*. Repression of inflammatory responses in the absence of DNA binding by the glucocorticoid receptor. *EMBO J* 2001; 20:7168–7173.

96. Reichardt HM, Kaestner KH, Tuckermann J, Kretz O, Wessely O, Bock R *et al*. DNA binding of the glucocorticoid receptor is not essential for survival. *Cell* 1998; 93:531–541.

97. Rahman I, Macnee W. Oxidative stress and regulation of glutathione in lung inflammation. *Eur Respir J* 2000; 16:534–554.

98. Chalmers GW, Macleod KJ, Little SA, Thomson LJ, McSharry CP, Thomson NC. Influence of cigarette smoking on inhaled corticosteroid treatment in mild asthma. *Thorax* 2002; 57:226–230.

99. Chaudhuri R, Livingston E, McMahon AD, Thomson L, Borland W, Thomson NC. Cigarette smoking impairs the therapeutic response to oral corticosteroids in chronic asthma. *Am J Respir Crit Care Med* 2003; 168:1308–1311.

100. Okamoto K, Tanaka H, Ogawa H, Makino Y, Eguchi H, Hayashi S et al. Redox-dependent regulation of nuclear import of the glucocorticoid receptor. *J Biol Chem* 1999; 274:10363–10371.

101. Matthews JG, Ito K, Barnes PJ, Adcock IM. Defective glucocorticoid receptor nuclear translocation and altered histone acetylation patterns in glucocorticoid-resistant patients. *J Allergy Clin Immunol* 2004; 113:1100–1108.

102. Wedzicha JA, Donaldson GC. Exacerbations of chronic obstructive pulmonary disease. *Respir Care* 2003; 48:1204–1213.

103. Bellettato C, Adcock IM, Ito K, Caramori G, Casolari P, Ciaccia A et al. Rhinovirus infection reduces glucocorticoid receptor nuclear translocation in airway epithelial cells. *Eur Respir J* 2003; 22(suppl):abstract 565S.

104. Adcock IM, Cosio B, Tsaprouni L, Barnes PJ, Ito K. Redox regulation of histone deacetylases and glucocorticoid-mediated inhibition of the inflammatory response. *Antioxid Redox Signal* 2005; 7(1–2):144–152.

105. Barnes PJ, Ito K, Adcock IM. Corticosteroid resistance in chronic obstructive pulmonary disease: inactivation of histone deacetylase. *Lancet* 2004; 363:731–733.

106. Ito K, Lim S, Caramori G, Chung KF, Barnes PJ, Adcock IM. Cigarette smoking reduces histone deacetylase 2 expression, enhances cytokine expression, and inhibits glucocorticoid actions in alveolar macrophages. *FASEB J* 2001; 15:1110–1112.

107. Ito K, Hanazawa T, Tomita K, Barnes PJ, Adcock IM. Oxidative stress reduces histone deacetylase 2 activity and enhances IL-8 gene expression: role of tyrosine nitration. *Biochem Biophys Res Commun* 2004; 315:240–245.

108. Barnes PJ. Therapeutic strategies for allergic diseases. *Nature* 1999; 402:31–38.

109. Henricks PA, Nijkamp FP. Reactive oxygen species as mediators in asthma. *Pulm Pharmacol Ther* 2001; 14(6):409–420.

110. Dekhuijzen PN. Antioxidant properties of N-acetylcysteine: their relevance in relation to chronic obstructive pulmonary disease. *Eur Respir J* 2004; 23(4):629–636.

111. Cazzola M, Di Lorenzo G, Di Perna F, Calderaro F, Testi R, Centanni S. Additive effects of salmeterol and fluticasone or theophylline in COPD. *Chest* 2000; 118:1576–1581.

112. Calverley P, Pauwels R, Vestbo J, Jones P, Pride N, Gulsvik A et al. Combined salmeterol and fluticasone in the treatment of chronic obstructive pulmonary disease: a randomised controlled trial. *Lancet* 2003; 361:449–456.

113. Calverley PM, Boonsawat W, Cseke Z, Zhong N, Peterson S, Olsson H. Maintenance therapy with budesonide and formoterol in chronic obstructive pulmonary disease. *Eur Respir J* 2003; 22:912–919.

114. Szafranski W, Cukier A, Ramirez A, Menga G, Sansores R, Nahabedian S et al. Efficacy and safety of budesonide/formoterol in the management of chronic obstructive pulmonary disease. *Eur Respir J* 2003; 21:74–81.

115. Ito K, Lim S, Caramori G, Cosio B, Chung KF, Adcock IM, Barnes PJ. A molecular mechanism of action of theophylline: Induction of histone deacetylase activity to decrease inflammatory gene expression. *Proc Natl Acad Sci USA* 2002; 99:8921–8926.

116. Adcock IM, Caramori G. Kinase targets and inhibitors for the treatment of airway inflammatory diseases: the next generation of drugs for severe asthma and COPD? *BioDrugs* 2004; 18:167–180.

117. Barnes PJ. New treatments for COPD. *Nat Rev Drug Discov* 2002; 1:437–446.

118. Martin RJ, Szefler SJ, Chinchilli VM, Kraft M, Dolovich M, Boushey HA et al. Systemic effect comparisons of six inhaled corticosteroid preparations. *Am J Respir Crit Care Med* 2002; 165:1377–1383.

119. Dolovich MB, Ahrens RC, Hess DR, Anderson P, Dhand R, Rau JL et al. Device selection and outcomes of aerosol therapy: evidence-based guidelines: American College of Chest Physicians/American College of Asthma, Allergy, and Immunology. *Chest* 2005; 127(1):335–371.

120. Hanania NA, Darken P, Horstman D, Reisner C, Lee B, Davis S, Shah T. The efficacy and safety of fluticasone propionate (250 microg)/salmeterol (50 microg) combined in the Diskus inhaler for the treatment of COPD. *Chest* 2003; 124:834–843.

121. Mahler DA, Wire P, Horstman D, Chang CN, Yates J, Fischer T, Shah T. Effectiveness of fluticasone propionate and salmeterol combination delivered *via* the Diskus device in the treatment of chronic obstructive pulmonary disease. *Am J Respir Crit Care Med* 2002; 166:1084–1091.

122. Rice KL, Rubins JB, Lebahn F, Parenti CM, Duane PG, Kuskowski M *et al*. Withdrawal of chronic systemic corticosteroids in patients with COPD: a randomized trial. *Am J Respir Crit Care Med* 2000; 162:174–178.

123. Aaron SD, Vandemheen KL, Hebert P, Dales R, Stiell IG, Ahuja J *et al*. Outpatient oral prednisone after emergency treatment of chronic obstructive pulmonary disease. *N Engl J Med* 2003; 348:2618–2625.

11

Corticosteroids: clinical use

P. M. A. Calverley

INTRODUCTION

Chronic obstructive pulmonary disease (COPD) is now defined not only by the presence of persistent airflow obstruction but by its association with chronic inflammation within the lungs [1], a finding now confirmed in a large series of lung resection specimens [2]. It is no surprise then that corticosteroids, our most successful anti-inflammatory therapy, have been used to treat COPD patients. These drugs have proven very valuable in the management of bronchial asthma, so successful in fact that some clinicians seem to believe that any COPD patient responding to corticosteroid treatment could not have had COPD in the first place but must really have been an asthmatic – no matter how typical the clinical presentation might have been! This redefinition of 'asthma' in COPD by the response to a specific therapy, although neither officially accepted nor intellectually sustainable, has become a shorthand way of making clinical decisions. It is an approach that makes the rational use of corticosteroids in COPD particularly difficult and despite its seductive simplicity it should be resisted.

This chapter will briefly review some of the background to corticosteroid use in COPD care and summarise current views about when these drugs should be considered in patient management. Data about the efficacy or lack of it when using corticosteroids has been helped by recent studies using the combination of inhaled corticosteroids and long-acting β-agonists, but this is dealt with in detail elsewhere in this volume and will only be touched on briefly here.

PHARMACOLOGY AND MECHANISMS OF ACTION

The glucocorticosteroids used therapeutically are synthetic compounds based on the naturally occurring cortisone molecule. The most commonly used preparations are listed in Table 11.1. Oral preparations have good bioavailability and a long half-life. Thus once daily dosing is sufficient to achieve a stable therapeutic effect. Inhaled preparations are usually given twice daily although once daily therapy appears to be possible with mometasone fumarate. A range of formulations is available and although triamcinolone has been given as 6 puffs twice daily to COPD patients [3], the other commonly used corticosteroids require only two actuations a day to deliver an adequate dose. The time of onset of action is difficult to assess and good studies of this phenomenon are lacking in COPD, reflecting the somewhat indefinite nature of the end points influenced by corticosteroid therapy. Since anti-inflammatory therapy is usually chronic rather than acute, this is not a significant

Peter M. A. Calverley, MB ChB, FRCP, FRCPE, Professor of Medicine (Pulmonary & Rehabilitation), Clinical Sciences Centre, University Hospital Aintree, Liverpool, UK.

Table 11.1   Most commonly used corticosteroid preparation

Drug	Route of administration	Daily dose	Regimen
Prednisolone	Oral	2.5–5 mg 30–40 mg daily in exacerbation	Once daily
Methylprednisone	IV	500 mg in exacerbation	6 hourly
Beclomethasone dipropionate	Inhaled – MDI, DPI	400–2,000 µg	12 hourly
Budesonide	Inhaled – MDI, DPI, NEB	400–1,600 µg 2,000 µg in exacerbation	12 hourly
Fluticasone propionate	Inhaled – MDI, DPI	200–1,000 µg	12 hourly
Triamcinolone acetonide	Inhaled – MDI, DPI	400–1,200 µg	12 hourly

MDI = Metered dose inhaler; DPI = dry powder inhaler; NEB = nebuliser.

Table 11.2   Side-effects of corticosteroids

Central obesity, moon-face, 'buffalo hump' Striae, thinning of skin Spontaneous bruising Glucose intolerance, diabetes mellitus Osteoporosis Avascular necrosis Fluid retention Peptic ulceration, gastrointestinal bleeding Cataracts Peripheral muscle myopathy Adrenal suppression Pharyngeal candidiasis* Dysphonia*
*Only with inhaled form.

draw back. Nonetheless, when used in treating exacerbations as COPD where lung function is the outcome, changes in FEV_1 occur within 24 h of the first dose [4]. Drug metabolism occurs in the liver and its rapidity varies with the drug used, being most complete with fluticasone propionate. However, this does not prevent some drug being available to systemic circulation since direct absorption after alveolar deposition can occur. This explains the significant short-term adrenal suppression seen with fluticasone in normal volunteers [5]. However, when drug particle deposition is more central, as occurs in both asthma and COPD [6], the effect of fluticasone is proportionately less [7, 8]. The main side-effects of corticosteroids are pharmacologically predictable and are listed in Table 11.2. These are most obvious when oral corticosteroids are used either as maintenance treatment or when frequent courses are administered because of exacerbations, a common problem in severe COPD. The deleterious effects of oral corticosteroids on muscle function have now been clearly demonstrated in COPD patients. Thus higher doses of oral maintenance therapy (>4 mg per day) are associated with significant reductions in quadriceps force, increased health costs [9] and a higher mortality, a finding related to total oral corticosteroid use [10] (Figure 11.1). Using oral corticosteroids in this way in COPD patients is now no longer acceptable [1]. Other side-effects, especially bruising and thinning of the skin, are predominantly seen in patients who have received oral corticosteroids and use of these agents complicates the interpretation of the true incidence of significant side-effects in those patients managed with inhaled therapy

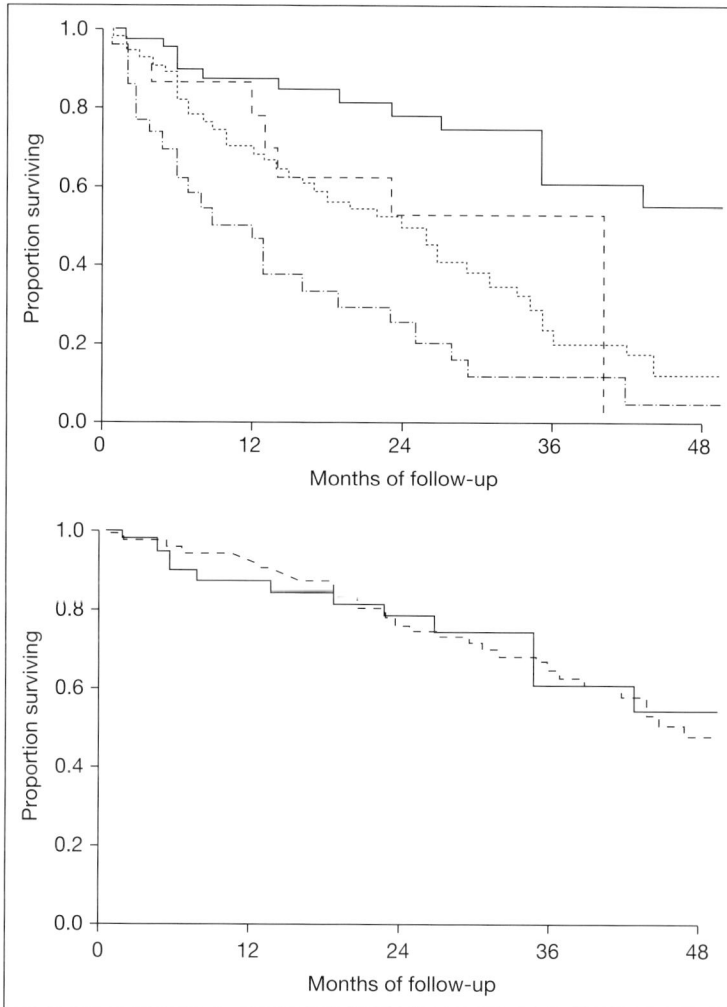

Figure 11.1 Kaplan-Meier survival plots of oral glucocorticoid users compared to similar patients not receiving maintenance therapy (solid line). There is a dose relationship with worse survival in those receiving 15 mg prednisolone daily (dash and dots) compared to 10 mg daily (dotted line) who are worse than the 5 mg daily group (dashed line) (above). Survival was uninfluenced by regular inhaled cortcosteroid use (below); dotted line is the inhaled steroid users. Reprinted with permission from reference [11].

alone. A further confounding factor is the unexpectedly high prevalence of osteoporosis in patients with more advanced COPD who have not received any form of corticosteroid. Prospective trials following the change in bone mineral density over time in patients randomised to inhaled corticosteroids or placebo are now underway. When these data become available in 2007, some of the current confusion surrounding the potential risks of maintenance therapy with inhaled corticosteroids should be resolved.

Selecting an appropriate dose of inhaled treatment for use in COPD remains difficult. The doses of inhaled corticosteroids conventionally used have tended towards the upper limit of the dosing range largely by extrapolating the results of retrospective data using oral corticosteroids (see below). There are limited data looking at lower and higher doses of corticosteroids with and without salmeterol, which suggest that the higher doses were associated with greater symptomatic benefit [11, 12]. However, similar studies have been conducted using modest doses of budesonide (total 800 µg per day) in more severe COPD and demonstrating reductions in exacerbations comparable to that seen with higher doses of fluticasone [13, 14]. Thus the high doses studied so far may not always be needed.

The mechanism of action of corticosteroids within the cell is complex, involving several different pathways, the relative importance of which is debated. Corticosteroid molecules combine with a soluble receptor within the cytoplasm and the subsequent complex binds to the nucleus leading to an increase in the number of β-2 receptors and a modulation of the transcription of pro-inflammatory proteins. Attention is now focused on the ability of these drugs to inhibit the unwinding of nuclear chromatin and hence the ease of access of the corticosteroid receptor complex to the nucleus. This process is mediated by the enzyme histone deacetylase. Failure of these drugs to interact with histone deacetylase 2 appears to be a relative specific feature of patients with COPD and this may relate to continuing oxidative stress in these patients [15]. How such changes relate to proposed markers of continuing inflammation in COPD remains controversial, as is the relevance of these processes to inflammation in other disorders like rheumatoid arthritis and inflammatory bowel disease. In COPD markers of respiratory inflammation in induced sputum such as interleukin-8 and TNF-α have not been modified by treatment with either inhaled or oral corticosteroids [16, 17]. However, other groups have suggested that inhaled corticosteroids can change chemotactic activity in the sputum [18] and even circulating levels of inflammatory markers like highly sensitive CRP or IL-6 [19]. Which, if any, of these changes relate to clinically important outcomes will need longer prospective studies to determine.

CORTICOSTEROIDS AS AN AID TO DIAGNOSIS

The belief that corticosteroid responsiveness was only seen in asthma lead to the use of the so-called 'trial of oral corticosteroids' as a diagnostic test for patients with stable COPD who might benefit from regular corticosteroid treatment. More widely used in Europe than North America, this concept extended to bronchodilator reversibility as well and influenced the patients included in the subsequent large clinical trials of corticosteroid treatment. The usual outcome is to report the change in FEV_1 either immediately after the bronchodilator drug or at some time, commonly 2 weeks, after taking a large dose of corticosteroids, usually the equivalent of 30–40 mg or oral prednisone [20]. Establishing criteria for what constitutes a significant pulmonary function change has proven difficult, particularly when changes are expressed as a percentage of the baseline value which itself declines as COPD worsens. Hence a small absolute change, which can fall within the between day reproducibility of the FEV_1, can appear significant and define a 'positive response' [21]. The day-to-day reproducibility of this type of testing is relatively poor [22] and neither the short-term bronchodilator nor oral corticosteroid response was found to relate to clinically important changes in lung function, exacerbation, frequency or health status irrespective of subsequent treatment [23]. This depressing conclusion has lead to the UK evidence-based COPD guidelines, abandoning routine testing with oral corticosteroids in the evaluation of COPD [24]. However, there may be times in specialist practice when a large response to bronchodilators can predict a significant improvement in lung function with corticosteroid treatment [25]. Moreover, the post-bronchodilator FEV_1 is a useful guide to future prognosis; so testing lung function in this way should not be abandoned entirely, even if small differences in spirometry are of very little value in making therapeutic decisions. A better appreciation of the natural day-to-day variation in airway calibre allows the experienced clinician to set these changes into context but also explains why we now place much more emphasis on changes in symptoms rather than small and potentially misleading changes in FEV_1 when evaluating the clinical impact of therapy.

CORTICOSTEROIDS IN ACUTE EXACERBATIONS OF COPD

Although short courses of oral corticosteroids have been used for the treatment of exacerbations of COPD for many years, clear evidence to support this practice has only been obtained recently. Albert *et al.* [26] noted a significant increase in pre-bronchodilator FEV_1 measured over the first 6h of admission in patients treated with corticosteroids compared to placebo, although the post bronchodilator FEV_1 effect was much smaller. In a carefully conducted but small (n = 17) study of out-patients with COPD, those whose exacerbations were treated with a tapering dose of oral prednisone (total dose 360 mg) had a significantly higher FEV_1 and PaO_2 at days 3 and 10 compared with the placebo-treated patients. Although symptomatic improvement appeared to be more rapid in the active treatment group this was not statistically significant for the whole admission [27]. Two larger studies of patients admitted to hospital with exacerbations have supported these findings. Niewoehner *et al.* [28] studied 271 patients using a treatment-failure end point (a combination of death, ventilation, re-admission or treatment intensification) and found that those who received oral corticosteroids were less likely to relapse than those given placebo. However, there was no difference between 2 weeks and 2 months of this intensive treatment. Post-bronchodilator FEV_1 increased more rapidly and hospital stay was shorter in the 56 patients studied by Davies *et al.* [4] (Figure 11.2). Although the change in FEV_1 was relatively modest, further analysis of the North American data showed that patients with the greatest FEV_1 improvement in the early stages of an exacerbation were less likely to relapse subsequently and confirmed the UK finding that this was more likely to be the case in the corticosteroid-treated individuals [29]. The total dose of oral corticosteroids (30 mg prednisolone daily for 2 weeks) in the UK study was significantly less than the cumulative doses used in the North American trial, but no clear difference in the magnitude of benefit was seen. Whether it is the dose or duration of treatment that produces these effects remains unclear. Further support for the role of oral corticosteroids in the treatment of exacerbations comes from a study of 147 Canadian patients discharged from the emergency room where treatment with prednisone for 10 days prolonged the time to relapse (p = 0.04) and reduced the overall relapse rate from 43 to 27% in the 30 days after discharge [30]. As with the earlier studies, the rate of recovery of FEV_1 was more rapid in those receiving corticosteroids as was the speed with which breathlessness improved when assessed by the transitional dyspnoea index.

A further Canadian study found that lung function could be improved to a similar degree with oral and nebulised corticosteroids, although whether this latter expensive therapy can be justified remains doubtful [31]. The logistical problems of examining different doses of oral corticosteroids remained formidable in this setting, the only small (and underpowered) study to address this finding that a slightly longer duration of treatment appeared to be beneficial [32]. However, in an environment of rapid patient throughput particular care is needed to ensure that oral corticosteroids are stopped after an appropriately brief exposure in case subsequent excessive side-effects develop. This may prove difficult when the patient perceives a significant symptomatic benefit while taking this high dose therapy but failure to stop therapy can be very deleterious (see above).

CORTICOSTEROIDS IN STABLE DISEASE

Throughout the 1990s a series of randomised controlled trials of varying length studied the question of whether inhaled corticosteroids could modify the rate of decline in FEV_1 typically seen in COPD. These studies gave conflicting results reflecting differences in patient selection and a limited duration of follow-up [33–36]. Probably the most intriguing data came from the Netherlands where the change in lung function 2 years before and after the institution of inhaled corticosteroids were monitored. The data suggested that the rate of decline in pre-bronchodilator FEV_1 was different to that after treatment was introduced.

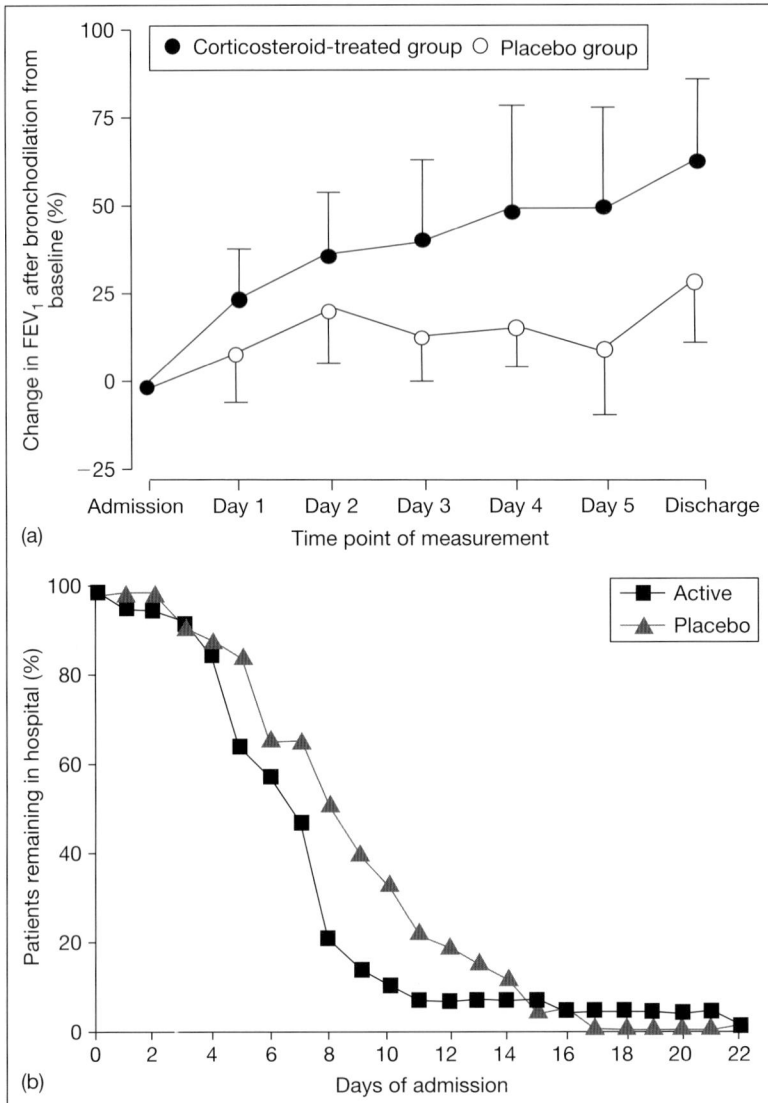

Figure 11.2 In this study post-bronchodilator FEV$_1$ improved significantly faster in patients receiving 30 mg oral prednisolone for 10 days than those getting placebo (a). The time to discharge from hospital was significantly shorter in the patients receiving oral corticosteroids for their non-acidotic COPD exacerbations (b). Redrawn with permission from reference [4].

However, this was not a properly randomised design and the changes in post-brochodilator lung function were less impressive [37].

In the last few years four large prospective randomised controlled trials, each of 3 years duration, studied whether or not the change in post-bronchodilator FEV$_1$, a more reliable guide to disease progression [38], is modified by inhaled corticosteroids [3, 8, 39, 40] (Table 11.3). These studies encompassed a wide range of COPD severity, ranging from individuals identified with mild disease in a prospective community sample to others with

Table 11.3   Randomised trials of one or more years comparing inhaled corticosteroids to placebo in stable COPD

Study	Duration	N	Drug/Dose	FEV₁ relative to placebo	Comment
CCLS	Three years	290	bud 400 µg bid	no change	no effect on FEV_1 decline
Euroscop	Three years	1,277	bud 400 µg bid	approx +40 ml	no effect on FEV_1 decline; increased bruising; no loss of bone density
LHSII	Three years	1,116	triamcinolone 600 µg bid	no change	no effect on FEV_1 decline; fewer unplanned visits with active therapy; accelerated loss of bone density
ISOLDE	Three years	751	FP 500 µg bid	+100 ml	no change in rate of decline in FEV_1; 25% reduction in exacerbation rate to 0.99/yr; reduced decline in health status
TRISTAN	One year*	735	FP 500 µg bid	+95 ml	19% reduction in exacerbation rate to 1.05/yr; no bruising
Szafranski	One year*	403	Bud 400 µg bid	+52 ml	no clinical effect
Calverley	One year*	513	Bud 400 µg bid	no change	Delayed time to first course of oral corticosteroid

*Decline in lung function not studied.
Bud = Budesonide; FP = fluticasone propionate.

symptomatic COPD attending regular hospital follow-up. They were biased towards current smokers as this was an entry requirement for Euroscop and the original Lung Health Study, although rather surprisingly smoking status did not appear to modify the outcome. In no trial was the rate of FEV_1 decline different over 3 years when placebo and active treatments were compared. The effect of inhaled corticosteroids in the most severely affected patients may have been harder to detect given the asymmetrical pattern of drop-out in this study i.e., patients on placebo were significantly more likely to be lost from the trial and they were the ones with the most rapid loss of lung function [41]. This could not explain the data in the other three studies where equivalent numbers of each group were available at the end of the trial for analysis. More recently meta-analyses of these studies have produced equally confusing conclusions. One group found no effect with the inhaled corticosteroids on rate of decline in the pooled data but did not discuss this finding in detail [42]. However, other workers, taking virtually the same data and modifying an error made by the first group in assigning the rate of change of lung function, now found a significant effect particularly in those who had received the more potent inhaled corticosteroids budesonide and fluticasone propionate (FP), amounting to around 10 ml per year reduction in the rate of decline [43]. As the original studies were not powered to detect this size of difference in rate of decline, the meta-analysis by Sutherland *et al.* [43] may be more relevant. More data preferably using harder clinical end points will be needed before this confusion is resolved.

THE EFFECT OF CORTICOSTEROIDS ON LUNG FUNCTION

If the data about inhaled corticosteroids and rate of decline in FEV_1 is contentious then that relating to the effects of corticosteroids on the change of lung function and specifically FEV_1 after bronchodilators is more consistent, although it is often overlooked. Interpreting change here is not easy as it does not appear immediately i.e., within 24 h, as is the case with acute bronchodilator drugs, but instead evolves over time. No convincing effects on post-bronchodilator FEV_1 were seen when placebo and inhaled corticosteroid data were compared in the Danish and US long-term studies [3, 39]. In subsequent studies FP 1,000 μg per day [8, 44] and even at 500 μg per day [12] have shown small but significant increases in post-bronchodilator spirometry weeks-to-month after the onset of treatment. These changes could not be identified in studies using budesonide where only post-dose lung function data where available [13, 14]. In general, these changes have been smaller in patients with more severe disease who were the ones recruited into the trials involving budesonide. Although these improvements in lung function are unlikely to be clinically important in themselves, they do provide a pointer to a biological effect of inhaled corticosteroids which may be more relevant when other non-spirometric effects are considered.

THE EFFECT ON HEALTH STATUS

Although spirometry is invaluable in confirming the diagnosis of COPD and as an aid to prognosis, it is only poorly related to the impact of the disease on the patients' well-being [45]. The development of disease-specific validated health-status questionnaires has shown that significant improvement in patient well-being can occur together with small changes in spirometry in stable patients [46]. Health status data has been collected almost exclusively in more severe disease (GOLD stages 3 and below), in patients rather than smokers with minimal symptomatology associated with their airflow obstruction and mostly, but not exclusively, using the St George's Respiratory Questionnaire (SGRQ). Treatment with inhaled corticosteroids in addition to short-acting bronchodilator therapy in the ISOLDE study did not change health status over the first 6 months of observation irrespective of whether oral corticosteroids were given during the run-in period. In this study, the only one to date with 3-year follow-up of patients, the rate of change of health status was modified in those patients receiving inhaled corticosteroids given by a mean of 3 units per year in the total SGRQ score, compared with placebo [47]. These changes were cumulative and suggest that the use of inhaled corticosteroids delays the time taken to reach a particular level of ill health rather than abolishing the progression of physical deterioration altogether. Similar data were seen in more severe patients when budesonide was used after an initial period of treatment with oral corticosteroids although this was influenced by the run-in protocols adopted [13, 14]. Withdrawing inhaled cortiosteroids was accompanied by worsening of health status in a further Dutch trial using fluticasone [48]. In a 6-month study of stable patients monitoring the change in breathlessness, inhaled corticosteroids were associated with a significant improvement in the transitional dyspnoea index compared to placebo, although this was not seen when a lower dose of FP was used [49].

THE EFFECT ON EXACERBATIONS

Although the definition of COPD exacerbation remains contentious [50], a similar definition of events has been used in most of the larger and longer (one year or more) clinical trials of symptomatic COPD patients [51]. The exception was the second Lung Health Study where regular treatment with triamcinolone was found to reduce the number of new symptoms and the frequency of unplanned clinic visits, a weak surrogate for exacerbation frequency [3]. In the other trials the use of oral corticosteroids and/or antibiotics prescribed by the patient's physician has been the primary defining characteristic of an exacerbation. These episodes are more frequent in patients with the worst lung function [52] (Figure 11.3) and unsurprisingly it is this group where inhaled corticosteroids have been shown to be most effective. Table 11.4 summarises the key findings from the recent trials in which the effect of inhaled corticosteroid on exacerbation rate has been reported. These studies were

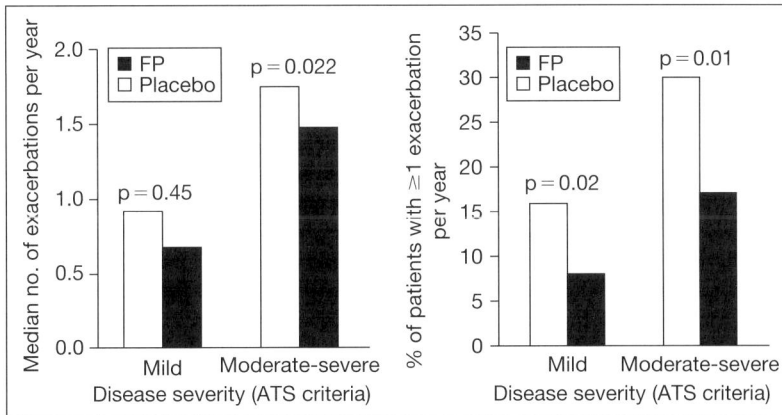

Figure 11.3 Effect of ICS therapy on exacerbations of COPD. In the ISOLDE trial, among patients with moderate or severe COPD (FEV$_1$ <50%), inhaled fluticasone proprionate significantly reduced the number of exacerbations per year and the number of patients who experienced at least one exacerbation. An effect of fluticasone on the number experiencing at least one exacerbation was present irrespective of baseline lung function (right) but was not observed if median exacerbation rate was the outcome variable (left). Adapted from Jones PW et al. [52].

selected because each had at least 12 months data which afforded a reasonable period in which exacerbations could occur and avoided issues of seasonality which might confound smaller, briefer studies.

Both the ISOLDE and TRISTAN studies involved very similar patient cohorts (mean pre-bronchodilator FEV$_1$ 44% predicted in each) and despite the TRISTAN participants all having a history of prior exacerbations, the exacerbation frequency during each study in patients receiving placebo was 1.3 events per year [8, 44]. Using FP in the same dose in each study reduced exacerbation rates by 20–25% suggesting that the routine use of inhaled corticosteroids can be effective in patients like this. Data with budesonide in patients with worse baseline lung function (mean FEV$_1$ 36% predicted) was much less impressive [13, 14] with the inhaled corticosteroid failing to have a statistically significant effect on the overall exacerbation rate, although the time to the first course of oral corticosteroids was delayed in one study [14]. Differences in exacerbation rate appear to be an important determinant of the rate of decline of health status which is slower in those who exacerbate less frequently. This effect may explain why inhaled corticosteroids had a beneficial effect in the ISOLDE study [53].

SIDE-EFFECTS

As noted above, regular use of inhaled corticosteroids is accompanied by a potentially important risk of side-effects, which might be more evident in older, frailer patients with COPD. In practice it has been very difficult to determine how great the risk of side-effects is in these patients as they have multiple co-morbidities which increase the chance of them presenting with these complications for reasons unrelated to inhaled corticosteroid use. The local side-effects of hoarseness, dryness of the mouth and candidiasis are undoubtedly reported more frequently in patients receiving inhaled corticosteroids and these may resolve spontaneously, settle with the use of a volume spacer device or stop when the treatment is discontinued. In the large number of patients in the randomised controlled trials there is evidence for a reduction in the morning cortisol levels, although these stay within the normal range in almost all individuals. Even those that do fall below the normal range on one

Table 11.4   One-year studies of the effect of inhaled corticosteroids (ICS) on COPD exacerbations

Study	N	Duration (years)	Mean FEV$_1$* % predicted	Comparison	Outcome	Side-effects
CCLS [39]	290	3	81	Budesonide 400 µg twice daily vs placebo	36 patients had temporary worsening in budesonide group, 34 in placebo group	None reported
LHS2 [3]	1116	3	64	Triamcinolone 600 µg twice daily vs placebo	Fewer physician visits on active drug (1.2 vs 2.1 per 100-person years)	Significant reduction in lumbar spine femoral density
ISOLDE [8]	751	3	43	Fluticasone 500 µg twice daily vs placebo	Exacerbations reduced significantly (1.32 vs 0.99 per year)	Bruising in 27 ICS patients, 15 on placebo; reduction in serum cortisol level with ICS but still in normal range
TRISTAN** [44]	735	1	44	Fluticasone 500 µg twice daily vs placebo	Significantly fewer exacerbations with ICS (1.3 vs 1.06 per year)	No difference in occurrence of observed bruising – local class-related side-effects
Szafranski** [13]	406	1	36	Budesonide 400 µg twice daily vs placebo	No significant change in exacerbation rate (budesonide 1.84 vs placebo 1.87 per year)	No reported bruising (details limited)
Calverley** [14]	513	1	36	Budesonide 400 µg twice daily vs placebo	Non-significant difference in exacerbation rate (1.8 vs 1.6 per year with ICS)	No excess of reported adverse events

N = Number of patients;
* = pre-bronchodilator value;
** = number refers to relevant comparison in the study.

reading are likely to spontaneously revert to the normal values subsequently and no direct ill-effects have been attributed to inhaled corticosteroid use over this duration of study [8, 44]. However, patients clearly have some systemic exposure to corticosteroids, which is thought to explain the increased prevalence of skin bruising in the Euroscop trial [40]. This was not seen in the subsequent TRISTAN study in patients with a lower baseline FEV$_1$, which may reflect a difference in the pattern of deposition and absorption but is more likely to reflect the greater concomitant use of oral corticosteroids which masks any effect of inhaled therapy. In general, use of inhaled corticosteroids in symptomatic patients with more advanced COPD appears to be relatively safe and preferable to further courses of oral corticosteroids. The widespread use of inhaled corticosteroids in patients with milder disease is much less desirable given the proportionately smaller benefits and the possibly greater risks of enhanced systemic absorption (see above). More data about the role of aerosol deposition and its relationship to systemic availability in COPD patients will be needed if we are to try and reliably predict the true exposure to inhaled corticosteroids experienced by our patients.

COMBINATION THERAPY

In general combining a long-acting β-agonist and an inhaled corticosteroid in the same inhaler on a regular basis appears to be beneficial compared with using either agent alone or in combination with short-acting β-agonists. Not all end points are superior to monotherapy but overall there are clear benefits best seen when treatment is used in more severe disease where exacerbations are occurring fairly regularly. Whether the combination requires to be given in a single inhaler is not clear. Likewise there is uncertainty about whether combining a long-acting inhaled anticholinergic would be as effective as the β-agonist and doubtless future studies will examine these issues. Certainly the additive effect of the inhaled corticosteroid is most dramatic with respect to exacerbations in the patients with more severe disease in the budesonide–formoterol combination trials. Giving formoterol from the dry powder reservoir had no impact on the mean exacerbation rate and budesonide alone was scarcely more effective. Combining the two did have a significant effect which was replicated in a further study. This is probably the best example of the potential for synergy that we have seen with these drugs in clinical practice.

CONCLUSIONS

There are now ample data to support the prescription of inhaled corticosteroids in patients with severe or very severe COPD, a fact recognised in a number of treatment guidelines [24, 54, 55]. The clearest benefits with respect to exacerbation frequency are seen in individuals with an FEV_1 below 50% predicted and a previous history of exacerbations. In these patients there is evidence of improvement in health status with a reduction in the number of courses of oral corticosteroids prescribed to control exacerbations. In this context these drugs may protect from rather than increase the risk of side-effects. Prescribing inhaled corticosteroids should be considered a second-line therapy for COPD patients and should not normally be used unless added on to regular bronchodilator treatment, the best data coming with the combination of long-acting β-agonists and inhaled corticosteroids. In the USA this combination is licensed for relief of breathlessness in patients with chronic bronchitis and further data are needed to determine in other settings whether this approach to treatment is better than using the newer long-acting inhaled bronchodilators alone.

The controversy over the role of inhaled corticosteroids in preventing hospitalisation and even mortality has been specifically avoided here as it has strong proponents [56] and opponents [57]. Much is dependent on the interpretation of information in large health databases, specifically the role of immortal time bias in influencing the conclusion. Even when this appears to have been adequately addressed [58] there are still concerns about methodology. One must be cautious about over defining information in these data as it is perfectly possible to eliminate a real finding of effect including patients with inappropriately mild disease. Certainly the identification in one negative trial of a control population of COPD patients managed by inhaled corticosteroids before receiving any bronchodilator treatment seems clinically unusual. Ultimately, there is no substitute for looking at outcomes like hospitalisation or mortality in individuals known to have spirometrically confirmed

COPD and randomly assigned to a treatment. A large prospective trial is now underway, which is doing just this and hopefully by 2006 when it reports we will have a clearer idea of whether this approach for treatment is of more than just symptomatic benefit [59].

Until then we do have information that inhaled corticosteroids have some value in specific circumstances which can be readily identified clinically. Whatever their risks, they are almost certainly lower than those associated with oral corticosteroid use which is not recommended as maintenance therapy by any guideline. Our task as physicians remains to use these drugs in an intelligent way, which maximises the advantages they offer our patients whilst reducing unnecessary risk.

REFERENCES

1. Pauwels RA, Buist AS, Calverley PMA, Jenkins CR, Hurd SS. Global strategy for the diagnosis, management and prevention of chronic obstructive pulmonary disease. *Am J Respir Crit Care Med* 2001; 163:1256–1276.
2. Hogg JC, Chu F, Utokaparch S, Woods R, Elliott WM, Buzatu L *et al*. The nature of small-airway obstruction in chronic obstructive pulmonary disease. *N Engl J Med* 2004; 350:2645–2653.
3. The Lung Health Study Research Group. Effect of inhaled triamcinolone on the decline in pulmonary function in chronic obstructive pulmonary disease. *N Engl J Med* 2000; 343:1902–1909.
4. Davies L, Angus RM, Calverley PMA. Oral corticosteroids in patients admitted to hospital with exacerbations of chronic obstructive pulmonary disease: a prospective randomised controlled trial. *Lancet* 1999; 354:456–460.
5. Wilson AM, Clark DJ, McFarlane L, Lipworth BJ. Adrenal suppression with high doses of inhaled fluticasone propionate and triamcinolone acetonide in healthy volunteers. *Eur J Clin Pharmacol* 1997; 53:33–37.
6. Kim CS, Kang TC. Comparative measurement of lung deposition of inhaled fine particles in normal subjects and patients with obstructive airway disease. *Am J Respir Crit Care Med* 1997; 155:899–905.
7. Nelson HS, Busse WW, DeBoisblanc BP, Berger WE, Noonan MJ, Webb DR *et al*. Fluticasone propionate powder: oral corticosteroid-sparing effect and improved lung function and quality of life in patients with severe chronic asthma. *J Allergy Clin Immunol* 1999; 103:267–275.
8. Burge PS, Calverley PM, Jones PW, Spencer S, Anderson JA, Maslen TK. Randomised, double blind, placebo controlled study of fluticasone propionate in patients with moderate to severe chronic obstructive pulmonary disease: the ISOLDE trial. *Br Med J* 2000; 320:1297–1303.
9. Decramer M, Gosselink R, Troosters T, Verschueren M, Evers G. Muscle weakness is related to utilization of health care resources in COPD patients. *Eur Respir J* 1997; 10:417–423.
10. Schols AM, Wesseling G, Kester AD, de Vries G, Mostert R, Slangen J *et al*. Dose dependent increased mortality risk in COPD patients treated with oral glucocorticoids. *Eur Respir J* 2001; 17:337–342.
11. Mahler DA, Wire P, Horstman D, Chang CN, Yates J, Fischer T *et al*. Effectiveness of fluticasone propionate and salmeterol combination delivered *via* the diskus device in the treatment of chronic obstructive pulmonary disease. *Am J Respir Crit Care Med* 2002; 166:1084–1091.
12. Hanania NA, Darken P, Horstman D, Reisner C, Lee B, Davis S *et al*. The efficacy and safety of fluticasone propionate (250 microg)/salmeterol (50 microg) combined in the Diskus inhaler for the treatment of COPD. *Chest* 2003; 124:834–843.
13. Szafranski W, Cukier A, Ramirez A, Menga G, Sansores R, Nahabedian S *et al*. Efficacy and safety of budesonide/formoterol in the management of chronic obstructive pulmonary disease. *Eur Respir J* 2003; 21:74–81.
14. Calverley PM, Boonsawat W, Cseke Z, Zhong N, Peterson S, Olsson H. Maintenance therapy with budesonide and formoterol in chronic obstructive pulmonary disease. *Eur Respir J* 2003; 22:912–919.
15. Barnes PJ, Ito K, Adcock IM. Corticosteroid resistance in chronic obstructive pulmonary disease: inactivation of histone deacetylase. *Lancet* 2004; 363:731–733.
16. Keatings VM, Collins PD, Scott DM, Barnes PJ. Differences in interleukin-8 and tumor necrosis factor-alpha in induced sputum from patients with chronic obstructive pulmonary disease or asthma. *Am J Respir Crit Care Med* 1996; 153:530–534.
17. Culpitt SV, Rogers DF, Shah P, De Matos C, Russell RE, Donnelly LE *et al*. Impaired inhibition by dexamethasone of cytokine release by alveolar macrophages from patients with chronic obstructive pulmonary disease. *Am J Respir Crit Care Med* 2003; 167:24–31.

18. Llewellyn-Jones CG, Harris TA, Stockley RA. Effect of fluticasone propionate on sputum of patients with chronic bronchitis and emphysema. *Am J Respir Crit Care Med* 1996; 153:616–621.

19. Sin DD, Lacy P, York E, Man SF. Effects of fluticasone on systemic markers of inflammation in chronic obstructive pulmonary disease. *Am J Respir Crit Care Med* 2004 Jun 30(e-pub).

20. Davies L, Nisar M, Pearson MG, Costello RW, Earis JE, Calverley PMA. Oral corticosteroid trials in the management of stable chronic obstructive pulmonary disease. *QJM* 1999; 92:395–400.

21. Brand PL, Quanjer PH, Postma DS, Kerstjens HA, Koeter GH, Dekhuijzen PN *et al.* Interpretation of bronchodilator response in patients with obstructive airways disease. The Dutch Chronic Non-Specific Lung Disease (CNSLD) Study Group. *Thorax* 1992; 47:429–436.

22. Calverley PM, Burge PS, Spencer S, Anderson JA, Jones PW. Bronchodilator reversibility testing in chronic obstructive pulmonary disease. *Thorax* 2003; 58:659–664.

23. Burge PS, Calverley PM, Jones PW, Spencer S, Anderson JA. Prednisolone response in patients with chronic obstructive pulmonary disease: results from the ISOLDE study. *Thorax* 2003; 58:654–658.

24. Chronic obstructive pulmonary disease. National clinical guideline on management of chronic obstructive pulmonary disease in adults in primary and secondary care. *Thorax* 2004; 59(suppl 1):1–232.

25. Nisar M, Earis JE, Pearson MG, Calverley PM. Acute bronchodilator trials in chronic obstructive pulmonary disease. *Am Rev Respir Dis* 1992; 146:555–559.

26. Albert RK, Martin TR, Lewis SW. Controlled clinical trial of methylprednisolone in patients with chronic bronchitis and acute respiratory insufficiency. *Ann Intern Med* 1980; 92:753–758.

27. Thompson WH, Nielson CP, Carvalho P, Charan NB, Crowley JJ. Controlled trial of oral prednisone in outpatients with acute COPD exacerbation. *Am J Respir Crit Care Med* 1996; 154:407–412.

28. Niewoehner DE, Erbland ML, Deupree RH, Collins D, Gross NJ *et al.* Effect of systemic glucocorticoids on exacerbations of chronic obstructive pulmonary disease. *N Engl J Med* 1999; 340:1941–1947.

29. Niewoehner DE, Collins D, Erbland ML. Relation of FEV(1) to clinical outcomes during exacerbations of chronic obstructive pulmonary disease. Department of Veterans Affairs Cooperative Study Group. *Am J Respir Crit Care Med* 2000; 161:1201–1205.

30. Aaron SD, Vandemheen KL, Hebert P, Dales R, Stiell IG, Ahuja J *et al.* Outpatient oral prednisone after emergency treatment of chronic obstructive pulmonary disease. *N Engl J Med* 2003; 348:2618–2625.

31. Maltais F, Ostinelli J, Bourbeau J, Tonnel AB, Jacquemet N, Haddon J *et al.* Comparison of nebulized budesonide and oral prednisolone with placebo in the treatment of acute exacerbations of chronic obstructive pulmonary disease: a randomized controlled trial. *Am J Respir Crit Care Med* 2002; 165:698–703.

32. Sayiner A, Aytemur ZA, Cirit M, Unsal I. Systemic glucocorticoids in severe exacerbations of COPD. *Chest* 2001; 119:726–730.

33. Renkema TE, Schouten JP, Koeter GH, Postma DS. Effects of long-term treatment with corticosteroids in COPD. *Chest* 1996; 109:1156–1162.

34. Paggiaro PL, Dahle R, Bakran I, Frith L, Hollingworth K, Efthimiou J. Multicentre randomised placebo-controlled trial of inhaled fluticasone propionate in patients with chronic obstructive pulmonary disease. International COPD Study Group [published erratum appears in *Lancet* 1998 Jun 27; 351:1968]. *Lancet* 1998; 351:773–780.

35. Bourbeau J, Rouleau MY, Boucher S. Randomised controlled trial of inhaled corticosteroids in patients with chronic obstructive pulmonary disease. *Thorax* 1998; 53:477–482.

36. Wempe JB, Postma DS, Breederveld N, Kort E, van der Mark TW, Koeter GH. Effects of corticosteroids on bronchodilator action in chronic obstructive lung disease. *Thorax* 1992; 47:616–621.

37. Dompeling E, Van Schayck CP, van Grunsven PM, van Herwaarden CL, Akkermans R *et al.* Slowing the deterioration of asthma and chronic obstructive pulmonary disease observed during bronchodilator therapy by adding inhaled corticosteroids. A 4-year prospective study. *Ann Intern Med* 1993; 118:770–778.

38. Hansen EF, Phanareth K, Laursen LC, Kok-Jensen A, Dirksen A. Reversible and irreversible airflow obstruction as predictor of overall mortality in asthma and chronic obstructive pulmonary disease. *Am J Respir Crit Care Med* 1999; 159:1267–1271.

39. Vestbo J, Sorensen T, Lange P, Brix A, Torre P, Viskum. Long-term effect of inhaled budesonide in mild and moderate chronic obstructive pulmonary disease: a randomised controlled trial. *Lancet* 1999; 353:1819–1823.

40. Pauwels RA, Lofdahl CG, Laitinen LA, Schouten JP, Postma DS, Pride NB *et al.* Long-term treatment with inhaled budesonide in persons with mild chronic obstructive pulmonary disease who continue smoking. *N Engl J Med* 1999; 340:1948–1953.

41. Calverley PM, Spencer S, Willits L, Burge PS, Jones PW. Withdrawal from treatment as an outcome in the ISOLDE study of COPD. *Chest* 2003; 124:1350–1356.

42. Alsaeedi A, Sin DD, McAlister FA. The effects of inhaled corticosteroids in chronic obstructive pulmonary disease: a systematic review of randomized placebo-controlled trials. *Am J Med* 2002; 113:59–65.

43. Sutherland ER, Allmers H, Ayas NT, Venn AJ, Martin RJ. Inhaled corticosteroids reduce the progression of airflow limitation in chronic obstructive pulmonary disease: a meta-analysis. *Thorax* 2003; 58:937–941.

44. Calverley P, Pauwels R, Vestbo J, Jones P, Pride N, Gulsvik A *et al.* Combined salmeterol and fluticasone in the treatment of chronic obstructive pulmonary disease: a randomised controlled trial. *Lancet* 2003; 361:449–456.

45. Jones PW, Quirk FH, Baveystock CM, Littlejohns P. A self-complete measure of health status for chronic airflow limitation. The St. George's Respiratory Questionnaire. *Am Rev Respir Dis* 1992; 145:1321–1327.

46. Vincken W, van Noord JA, Greefhorst AP, Bantje TA, Kesten S, Korducki L *et al.* Improved health outcomes in patients with COPD during 1 yr's treatment with tiotropium. *Eur Respir J* 2002; 19:209–216.

47. Spencer S, Calverley PMA, Burge PS, Jones PW. Health status deterioration in patients with chronic obstructive pulmonary disease. *Am J Respir Crit Care Med* 2001; 163:122–128.

48. van der Valk, Monninkhof E, van der Palen J, Zielhuis G, van Herwaarden C. Effect of discontinuation of inhaled corticosteroids in patients with chronic obstructive pulmonary disease: the COPE study. *Am J Respir Crit Care Med* 2002; 166:1358–1363.

49. Mahler DA, Wire P, Horstman D, Chang CN, Yates J, Fischer T *et al.* Effectiveness of fluticasone propionate and salmeterol combination delivered *via* the Diskus device in the treatment of chronic obstructive pulmonary disease. *Am J Respir Crit Care Med* 2002; 166:1084–1091.

50. Pauwels R, Calverley P, Buist AS, Rennard S, Fukuchi Y, Stahl E *et al.* COPD exacerbations: the importance of a standard definition. *Respir Med* 2004; 98:99–107.

51. Rodriguez-Roisin R. Toward a consensus definition for COPD exacerbations. *Chest* 2000; 117:398S–401S.

52. Jones PW, Willits LR, Burge PS, Calverley PM. Disease severity and the effect of fluticasone propionate on chronic obstructive pulmonary disease. *Eur Respir J* 2003; 21:68–73.

53. Spencer S, Calverley PM, Burge PS, Jones PW. Impact of preventing exacerbations on deterioration of health status in COPD. *Eur Respir J* 2004; 23:698–702.

54. Global Initiative for Chronic Obstructive Lung Disease. Global strategy for the diagnosis, management and prevention of chronic obstructive pulmonary disease. NHLBI/WHO workshop report. NIH Publication No 2701,1–100. 2001. Bethesda, National Heart Blood and Lung Institute. Updated July 2004.

55. Celli BR, MacNee W. Standards for the diagnosis and treatment of patients with COPD: a summary of the ATS/ERS position paper. *Eur Respir J* 2004; 23:932–946.

56 Sin DD, Tu JV. Inhaled corticosteroids and the risk of mortality and readmission in elderly patients with chronic obstructive pulmonary disease. *Am J Respir Crit Care Med* 2001; 164:580–584.

57. Suissa S. Effectiveness of inhaled corticosteroids in chronic obstructive pulmonary disease: immortal time bias in observational studies. *Am J Respir Crit Care Med* 2003; 168:49–53.

58. Soriano JB, Vestbo J, Pride NB, Kiri V, Maden C, Maier WC. Survival in COPD patients after regular use of fluticasone propionate and salmeterol in general practice. *Eur Respir J* 2002; 20:819–825.

59. Vestbo J. TORCH Study Group The TORCH (TOwards a Revolution in COPD Health) Survival Study protocol. *Eur Respir J* 2004; 24:206–210.

12

The pharmacology of combination therapy with long-acting β-adrenoceptor agonists and glucocorticoids in COPD

J. Lötvall, A. Lindén

INTRODUCTION

COPD is increasingly understood to be a chronic inflammatory disease, affecting mainly the peripheral airways (i.e., bronchiolitis) through remodeling and the lung parenchyma by degradation of the alveoli (i.e., emphysema) [1]. The inflammatory processes in COPD typically display periods of worsening (exacerbations), which frequently relate to bacterial infection. Several inflammatory cells are increased in the bronchial tissue of patients with COPD, including macrophages, neutrophils and T-lymphocytes (especially CD8 cells). In some reports on COPD, eosinophils are observed in bronchial biopsies or sputum; patients with COPD may thus display a type of pathology normally associated with asthma [2]. COPD may even be associated with atopy according to a recent report [3], even though it must be remembered that a number of patients have a combination of asthma and COPD, resulting in a more complex pathology.

Both inhaled glucocorticoids (GCs) and long-acting β-adrenoceptor agonists (BAs) demonstrate clinical efficacy in patients with COPD. In general, GCs are weak in their effects when given as monotherapy, and long-acting BA are primarily symptom-relieving drugs. However, combination therapy with these two classes of drugs, given *via* inhalation, has recently been proven to be effective in COPD, especially in terms of reducing the frequency of exacerbations [4]. Whether this is due to an additive or synergistic effect of the two drugs in the clinical situation is not yet known. This chapter focuses on the experimental and clinical evidence for beneficial effects of combination therapy in COPD.

GLUCOCORTICOIDS

CLINICAL EFFECTS OF GLUCOCORTICOIDS IN COPD

Long-term treatment with oral GCs is generally not recommended for use in patients with COPD, primarily because of weak efficacy and severe systemic side-effects [5]. However, high-dose inhaled GCs have proven some efficacy in several large multi-centre long-term studies with COPD, although the gradual decline in lung function is 'right-shifted' rather

Jan Lötvall, MD, PhD, Professor of Allergy, Head of Department, Department of Respiratory Medicine and Allergology, Göteborg University, Göteborg, Sweden.

Anders Lindén, MD, PhD, Associate Professor, Certified Specialist in Respiratory Medicine and Allergology, Lung Pharmacology Group, Department of Respiratory Medicine and Allergology, Göteborg, Sweden.

than reduced [6, 17]. Thus, some improvement in lung function can be observed, compared to placebo, over time. Probably more important, inhaled GCs slightly reduce the frequency of exacerbations in COPD, and may also to some degree improve symptoms and quality of life [5–10]. It seems that patients with COPD that have a pathology somewhat similar to asthma patients may show a greater response to inhaled GCs [2].

A problem with treating COPD patients with GCs, is that ongoing smoking may counteract the beneficial effects of both inhaled and oral GCs over time, at least as indicated in patients with asthma [11–13]. Consequently, it can be speculated that patients with a combination of asthma and COPD would experience a better response to inhaled GCs if they stop smoking [2].

MECHANISMS OF ACTION FOR GLUCOCORTICOIDS IN IN VITRO MODELS

It is widely accepted that the primary anti-inflammatory actions of GCs arise by activation of specific GC Receptors (GR), which are found in the cytoplasm of most mammalian cell types [14, 15]. GR belongs to a superfamily of nuclear receptors, including the receptors for mineralocorticoids, sexual and thyroid hormones, retinoic acid and vitamin D. The detailed molecular mechanisms of the GC-GR interaction are currently becoming better understood. Briefly, without a GC ligand, the GR subunits are each bound to two molecules of heat shock protein-90 (HSP90). When the GC ligand interacts with the GR, the HSP90 molecules are detached, resulting in a conformational change and formation of a GR dimer [14, 16]. The dimer GR complex binds to specific sequences of DNA within promoter regions of several genes. These regions of DNA are called GC response elements (GRE). The referred interaction with GRE will either up- or down-regulate gene expression, thus influencing the amount of mRNA being produced from each of the involved genes. This process is also active when DNA is densely packaged around histone proteins because GREs are located on the surface of the DNA, and are therefore available for interactions with the GR.

Another mechanism by which GRs may influence inflammatory processes in COPD is the interaction with the key transcription factor NF-κB (nuclear factor kappa B) (Figure 12.1). NF-κB is up-regulated in many cell types during inflammatory processes, and favours the expression of pro-inflammatory genes. Specifically, it is known that NF-κB is involved in several inflammatory diseases in the lungs and airways, including COPD [16]. For example, exposure to tobacco smoke is linked to NF-κB expression, and this mechanism may thus in part contribute to bronchial inflammation in tobacco smokers [17]. GRs can directly bind to NF-κB, and thereby neutralise this pro-inflammatory molecule, as well as its pro-inflammatory effects [14]. GR-mediated processes can also increase the production of a NF-κB inhibitory protein in some cells [18, 19].

Exposure to tobacco smoke reduces the expression of histone deacetylase (HDAC)-2 [20], and this effect may lead to reduced effects of GCs, since GCs require HDAC activity. Whether this is the sole mechanism of the weak effect of GCs in patients with COPD is not known.

On a cellular level, GCs have shown inhibitory effects on a multitude of different mechanisms that can be related to COPD on a hypothetical basis. Thus, GCs regulate the expression of many cytokines, chemokines, and enzymes [16, 21]. In addition, macrophages from patients with COPD release more matrix metalloproteinase-9, and this proteinase release is attenuated by a GC (dexamethasone) *in vitro* [22]. GCs could also improve the host defence against bacterial infection, since a GC (dexamethasone) enhances the expression of Toll-like receptor 2 (TLR2) on airway epithelial cells [23], and bacterial infections may enhance the progression of COPD [24].

In reality, the potentially beneficial effects of GCs on inflammatory events demonstrated in cellular studies may be weak. For example, a prospective double-blind study on the effect of an inhaled GC (fluticasone) in patients with COPD revealed very little improvement of inflammatory end points in bronchial tissue [25]. Of note, though, a reduction in the CD8:CD4

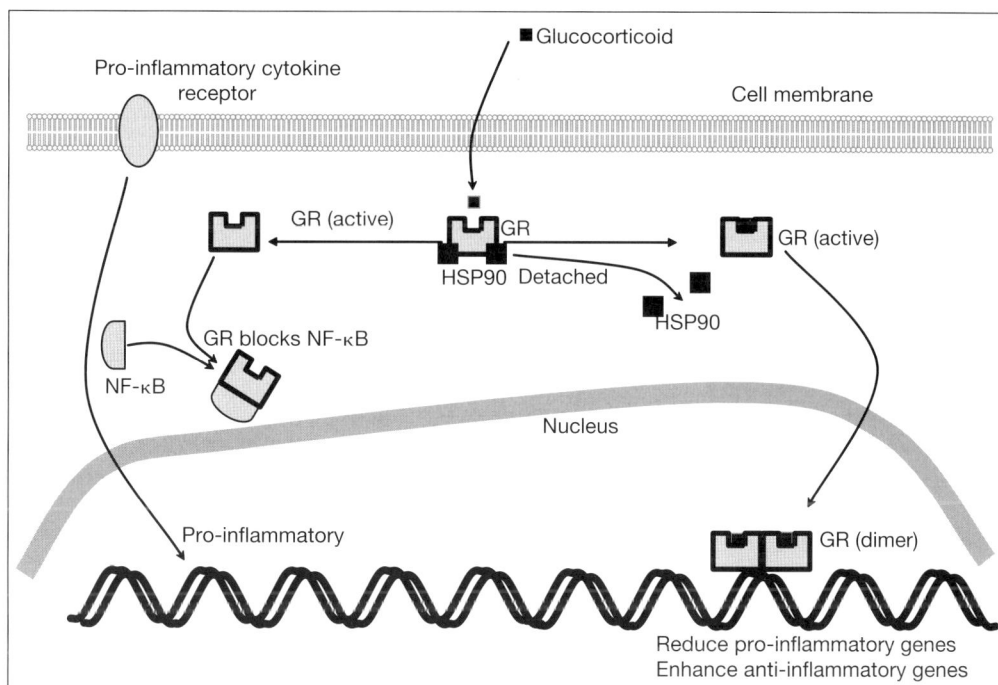

Figure 12.1 Principles of action of anti-inflammatory effects of glucocorticoids through the conformational change of glucocorticoid receptors in the cytoplasm, and subsequent effects on gene expression [adapted from 16].

ratio within the epithelium was observed, as well as a reduced number of mast cells in the subepithelial layer. These events paralleled reduced symptoms and fewer exacerbations in the subjects treated with the inhaled GC. In line with these observations in bronchial tissue, similar analyses in induced sputum and BAL fluid indicate weak overall effects of inhaled GCs [26–29].

β_2-SELECTIVE ADRENOCEPTOR AGONISTS

CLINICAL EFFECTS OF β_2-AGONISTS IN COPD

Short-acting and β_2-selective BAs such as salbutamol are utilized for symptom relief among patients with COPD. However, in recent years, data have emerged showing that regular twice-daily treatment with long-acting and β_2-selective BAs such as salmeterol and formoterol (Figure 12.2), provides clinically important improvements in patients with COPD [30–36]. These improvements may not solely depend on the prolonged bronchodilating effects of these drugs, since they can be demonstrated in patients with very little or no reversibility. The clearest effects are observed on the subjective symptoms of COPD, with significant reduction in dyspnoea and improved quality of life. Adding an inhaled anticholinergic such as ipratropium bromide to a long-acting β_2-selective BA generally results in little or no additional clinical effect (Figure 12.3). In fact, there is evidence that long-acting and β_2-selective BAs are similarly or more effective than ipratropium bromide [37], but so far no full-scale comparison with the once-daily administered long-acting anticholinergic tiotropium has been published. One smaller study suggest that there may be a benefit of

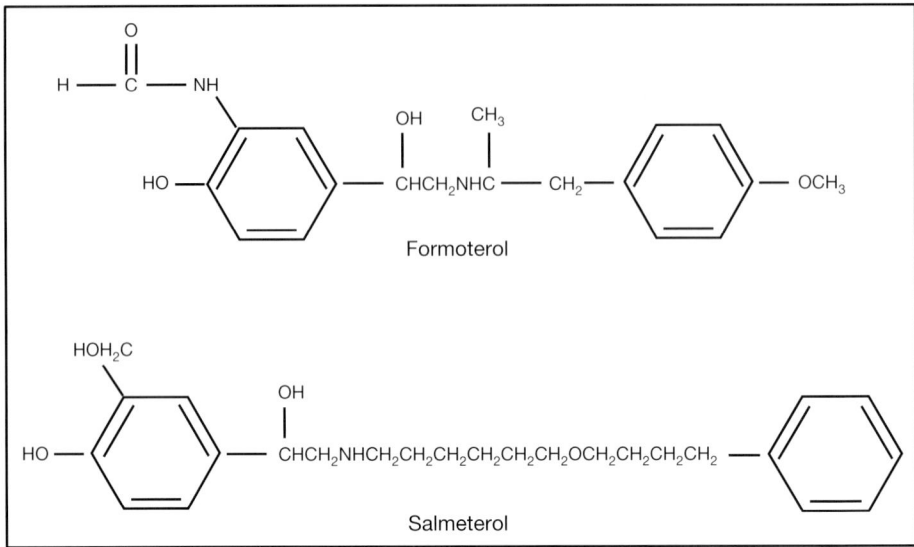

Figure 12.2   The chemical structure of formoterol and salmeterol.

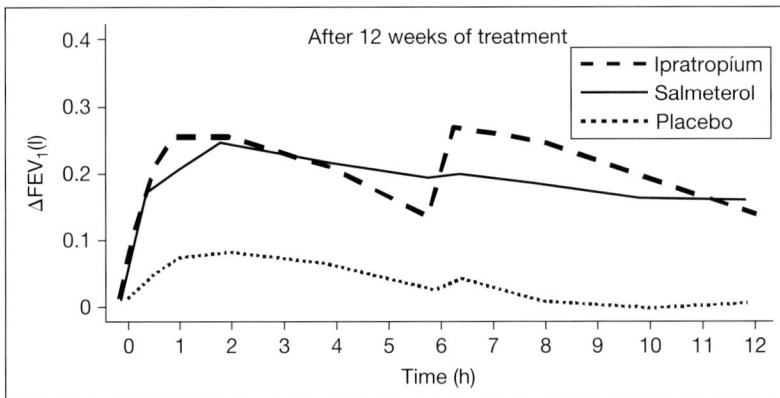

Figure 12.3   Time-course of mean FEV_1 in patients with COPD with some reversibility, after regular inhalation of formoterol or ipratropium bromide [adapted from 35].

combining tiotropium with a long-acting and β_2-selective BA [38], although this treatment should probably be given as a twice-daily regimen.

MECHANISMS OF ACTION FOR β_2-AGONISTS IN *IN VITRO* MODELS

When binding to the β_2-receptor (β_2-R), a β_2-selective BA forms hydrogen bonds to specific amino acids, and thereby induces a change in the three-dimensional structure of the β_2-R. This process enables the receptor to interact with intracellular G-proteins (Gs) [39, 40], which in turn stimulate the production of intracellular cyclic adenosine monophosphate (cAMP). Production of cAMP leads to activation of protein kinase A (PKA), which leads to the phosphorylation of several intracellular proteins, resulting in bronchial smooth muscle relaxation by inhibition of myosin-actin interaction. Additional mechanisms of action of β_2-selective BAs that are independent of cAMP have also been suggested, including K^+ channel activation via a subunit of the Gs. Importantly, β_2-selective BAs are functional antagonists. Thus, they cause relaxation of the smooth muscle, seemingly regardless of the extra- or intracellular stimulus causing the contraction.

There is no question that β_2-selective BAs evoke important clinical effects by relaxing the bronchial smooth muscle, thus reducing the subjective symptoms of airway obstruction. This is true for short- and long-acting β_2-selective BAs. In addition to the smooth muscle relaxation, all β_2-selective BAs may have other functional effects, such as attenuation of mast cell mediator release, reduction of plasma exudation and reduced activation of sensory nerves [41–43]. More functional effects include enhancement of mucociliary transport, inhibition of plasma exudation, reduction of neutrophil traffic, attenuation of chemokine release, and inhibition of bronchial smooth muscle cell proliferation [44, 45]. Interestingly, a long-acting β_2-selective BA (salmeterol) has also shown protective effect on experimental bacterial infection in one in vitro model, with reduced mucosal damage and significantly better preservation of ciliated cells under such conditions [46]. Whether any such effects would lead to clinically important anti-inflammatory effects in vivo in man is not known.

SIMILARITIES AND DIFFERENCES OF LONG-ACTING AND β_2-SELECTIVE β-ADRENOCEPTOR AGONISTS

During the last 10 years, we have had access to long-acting β_2-selective BAs but, short-acting BAs are still used extensively as symptom-relieving drugs in both asthma and COPD, even though they are not recommended for regular dosing. The two long-acting and β_2-selective BAs salmeterol and formoterol have extended duration of action, with a substantially maintained effect 12 h after inhalation of a single dose, and this prolonged effect may hypothetically represent a shared therapeutic advantage. In fact, bronchodilating effects have been demonstrated up to 24 h after the administration of these drugs in patients with asthma, although the full duration of these drugs has not been compared in patients with COPD.

Salmeterol and formoterol also behave differently in several ways. Even though both drugs are lipophilic (Figure 12.2), salmeterol is clearly more lipophilic than formoterol. At the level of the airway smooth muscle, when evaluated in in vitro models, the onset of action of salmeterol is substantially slower than both salbutamol and formoterol, whereas the onset of action of formoterol is as rapid as the short-acting and β_2-selective BA salbutamol. In line with this, clinical studies show that salmeterol and formoterol have different onset of action, with formoterol being much more rapid [47, 48], in common with salbutamol [49]. Clinically, salmeterol and formoterol have very parallel durations of action in patients with asthma, despite the fact that formoterol has a slightly shorter duration of action than salmeterol does in vitro.

Salmeterol and formoterol also differ in their ability to produce maximal effect (i.e., efficacy). Several studies on airway smooth muscle in vitro indicate that salmeterol is a partial agonist at the β_2-R [50]. Thus, salmeterol will not fully reverse severe, induced smooth muscle contraction, unlike the more effective short- and long-acting β_2-selective BAs such as terbutaline, fenoterol, salbutamol or formoterol [50]. In contrast, the long-acting β_2-selective BA formoterol is a full agonist, and has been shown to be more effective and have a greater maximal effect than salmeterol in patients with asthma in vivo [51]. Hypothetically, this implies that formoterol is better for bronchodilation in patients with acute, severe airflow obstruction but this question needs to be addressed further in clinical studies on COPD [52, 53].

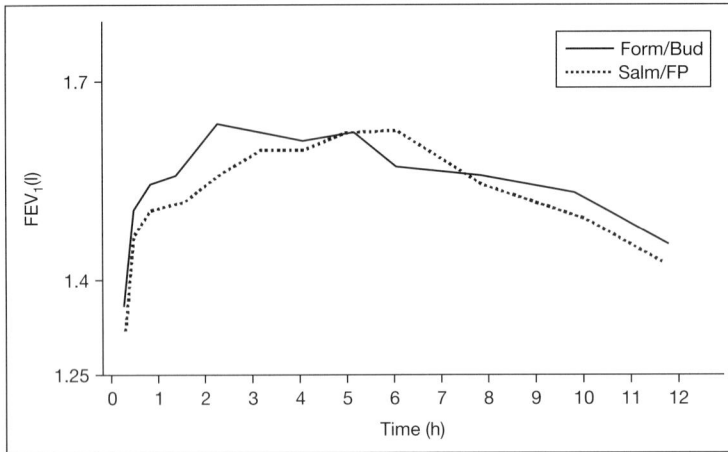

Figure 12.4 Time course of mean FEV$_1$ in patients with COPD with some reversibility after inhalation of 50 μg salmeterol/250 μg futicasone (Salm/FP) combination or a 12 μg formoterol/400 mg budesonide (Form/Bud). A significant difference between the two treatments could only be seen at the two-hour time point (in favour of Bud/Form, possibly due to the slightly more rapid onset of action of formoterol, or the higher efficacy of this drug; [48, 52]). The figure is adapted from Cazzola et al., 2004 [38].

A common feature of all β$_2$-selective BAs is their ability to evoke some tolerance at the level of β$_2$-R. Thus, the first dose is generally more effective than subsequent doses. In the airways, this has been primarily documented as a tolerance to the bronchoprotective effect on provocations, such as methacholine, allergen or exercise [48]. Of clinical importance, the tolerance to the systemic effects of β$_2$-agonists does seem to be more pronounced than the tolerance to the bronchodilatation [54]. The clinical relevance of the tolerance in the airways by regular daily treatment in patients with COPD remains uncertain.

It seems reasonable to assume that despite certain clinical benefits of monotherapy with long-acting β$_2$-selective BAs in patients with COPD, these drugs should be used primarily as symptom-relieving drugs. However, when given as combination therapy together with inhaled GCs, there is now evidence that these drugs may be used to control COPD.

COMBINATION THERAPY

CLINICAL EFFECTS OF COMBINATION THERAPY IN COPD

Increasing evidence argues that combining a long-acting β$_2$-selective BA with an inhaled GC may target both the symptomatic airway obstruction as well as certain aspects of the local inflammatory process in patients with COPD. Consequently, the combination products of salmeterol/fluticasone (Seretide®) and formoterol/budesonide (Symbicort®) have undergone extensive evaluation in COPD patients, and have been approved for clinical use in many countries (Figure 12.4) [55–63]. A meta-analysis of studies on either combination therapy demonstrates that the frequency of exacerbations is significantly reduced compared with placebo and the long-acting β$_2$-selective BA alone, but not necessarily when compared with GC treatment alone. On average, one exacerbation per 2–4 years of treatment per patient can be prevented using this combination therapy [4]. Compared with placebo, the combination therapy also resulted in a clinically meaningful improvement in quality of life, symptoms and exacerbations, perhaps due to smooth muscle effects of the long-acting β$_2$-selective BA.

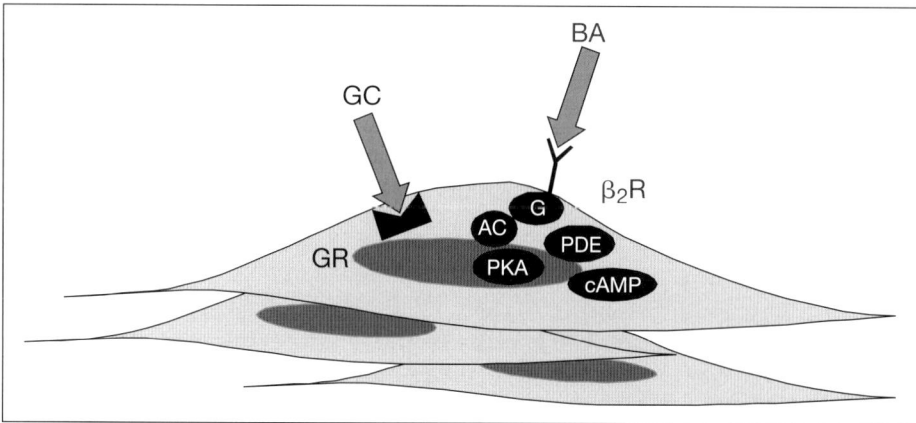

Figure 12.5 Experimentally confirmed sites of interactions during co-stimulation of airway smooth muscle cells with glucocorticoids (GC) and β_2-selective adrenoceptor agonists (BA). GC and BA act on and interact at the level of glucocorticoid receptors (GR) and β_2-adrenoceptors (β_2R), respectively, and this co-stimulation potentiates the activation of G-protein (G), adenylyl cyclase (AC), phosphodiesterase (PDE), and phosphokinase A (PKA), leading to increased production of cyclic AMP (cAMP).

It has been shown that treatment with long-acting β_2-selective BAs alone, or in combination with an inhaled GC, is at least as effective as ipratropium bromide given three times daily [35, 37]. However, more extensive comparisons of combinations of inhaled long-acting β_2-selective BAs and GCs with the ultra-long-acting anticholinergic tiotropium bromide are required to gain clinically useful information [38]. On a hypothetical basis, it seems plausible that at least in some patients, a triple combination can be beneficial.

MECHANISMS OF ACTION FOR COMBINATION THERAPY IN IN VITRO MODELS

Very few mechanistic studies on combination therapy have been conducted on tissue or isolated cells from patients with COPD. Therefore, studies on tissue or isolated cells from either healthy human donors, patients with other types of lung disease or rodents constitute the current basis for evaluating putative cellular mechanisms that may explain synergistic or additive clinical effects of combination therapy in COPD.

Airway Smooth Muscle

Several studies have addressed potentially beneficial effects of co-stimulation with a GC and a BA in airway smooth muscle *in vitro* [64]. For example, one study on human airway smooth muscle from patients with cancer or lung transplant donors demonstrates that a combination of BA and GC synergistically activates the GR and stimulates transcription factors, which leads to an additive inhibition of serum-induced proliferation (Figure 12.5) [65]. The protein kinase inhibitor p21 seems to be crucial in this context and, of some note, BAs and GCs may be effective at much lower concentrations when co-stimulating the airway smooth muscle than when stimulating as single drugs. In another example, spontaneous (but not induced) migration of isolated airway smooth muscle from lung transplant donors is inhibited by a long-acting BA and by other cAMP-elevating stimuli [66]. In the same model, stimulation with a long-acting BA plus a GC further inhibits induced cell migration. It seems likely that the synergism achieved by adding a GC is related to an augmentation of the BA-induced cAMP/protein kinase-dependent gene transcription.

It is also known that co-stimulation with a GC and a short- or long-acting β_2-selective BA synergistically inhibits the release of the neutrophil chemoattractant, interleukin-8 (IL-8) caused by the pro-inflammatory cytokine, tumour necrosis factor alpha (TNF-α) in isolated human airway smooth muscle [67]. Of mechanistic interest, this potentially beneficial effect of combination therapy can be mimicked by replacing the BA with a direct stimulator of adenylyl cyclase, a selective protein kinase A inhibitor or a phosphodiesterase inhibitor. Paradoxically, the referred synergistic inhibitory effect on IL-8 achieved by co-stimulation is observed in spite of the short- and long-acting BA *per se* actually increasing IL-8 release in unstimulated airway smooth muscle cells [67]. Yet another example of a mechanism that may underlie synergism for combination therapy is provided by a study on airway smooth muscle from cows [68]. In this *in vitro* model, a GC increases the density of β-adrenoceptors as well as both high- and low-affinity binding of a BA. Furthermore, a GC elevates intracellular G-protein, leading to a substantial increase in the maximal cAMP generation caused by a non-selective BA [68]. Supportive evidence regarding the impact of a BA on the affinity and density of β-adrenoceptors as well as a reduced inducible adenylate cyclase activity has also been generated in an airway smooth muscle cell line from rodents [69]. Interestingly, these events appear reversible if stimulation with a BA is removed or if stimulation with a GC is added.

Currently, it is not known what effect a GC exerts on the up-regulation of histamine (H1) receptors exerted by a BA in airway smooth muscle from cows [70]. It has also been shown that adding a long-acting GC does not completely inhibit the BA-induced potentiation of TNF-α-induced IL-6 release in airway smooth muscle, when using cells from lung transplant donors [71].

Bronchial Epithelial Cells

The finding that a β_2-selective and a non-selective short-acting BA, respectively, can increase the release of IL-8 in isolated and transformed bronchial epithelial cells from humans indicates a potentially pro-inflammatory, detrimental effect involving the epithelium and neutrophils as well [72]. However, it has also been shown that, whereas two different long-acting and β_2-selective BAs can also increase IL-8 in primary bronchial epithelial cells from humans, this effect is abolished if a GC is added for simultaneous stimulation [73].

Inflammatory Cells

There are studies on isolated inflammatory cells indicating that BAs and GCs may interact in a beneficial manner in terms of modulating inflammatory cells. Thus, co-stimulation with a BA plus a GC synergistically does inhibit expression of the adhesion-facilitating surface antigen CD11b in isolated neutrophils from cow blood [74]. However, there are observations from isolated inflammatory cells providing evidence for detrimental effects of adding stimulation with a BA to that of a GC. Thus, long-term exposure to a BA increases fMLP-induced respiratory burst and counteracts the potentially beneficial GC-induced apoptosis in isolated eosinophils obtained from healthy human donors [75].

It also seems that stimulation with a GC does not counteract BA-induced desensitisation of β-adrenoceptors in alveolar macrophages from healthy smoking human volunteers [76]. This latter observation contrasts with earlier observations on rat lung membranes *in vitro*; stimulation with a GC can restore the reduction in β-adrenoceptor number, agonist affinity and related adenylate cyclase activity that is observed after BA stimulation in rat lung membranes *in vitro* [77]. Similarly, stimulation with a BA decreases the number of binding sites for BAs in isolated human lymphocytes from blood and this effect is counteracted by a GC [78].

Tentatively, the reviewed experimental studies on isolated cells of relevance for airway and lung function indicate that the potentially beneficial effects of combination therapy with a BA and a GC involve such diverse targets as the regulation of the affinity and density of β-adrenoceptors, the linked control of G-protein, adenylyl cyclase, protein kinase A, phosphodiesterases and cyclic AMP. There is also evidence that this type of co-treatment exerts an impact on the activation of the GR as well as the transcription of cytokines and growth factors.

MECHANISMS OF ACTION BEHIND COMBINATION THERAPY IN IN VIVO MODELS

Very few studies on animals *in vivo* have specifically addressed the mechanisms behind the potentially beneficial synergism between BAs and GCs in the airways and lungs. There is one study of particular interest conducted on rat lungs *in vivo* [79]. This study demonstrates that a GC restores the number and the mRNA of β-2- but not β-1-adrenoceptors during stimulation with a BA [79]. These findings may relate to the GC-induced reversal of a BA-induced decrease in activity of the cyclic AMP-responsive binding protein [79]. In the same study, a GC enhanced the transcription rate of the gene for β_2-R. Clearly, these findings support the theory that a GC can prevent BA-induced desensitisation of β_2-R in the airways and lungs. Also, of potential clinical relevance, a recent study on mice *in vivo* provided evidence that adding a short-acting BA can counteract the detrimental effects on skeletal muscle caused by long-term treatment with a GC, including myosin heavy chain loss and the loss of muscle fibre cross-sectional area [80].

No recent and relevant observations on combination therapy and anti-inflammatory effects *in vivo* have been published. This means, for example, that it remains unclear whether a GC potentiates the inhibitory effect of a BA on neutrophil accumulation in rodent airways caused by either the pro-inflammatory cytokine IL-1β or by endotoxin *in vivo* [46, 81].

The limited work on the mechanisms underpinning co-treatment in animal *in vivo* models thus supports the theory that one level of interaction may be the control of the density of β_2-R. However, many other mechanisms that have been identified in *in vitro* studies remain to be evaluated *in vivo*.

CONCLUSIONS

There is certain clinical and experimental evidence that COPD, with its mobilisation of macrophages, neutrophils and certain T-lymphocytes, responds more beneficially to combination therapy with a GC and a long-acting and β_2-selective BA than it does to monotherapy with either of these two classes of drugs. However, the response to combination therapy seems to be restricted to a reduced number of exacerbations, and it is unclear whether this is due to synergism or an additive effect of the key pharmacological actions of GCs and long-acting, β_2-selective BAs. It thus remains uncertain whether this type of combination therapy exerts any truly beneficial long-term effects on the course of bronchiolitis or emphysema – the two pathological hallmarks of COPD.

REFERENCES

1.   Vignola AM, Paganin F, Capieu L, Scichilone N, Bellia M, Maakel L et al. Airway remodelling assessed by sputum and high-resolution computed tomography in asthma and COPD. *Eur Respir J* 2004; 24:910–917.
2.   Chanez P, Vignola AM, O'Shaugnessy T, Enander I, Li D, Jeffery PK et al. Corticosteroid reversibility in COPD is related to features of asthma. *Am J Respir Crit Care Med* 1997; 155:1529–1534.
3.   Sitkauskiene B, Sakalauskas R, Malakauskas K, Lötvall J. Reversibility to a beta2-agonist in COPD: relationship to atopy and neutrophil activation. *Respir Med* 2003; 97:591–598.
4.   Nannini L, Cates CJ, Lasserson TJ, Poole P. Combined corticosteroid and long acting beta-agonist in one inhaler for chronic obstructive pulmonary disease. *Cochrane Database Syst Rev* 2004; CD003794.
5.   Pauwels RA, Buist AS, Ma P, Jenkins CR, Hurd SS. Global strategy for the diagnosis, management, and prevention of chronic obstructive pulmonary disease: National Heart, Lung, and Blood Institute and World Health Organization Global Initiative for Chronic Obstructive Lung Disease (GOLD): executive summary. *Respir Care* 2001; 46:798–825.

6.   Burge PS, Calverley PM, Jones PW, Spencer S, Anderson JA, Maslen TK. Randomised, double blind, placebo controlled study of fluticasone propionate in patients with moderate to severe chronic obstructive pulmonary disease; the ISOLDE trial. *Br Med J* 2000; 320:1297–1303.

7.   Pauwels RA, Lofdahl CG, Laitinen LA *et al*. Long-term treatment with inhaled budesonide in persons with mild chronic obstructive pulmonary disease who continue smoking. European Respiratory Society Study on Chronic Obstructive Pulmonary Disease. *N Engl J Med* 1999; 340:1948–1953.

8.   Vestbo J, Sorensen T, Lange P, Brix A, Torre P, Viskum K. Long-term effect of inhaled budesonide in mild and moderate chronic obstructive pulmonary disease: a randomised controlled trial. *Lancet* 1999; 353:1819–1823.

9.   Spencer S, Calverley PMA, Burge PS, Jones PW and for the ISOLDE Study Group. Health status deterioration in patients with chronic obstructive pulmonary disease. *Am J Respir Crit Care Med* 2001; 163:122–128.

10. Sin DD, Tu JV. Inhaled corticosteroids and the risk of mortality and readmission in elderly patients with chronic obstructive pulmonary disease. *Am J Respir Crit Care Med* 2001; 164:580–584.

11. Pedersen B, Dahl R, Karlström R, Peterson CG, Venge P. Eosinophil and neutrophil activity in asthma in a one-year trial with inhaled budesonide: the impact of smoking. *Am J Respir Crit Care Med* 1996; 153:1519–1529.

12. Chalmers GW, Macleod KJ, Little SA, Thomson LJ, McSharry CP, Thomson NC. Influence of cigarette smoking on inhaled corticosteroid treatment in mild asthma. *Thorax* 2002; 57:226–230.

13. Chaudhuri R, Livingston E, McMahon AD, Thomson L, Borland W, Thomson NC. Cigarette smoking impairs the therapeutic response to oral corticosteroids in chronic asthma. *Am J Respir Crit Care Med* 2003; 168:1308–1311.

14. Di Stefano A, Caramori G, Ricciardolo FL, Capelli A, Adcock IM, Donner CF. Cellular and molecular mechanisms in chronic obstructive pulmonary disease: an overview. *Clin Exp Allergy* 2004; 34:1156–1167.

15. Adcock I, Gilbey T, Gelder CM, Chung KF, Barnes PJ. Glucocorticoid receptor localization in normal and asthmatic lung. *Am J Respir Crit Care Med* 1996; 154:771–782.

16. Caramori G, Adcock IM, Ito K. Anti-inflammatory inhibitors of IkappaB kinase in asthma and COPD. *Curr Opin Investig Drugs* 2004; 5:1141–1147.

17. Hellermann GR, Nagy SB, Kong X, Lockey RF, Mohapatra SS. Mechanism of cigarette smoke condensate-induced acute inflammatory response in human bronchial epithelial cells. *Respir Res* 2002; 3:22.

18. Auphan N, Didonato JA, Rosette C, Helmberg A, Karin M. Immunosuppression by glucocorticoids: inhibition of NF-kappa B activity through induction of I kappa B synthesis. *Science* 1995; 270:286–290.

19. Scheinman R, Cogswell PC, Lofquist AK, Baldwin AS Jr. Role of transcriptional activation of I kappa B alpha in mediation of immunosuppression by glucocorticoids. *Science* 1995; 270:283–286.

20. Ito K, Lim S, Caramori G, Chung KF, Barnes PJ, Adcock IM. Cigarette smoking reduces histone deacetylase 2 expression, enhances cytokine expression, and inhibits glucocorticoid actions in alveolar macrophages. *FASEB J* 2001; 15:1110–1112.

21. Pelaia G, Vatrella A, Cuda G, Maselli R, Marsico SA. Molecular mechanisms of corticosteroid actions in chronic inflammatory airway diseases. *Life Sci* 2003; 72:1549–1561.

22. Russell RE, Culpitt SV, DeMatos C, Donnelly L, Smith M, Wiggins J *et al*. Release and activity of matrix metalloproteinase-9 and tissue inhibitor of metalloproteinase-1 by alveolar macrophages from patients with chronic obstructive pulmonary disease. *Am J Respir Cell Mol Biol* 2002; 26:602–609.

23. Homma T, Kato A, Hashimoto N, Batchelor J, Yoshikawa M, Imai S *et al*. Corticosteroid and cytokines synergistically enhance toll-like receptor 2 expression in respiratory epithelial cells. *Am J Respir Cell Mol Biol* 2004; 31:463–469.

24. Soler N, Torres A, Ewig S, Gonzalez J, Celis R, El-Ebiary M *et al*. Related bronchial microbial patterns in severe exacerbations of chronic obstructive pulmonary disease (COPD) requiring mechanical ventilation. *Am J Respir Crit Care Med* 1998; 157(5 Pt 1):1498–1505.

25. Hattotuwa KL, Gizycki MJ, Ansari TW, Jeffery PK, Barnes NC. The effects of inhaled fluticasone on airway inflammation in chronic obstructive pulmonary disease: a double-blind, placebo-controlled biopsy study. *Am J Respir Crit Care Med* 2002; 165:1592–1596.

26. Confalonieri M, Mainardi E, Della Porta R *et al*. Inhaled corticosteroids reduce neutrophilic bronchial inflammation in patients with chronic obstructive pulmonary disease. *Thorax* 1998; 53:583–585.

27. Keatings VM, Jatakanon A, Worsdell YM, Barnes PJ. Effects of inhaled and oral glucocorticoids on inflammatory indices in asthma and COPD. *Am J Respir Crit Care Med* 1997; 155:542–548.

28. Thompson AB, Mueller MB, Heires AJ *et al.* Aerosolized beclomethasone in chronic bronchitis. Improved pulmonary function and diminished airway inflammation. *Am Rev Respir Dis* 1992; 146:389–395.

29. Balbi B, Majori M, Bertacco S *et al.* Inhaled corticosteroids in stable COPD patients: do they have effects on cells and molecular mediators of airway inflammation? *Chest* 2000; 117:1633–1637.

30. Cazzola M, Santangelo G, Piccolo A, Salzillo A, Matera MG, D'Amato G *et al.* Effect of salmeterol and formoterol in patients with chronic obstructive pulmonary disease. *Pulm Pharmacol* 1994; 7:103–107.

31. Matera MG, Cazzola M, Vinciguerra A, Di Perna F, Calderaro F, Caputi M *et al.* A comparison of the bronchodilating effects of salmeterol, salbutamol and ipratropium bromide in patients with chronic obstructive pulmonary disease. *Pulm Pharmacol* 1995; 8:267–271.

32. Ayers ML, Mejia R, Ward J, Lentine T, Mahler DA. Effectiveness of salmeterol versus ipratropium bromide on exertional dyspnoea in COPD. *Eur Respir J* 2001; 17:1132–1137.

33. Jarvis B, Markham A. Inhaled salmeterol: a review of its efficacy in chronic obstructive pulmonary disease. *Drugs Aging* 2001; 18:441–472.

34. Ramirez-Venegas A, Ward J, Lentine T, Mahler DA. Salmeterol reduces dyspnea and improves lung function in patients with COPD. *Chest* 1997; 112:336–340.

35. Rennard SI, Anderson W, ZuWallack R, Broughton J, Bailey W, Friedman M *et al.* Use of a long-acting inhaled beta2-adrenergic agonist, salmeterol xinafoate, in patients with chronic obstructive pulmonary disease. *Am J Respir Crit Care Med* 2001; 163:1087–1092.

36. Appleton S, Smith B, Veale A, Bara A. Long-acting beta2-agonists for chronic obstructive pulmonary disease. *Cochrane Database Syst Rev* 2000; CD001104.

37. Dahl R, Greefhorst LA, Nowak D, Nonikov V, Byrne AM, Thomson MH *et al*; Formoterol in Chronic Obstructive Pulmonary Disease I Study Group. Inhaled formoterol dry powder versus ipratropium bromide in chronic obstructive pulmonary disease. *Am J Respir Crit Care Med* 2001; 164:778–784.

38. Cazzola M, Centanni S, Santus P, Verga M, Mondoni M, di Marco F *et al.* The functional impact of adding salmeterol and tiotropium in patients with stable COPD. *Respir Med* 2004; 98:1214–1221.

39. Johnson M. The beta-adrenoceptor. *Am J Respir Crit Care Med* 1998; 158(5 Pt 3):S146–S153. Review.

40. Liggett SB. Update on current concepts of the molecular basis of beta2-adrenergic receptor signaling. *J Allergy Clin Immunol* 2002; 110(suppl):S223–S227.

41. Tomioka K, Yamada T, Ida H. Anti-allergic activities of the beta-adrenoceptor stimulant formoterol (BD 40A). *Arch Int Pharmacodyn Ther* 1981; 250:279–292.

42. Tokuyama K, Lotvall JO, Lofdahl CG, Barnes PJ, Chung KF. Inhaled formoterol inhibits histamine-induced airflow obstruction and airway microvascular leakage. *Eur J Pharmacol* 1991; 193:35–39.

43. Skoogh BE, Svedmyr N. Beta2-adrenoceptor stimulation inhibits ganglionic transmission in ferret trachea. *Pulm Pharmacol* 1989; 1:167–172.

44. Johnson M, Rennard S. Alternative mechanisms for long-acting beta(2)-adrenergic agonists in COPD. *Chest* 2001; 120:258–270. Review.

45. Miyamoto M *et al.* Beta-adrenoceptor stimulation and neutrophils in mouse airways. *Eur Respir J* 2004; 24:231–237

46. Dowling RB, Rayner CF, Rutman A *et al.* Effect of salmeterol on *Pseudomonas aeruginosa* infection of respiratory mucosa. *Am J Respir Crit Care Med* 1997; 155:327–336.

47. Palmqvist M, Persson G, Lazer L, Rosenborg J, Larsson P, Lotvall J. Inhaled dry-powder formoterol and salmeterol in asthmatic patients: onset of action, duration of effect and potency. *Eur Respir J* 1997; 10:2484–2489.

48. Sears MR, Lotvall J. Past, present and future—beta2-adrenoceptor agonists in asthma management. *Respir Med* 2005, 99.152–170.

49. Seberova E, Andersson A. Oxis (formoterol given by Turbuhaler) showed as rapid an onset of action as salbutamol given by a pMDI. *Respir Med* 2000; 94:607–611.

50. Linden A, Bergendal A, Ullman A, Skoogh BE, Lofdahl CG. Salmeterol, formoterol, and salbutamol in the isolated guinea-pig trachea: differences in maximum relaxant effect and potency but not in functional antagonism. *Thorax* 1993; 48:547–553.

51. Palmqvist M, Ibsen T, Mellen A, Lötvall J. Comparison of the relative efficacy of formoterol and salmeterol in asthmatic patients. *Am J Respir Crit Care Med* 1999; 160:244–249.

52. Pauwels RA, Sears MR, Campbell M, Villasante C, Huang S, Lindh A, *et al*; RELIEF Study investigators. Formoterol as relief medication in asthma: a worldwide safety and effectiveness trial. *Eur Respir J* 2003; 22:787–794.

53. Malolepszy J, Boszormenyi Nagy G, Selroos O, Larsso P, Brander R. Safety of formoterol Turbuhaler at cumulative dose of 90 microg in patients with acute bronchial obstruction. *Eur Respir J* 2001; 18:928–934.

54. Svedmyr NL, Larsson SA, Thiringer GK. Development of 'resistance' in beta-adrenergic receptors of asthmatic patients. *Chest* 1976; 69:479–483.

55. Donohue JF, Kalberg C, Emmett A, Merchant K, Knobil K. A short-term comparison of fluticasone propionate/salmeterol with ipratropium bromide/albuterol for the treatment of COPD. *Treat Respir Med* 2004; 3:173–181.

56. Fenton C, Keating GM. Inhaled salmeterol/fluticasone propionate: a review of its use in chronic obstructive pulmonary disease. *Drugs* 2004; 64:1975–1996.

57. Cazzola M, Santus P, Di Marco F, Boveri B, Castagna F, Carlucci P et al. Bronchodilator effect of an inhaled combination therapy with salmeterol + fluticasone and formoterol + budesonide in patients with COPD. *Respir Med* 2003; 97:453–457.

58. Cazzola M, Noschese P, Centanni S, Santus P, Di Marco F, Spicuzza L et al. Salmeterol/fluticasone propionate in a single inhaler device versus theophylline + fluticasone propionate in patients with COPD. *Pulm Pharmacol Ther* 2004; 17:141–145.

59. Hanania NA, Darken P, Horstman D, Reisner C, Lee B, Davis S et al. The efficacy and safety of fluticasone propionate (250 microg)/salmeterol (50 microg) combined in the diskus inhaler for the treatment of COPD. *Chest* 2003; 124:834–843.

60. Calverley P, Pauwels R, Vestbo J, Jones P, Pride N, Gulsvik A et al. TRial of Inhaled STeroids ANd long-acting beta2 agonists study group. Combined salmeterol and fluticasone in the treatment of chronic obstructive pulmonary disease: a randomised controlled trial. *Lancet* 2003; 361:449–456.

61. Calverley PM, Boonsawat W, Cseke Z, Zhong N, Peterson S, Olsson H. Maintenance therapy with budesonide and formoterol in chronic obstructive pulmonary disease. *Eur Respir J* 2003; 22:912–919.

62. Mahler DA, Wire P, Horstman D, Chang CN, Yates J, Fischer T et al. Effectiveness of fluticasone propionate and salmeterol combination delivered *via* the Diskus device in the treatment of chronic obstructive pulmonary disease. *Am J Respir Crit Care Med* 2002; 166:1084–1091.

63. Szafranski W, Cukier A, Ramirez A, Menga G, Sansores R, Nahabedian S et al. Efficacy and safety of budesonide/formoterol in the management of chronic obstructive pulmonary disease. *Eur Respir J* 2003; 21:74–81. Erratum in: *Eur Respir J* 2003; 21:912.

64. Howarth PH et al. Synthetic responses in airway smooth muscle. *J Allergy Clin Immunol* 2004; 114:S32–S50.

65. Roth M et al. Interaction between glucocorticoids and β2-agonists on bronchial airway smooth muscle cells through synchronized cellular signaling. *Lancet* 2002; 360:1293–1299.

66. Goncharova EA et al. Cyclic AMP-mobilizing agents and glucocorticoids modulate human smooth muscle cell migration. *Am J Respir Cell Mol Biol* 2003; 29:19–27.

67. Pang L, Knox AJ. Synergistic inhibition by β2-agonists and corticosteroids on tumor necrosis factor-α-induced interleukin-8 release from cultured human airway smooth muscle cells. *Am J Respir Cell Mol Biol* 2000; 23:79–85.

68. Kalavantavich K, Schramm CM. Dexamethasone potentiates high-affinity B-agonist binding and Gsa protein expression in airway smooth muscle. *Am J Physiol Lung Cell Mol Physiol* 2000; 278:L1101–L1106.

69. Scarpace PJ et al. Desensitisation and resensitization of beta-adrenergic receptors in a smooth muscle cell line. *Mol Pharmacol* 1985; 28:495–501.

70. Mak JC et al. Up-regulation of airway smooth muscle histamine H1 receptor mRNA, protein, and function by B2-adrenoceptor activation. *Mol Pharmacol* 2000; 57:857–864.

71. Ammit AJ et al. Tumor necrosis factor-α-induced secretion of RANTES and interleukin-6 from human airway smooth muscle cells. *Am J Respir Cell Mol Biol* 2002; 26:465–474.

72. Lindén A. Increased interleukin-8 release by beta-adrenoceptor activation in human transformed bronchial epithelial cells. *Br J Pharmacol* 1996; 119:402–406.

73. Korn SH, Brattsand R. Effects of formoterol and budesonide on GM-CSF and IL-8 secretion by triggered human bronchial epithelial cells. *Eur Respir J* 2001; 17:1070–1077.

74. Diez-Fraile A et al. Effect of isoproterenol and dexamethasone on the lipopolysaccharide induced expression of CD11b on bovine neutrophils. *Vet Immunol Immunopathol* 2000; 76:151–156.

75. Nielson CP, Hadjokas NE. Beta-adrenceptor agonists block corticosteroid inhibition in eosinophils. *Am J Respir Crit Care Med* 1998; 157:184–191.

76. Zetterlund A *et al*. Beta2-adrenoceptor desensitisation in human alveolar macrophages induced by inhaled terbutaline *in vivo* is not counteracted by budesonide. *Clin Sci* 2001; 100:451–457.

77. Scarpace PJ, Abrass IB. Desensitisation of adenylate cyclase and down regulation of beta-adrenergic receptors after *in vivo* administration of beta agonist. *J Pharmacol Exp Ther* 1982; 223:327–331.

78. Hui KK *et al*. Reversal of human lymphocyte beta-adrenoceptor desensitization by glucocorticoids. *Clin Pharmacol Ther* 1982; 32:566–571.

79. Mak JC *et al*. Protective effects of a glucocorticoid on downregulation of pulmonary B2-adrenergic receptors *in vivo*. *J Clin Invest* 1995; 96:99–106.

80. Pellegrino MA *et al*. Clenbuterol antagonizes glucocorticoid-induced atrophy and fibre type transformation in mice. *Exp Physiol* 2004; 89:89–100.

81. Sergejeva S *et al*. A synthetic VIP analogue inhibits neutrophil recruitment in rat airways *in vivo*. *Regul Pept* 2004; 117:149–154.

13

The role of inhaled combination therapy with corticosteroids and long-acting β₂-agonists in the management of COPD

R. Dahl, M. Cazzola

INTRODUCTION

Long-acting β₂-agonists (LABA) and inhaled corticosteroids (ICSs) treat different aspects of COPD [1]. LABAs have both bronchodilator and non-bronchodilator properties, whereas ICSs are potent anti-inflammatory agents. Combining two therapies that possess different modes of action could be expected to have a greater benefit in the management of COPD. Furthermore, when a LABA is added to an ICS, it has the potential for countering some of the possible negative effects of the corticosteroid [2].

It is not surprising, therefore, that use of ICS with LABA may be associated with a reduction of rehospitalisation or death in COPD patients. Soriano *et al.* [3] in a retrospective analysis investigated the survival rates of COPD patients receiving different types of medication, using records available from the UK General Practice Research Database. In total, 1,045 COPD patients who were prescribed fluticasone and salmeterol were identified and their 3-year mortality rates were analysed in comparison to 3,620 individuals with the same diagnosis who were treated with bronchodilators, but not ICSs or LABAs. The researchers found that patients receiving fluticasone and salmeterol had better 3-year survival rates compared to the reference group (78.6% vs. 63.6%, respectively). Individuals receiving combination therapy had the lowest mortality rates followed by those using fluticasone alone, salmeterol alone and finally users of alternative types of medication. Greater numbers of prescriptions for both drugs were also associated with increased survival. The same group of researchers [4] also documented that prescription of ICSs after a hospital admission for COPD reduced the risk of readmission or death in the subsequent year compared with COPD patients who did not receive ICSs. However, the reduction in risk of readmission or death was much larger if the combination of ICSs and LABAs was prescribed (42%) than when only ICSs were given (16%).

There is an exciting possibility that the potential benefit in combining these two classes of drugs might be due to a synergistic interaction, the resulting synergetic effect being greater than the sum of responses achieved from each drug alone. However, the basic molecular mechanism of such an interaction is still to be fully identified. Recent *in vitro* and

Ronald Dahl, MD, Dr.med.sci. Professor of Respiratory Medicine, Department of Respiratory Diseases, Aarhus University Hospital, Aarhus, Denmark.

Mario Cazzola, MD, Consultant in Respiratory Medicine, Chief of Respiratory Medicine, Unit of Pneumology and Allergology, Department of Respiratory Medicine, A. Cardarelli Hospital, Naples, Italy.

in vivo evidence suggests a mechanistic interaction at the molecular level between ICSs and LABAs. Corticosteroids have been shown to up-regulate the β_2-adrenoceptor in human airways, which may provide more receptors for β_2-agonists to activate [5, 6]. On the other side, LABAs may potentiate the molecular mechanism of corticosteroid actions, with increased nuclear localisation of glucocorticoid receptors and additive or sometimes synergistic suppression of inflammatory mediator release [7–10].

CLINICAL EFFECTS IN ADDING AN ICS TO A LABA

The capacity of corticosteroids to prevent homologous down-regulation of β_2-adrenoceptor number and induce an increase in the rate of synthesis of these receptors may be critical when a patient is receiving regular treatment with a LABA. The addition of an ICS to a LABA was initially studied in a 3-month trial that enrolled 80 COPD patients. The combination therapy progressively improved lung function over the 3-month period compared to the long-acting bronchodilator treatment alone, although the difference was not statistically significant [11]. However, the combination of salmeterol (50 µg twice daily) with fluticasone (250 or 500 µg twice daily) allowed a significantly greater improvement in lung function after salbutamol than salmeterol (50 µg twice daily) alone. It is likely that this effect was due to prevention of the homologous down-regulation of β_2-adrenoceptors and induction of an increase in the rate of synthesis of receptors through a process of increased β_2-adrenoceptor gene transcription elicited by fluticasone. This may be considered clinically important, because when airway obstruction becomes more severe the preferred therapeutic option is to add a fast-acting inhaled β_2-agonist as rescue medication to produce rapid relief of bronchospasm.

The capacity of ICS to influence the onset of action of a LABA, however, might be explained by actions that can broadly be termed nongenomic [12]. A recent small study, in fact indicated that the addition of budesonide influences the fast onset of action of formoterol without induction of systemic effects, in patients with COPD [13]. Serial measurements of FEV_1 were performed over 60 min in 20 subjects. Budesonide/formoterol combination (BFC) elicited a significantly larger mean FEV_1-$AUC_{0–15 min}$ than formoterol alone. Also the change in FEV_1 15 min after inhalation of BFC (0.197 l; 95% CI: 0.142–0.252) was greater than that induced by formoterol alone (0.147 l; 95% CI: 0.092–0.201). The mean increases in FEV_1 were always higher after BFC than formoterol alone, although both treatments induced a significant improvement over baseline at each explored time point. Even the FEV_1-$AUC_{0–60 min}$ after BFC was significantly larger than that after formoterol. Both treatments did not alter heart rate in a statistically significant manner ($p > 0.05$). In any case, the results of this study suggest that the use of the BFC combination is preferable to that of formoterol alone when a rescue action is needed, as in the case of acute exacerbations of COPD. It is likely, in fact, that the faster onset of action might influence the control of symptoms in such a pathological condition.

Delivery of these medications together, administered as one inhalation twice daily, may help simplify treatment regimens and may also improve patient adherence compared with currently available COPD treatments. For this reason, there is a real interest in use of ICS/LABA combination by a single inhaler.

The value of regular combination therapy with ICSs and LABAs delivered *via* a single inhaler to COPD patients has repeatedly been documented (Table 13.1). Thus, the impact on lung function of a combination with fluticasone propionate and salmeterol (FSC) has been studied both using a dose of fluticasone 500 µg and salmeterol 50 µg, and fluticasone 250 µg and salmeterol 50 µg twice daily for 6 months or 12 months. In particular, Hanania *et al.* [14] compared the efficacy and safety of 24 weeks' treatment with fluticasone 250 µg and salmeterol 50 µg, administered together twice daily in a single inhaler device, with that of placebo and the individual agents alone in 723 patients with COPD and a mean baseline FEV_1 of

Table 13.1 Long-term effect of combination therapy in COPD

Study	Number of patients enrolled, drugs examined, study duration	Outcomes
Fluticasone/salmeterol (FSC)		
Hanania *et al.* [14]	723 patients with COPD (mean baseline FEV_1 42% of predicted values). F/S 250/50 µg, fluticasone 250 µg, salmeterol 50 µg, placebo, all given twice daily. F/U: 24 weeks.	Primary outcomes: morning pre-dose FEV_1 for FSC compared with salmeterol and 2-hour post-dose FEV_1 for FSC compared with fluticasone. Secondary outcomes: morning PEF; use of reliever medication, TDI; HRQL (CRDQ); COPD symptoms score (CBSQ); exacerbations.
Mahler *et al.* [15]	691 patients with moderate to severe COPD (FEV_1 41% of predicted value). F/S 500/50 µg, fluticasone 500 µg, salmeterol 50 µg, placebo, all given twice daily. F/U: 24 weeks.	Primary outcomes: morning pre-dose FEV_1 for FSC compared with salmeterol and fluticasone with placebo, and 2-hour post-dose FEV_1 for FSC compared with fluticasone and salmeterol with placebo. Secondary outcomes: morning PEF; use of reliever medication, TDI; HRQL (CRDQ); COPD symptoms score (CBSQ).
Dal Negro *et al.* [16]	18 patients with moderate to severe COPD (mean FEV_1 49.1% of predicted value). FSC 250/50 µg, salmeterol 50 µg, placebo, all given twice daily. F/U: 52 weeks.	Number of exacerbations, lung function.
Calverley *et al.* (TRISTAN study) [17]	1,465 patients with moderate to severe COPD (mean FEV_1 45% of predicted value). FSC 500/50 µg, fluticasone 500 µg, salmeterol 50 µg, placebo, all given twice daily. F/U: 52 weeks.	Primary outcome: pre-treatment FEV_1 Secondary outcomes: other lung function measurements, COPD symptoms score, use of reliever medication, number of exacerbations, patient withdrawals, HRQL (SGRQ).
Budesonide/formoterol (BFC)		
Szafranski *et al.* [18]	812 patients with moderate to severe COPD (mean FEV_1 36% of predicted value). BFC 400/12 µg, budesonide 400 µg, formoterol 12 µg or placebo, all given twice daily. F/U: 52 weeks.	Primary outcomes: number of severe exacerbations and change in post-medication FEV_1. Secondary outcomes: VC, HRQL (SGRQ), COPD symptoms score, PEF, use of reliever medication, number of mild exacerbations.
Calverley *et al.* [19]	1,022 patients with moderate to severe COPD (mean FEV_1 36% of predicted value). Initially, formoterol (12 µg twice daily) and oral prednisolone (30 mg once daily) for 2 weeks. After, BFC 400/12 µg, budesonide 400 µg, formoterol 12 µg or placebo, all given twice daily for 12 months. F/U: 2+52 weeks.	Primary outcomes: time to first exacerbation and change in post-medication FEV_1. Secondary outcomes: number of exacerbations, time to and number of oral corticosteroid treated episodes, morning and evening PEF, slow VC, HRQL (SGRQ), symptom score, use of reliever medication, acute events.

42% predicted. Mahler *et al.* [15] weighted the use of fluticasone 500 μg and salmeterol 50 μg in combination twice daily, against the individual components alone at the same doses, or placebo for 24 weeks in 691 patients with COPD and a mean baseline FEV_1 of 41% predicted. Dal Negro *et al.* [16] compared fluticasone 250 μg and salmeterol 50 μg in combination twice daily *via* a single inhaler with salmeterol 50 μg twice daily alone, and placebo in a 52-week study that enrolled a small group of ICS naïve patients with moderate COPD, already treated with theophylline 400 mg/day and an inhaled short-acting β_2-agonist on demand. A 52-week, multicentre, randomised, double-blind, placebo-controlled trial (TRial of Inhaled STeroids ANd long-acting β_2-agonists or TRISTAN) compared the safety and efficacy of the fluticasone 500 μg/salmeterol 50 μg combination twice daily with that of the individual drugs alone in 1,465 patients with COPD (mean FEV_1 45% predicted) [17]. Also, the effects of BFC treatment in COPD patients have been investigated. In a 12-month, randomised, double-blind, placebo-controlled, parallel-group, multicentre study, 812 adults with moderate to severe COPD (mean age 64 years; mean FEV_1 36% predicted) received two inhalations of either budesonide 200 μg/formoterol 6 μg, budesonide 200 μg alone, formoterol 6 μg alone, or placebo twice daily [18]. In a more recent trial [19], 1,022 COPD patients (mean FEV_1 36% predicted) initially received formoterol (12 μg twice daily) and oral prednisolone (30 mg once daily) for 2 weeks. After this time, patients were randomised to twice daily inhaled budesonide/formoterol 400/12 μg, budesonide 400 μg, formoterol 12 μg or placebo for 12 months.

The overall goals for improving clinical outcomes are to reduce symptoms, especially dyspnoea, reduce exacerbations and the possible need for hospitalisation, and enhance health status [20]. Therefore, the different trials have not only evaluated the efficacy of combination therapy on lung function, but also its impact on these other clinical outcomes.

EVALUATION OF IMPACT ON LUNG FUNCTION

Changes in lung function induced by long-term treatment with combined therapy are illustrated in Table 13.2.

At the end of Hanania trial [14], a significantly greater increase in morning pre-dose FEV_1 was observed following treatment with FSC (165 ml) compared with treatment with salmeterol alone (91 ml; p = 0.012) and placebo (1 ml; p < 0.001). A significantly greater increase in pre-dose FEV_1 was observed for treatment with fluticasone (109 ml) vs. placebo (1 ml; p < 0.001). The increase in pre-dose FEV_1 following treatment with FSC was 16.6% over baseline. Estimated differences between treatment groups were 161 ml FSC vs. placebo, 49 ml FSC vs. fluticasone, 69 ml FSC vs. salmeterol, 112 ml fluticasone vs. placebo, and 92 ml salmeterol vs. placebo. Only the difference between FSC and fluticasone was not statistically significant (p > 0.05). At end point, there was a significantly greater improvement in 2-hour post-dose FEV_1 in patients taking FSC (27%, 281 ml) compared with those taking salmeterol (19%, 200 ml), fluticasone (14%, 147 ml) or placebo (6%, 58 ml). The magnitude of responses in lung function for patients who demonstrated reversibility of airflow obstruction after salbutamol inhalation was higher compared with nonreversible patients. Importantly, the effect was clinically meaningful in both subgroups.

Mahler *et al.* [15] reported an improvement in pre-dose FEV_1 in the group treated with FSC vs. placebo (156 ml vs. −4 ml, respectively; p < 0.001). There was also a significant increase in those treated with FSC vs. those treated with salmeterol and fluticasone (156 ml vs. 107 ml and 109 ml, respectively; FSC vs. salmeterol, p = 0.012; FSC vs. fluticasone, p = 0.038). The increase in pre-dose FEV_1 corresponded to a 14.5% increase over baseline values. Interestingly, no significant differences were observed in a subgroup analysis stratified according to partial and no reversibility after inhaled short-acting β_2-agonist and reversibility defined a priori as an increase of 12% or more and 200 ml in FEV_1.

Table 13.2 Long-term effect on lung function of combination therapy in COPD

Study	Changes in functional parameter
Hanania et al. [14]	Significantly (p < 0.012) greater increase in morning pre-dose FEV_1 (165 ml) with FSC compared with salmeterol (91 ml) and placebo (1 ml), and significantly (p < 0.001) greater increase in the 2-hour post-dose FEV_1 (281 ml) compared with fluticasone (147 ml) and placebo (58 ml).
	Improvements in lung function with FSC compared with fluticasone and salmeterol, and with fluticasone and salmeterol compared with placebo, as measured by the average daily morning PEF, observed within approximately 24 h after the initiation of treatment (p < 0.034).
Mahler et al. [15]	Significantly greater increase in pre-dose FEV_1 after FSC (156 ml) compared with salmeterol (107 ml, p = 0.012) and placebo (−4 ml, p < 0.0001). Significantly greater increase in 2-hour post-dose FEV_1 after FSC (261 ml) compared with fluticasone (138 ml, p < 0.001) and placebo (28 ml, p < 0.001).
	Increases in morning PEF on Day 2, greater for FSC compared with fluticasone, salmeterol, and placebo, (p < 0.005). Greater increases in morning PEF throughout the 24-week treatment period with FSC compared with fluticasone, salmeterol, and placebo, respectively.
Dal Negro et al. [16]	Patients receiving FSC with the highest mean improvement in FEV_1 (+7.3% ± 3.3; p = 0.001) over the baseline pre-treatment value after 36 weeks of treatment, being FEV_1 unchanged after 52 weeks of treatment in salmeterol group (+0.33% ± 2.4) and with a substantial decrease following placebo (−2.6% ± 1.2; p = 0.001).
	Morning PEF (L/min) increased in subjects treated with FSC (p < 0.001), but unchanged in salmeterol and placebo group (in both, p = ns).
Calverley et al. (TRISTAN study) [17]	Significant increase in FEV_1 with all active treatments compared with placebo (FSC p < 0.0001; salmeterol p < 0.0001; fluticasone p = 0.0063) evident by Week 2 and was sustained throughout treatment.
	Rise in FEV_1 associated with combination therapy significantly greater than with either of its components separately (FSC vs. salmeterol: 73 ml (95% CI: 46–101), p < 0.001; FSC vs. fluticasone: 95 ml (95% CI: 67–122), p < 0.001; FSC vs. placebo: 133 (95% CI: 105–161), p < 0.001).
Szafranski et al. [18]	FEV_1 increased with BFC by 15% vs. placebo and 9% vs. budesonide. VC improved by all active treatments compared with placebo (9%, p < 0.001; 4%, p < 0.05; 11%, p < 0.001 for BFC, budesonide and formoterol, respectively).
	Morning PEF with BFC improved significantly on Day 1 vs. placebo and budesonide, after 1 week, morning PEF vs. placebo, budesonide and formoterol. Improvements in morning and evening PEF vs. comparators maintained over 12 months.
Calverley et al. [19]	After the optimisation period, improvement in FEV_1 seen during run-in maintained with BFC treatment throughout the study, but declined greatly and rapidly with all other treatments. Difference significant with BFC vs. placebo (14%), budesonide (11%) and formoterol (5%), and with formoterol vs. placebo (8%), but not with budesonide vs. placebo (2%).
	Changes in VC similar to those in FEV_1. BFC associated with higher morning PEF compared with all other treatments, and higher evening PEF compared with placebo and budesonide.

In the Dal Negro study [16], patients receiving FSC showed the highest mean improvement in FEV_1 (+6.6% ± 2.4) over the baseline pre-treatment value (p < 0.001), FEV_1 being unchanged after 52 weeks of treatment in the salmeterol group (+0.3% ± 0.9) and with a substantial decrease following placebo (−2.6% ± 0.5; p < 0.001).

The TRISTAN study [17] reported an increase in pre-dose FEV_1 in those treated with FSC vs. comparators (treatment difference for adjusted means averaged over 52 weeks: FSC vs. salmeterol: 73 ml (95% CI: 46–101), p < 0.001; FSC vs. fluticasone: 95 ml (95% CI: 67–122), p < 0.001; FSC vs. placebo: 133 ml (95% CI: 105–161), p < 0.001.

Szafranski et al. [18] demonstrated that all active treatments increased FEV_1 vs. placebo; BFC also increased FEV_1 vs. budesonide. The improvements in FEV_1 were sustained with BFC throughout the study period compared with budesonide (by 9%, p < 0.001), and placebo (by 15%, p < 0.001). The difference vs. formoterol was not significant (1%). After one week, BFC increased morning PEF by 15.6 l/min, compared with a mean increase in placebo treated participants of 1.1 l/min (p < 0.001), an increase in budesonide-treated participants of 3.4 l/min, (p < 0.001) and an increase in the formoterol group of 8.8 l/min, (p < 0.002). At 12 months, morning PEF was improved by 26.4 l/min from baseline in the BFC group, compared with improvements of 2.4 l/min in the placebo group (p < 0.001), 10.6 l/min in the budesonide group (p < 0.001) and 14.7 l/min in the formoterol group (p < 0.001).

In the Calverley study [19], after the optimisation period, the improvement in FEV_1 seen during run-in was maintained with BFC treatment throughout the study. In contrast, FEV_1 declined greatly and rapidly (by 1 month in patients treated with either placebo or budesonide) with all other treatments. This difference was significant with BFC compared with placebo (14%), budesonide (11%) and formoterol (5%), and with formoterol vs. placebo (8%), but not with budesonide vs. placebo (2%).

EVALUATION OF IMPACT ON SYMPTOMS

Table 13.3 reports the influence on symptoms of long-term treatments with combined therapy.

In the Hanania study [14], the mean Transition Dyspnoea Index (TDI) score for treatment with FSC (+1.7) was significantly greater than that following treatment with placebo (+1.0; p = 0.023). Moreover, TDI scores were numerically greater for salmeterol treatment alone (+1.6; p = 0.043) and fluticasone treatment alone (+1.7; p = 0.057) compared with placebo. Estimated differences between treatment groups were 0.8 FSC vs. placebo, 0.1 FSC vs. fluticasone, 0.1 FSC vs. salmeterol, 0.7 fluticasone vs. placebo, and 0.7 salmeterol vs. placebo. These estimated differences did not exceed the predefined criteria for clinical importance of 1 unit or more [21]. Improvements in Chronic Bronchitis Symptom Questionnaire (CBSQ) with fluticasone (2.2) and FSC (2.1) were significantly greater compared with placebo (1.4; p ≤ 0.017). The mean change from baseline was also numerically greater with FSC compared with salmeterol throughout the study. Similar mean changes in CBSQ were observed for FSC and fluticasone throughout the study.

In the Mahler study [15], the mean TDI score for treatment with FSC (2.1) was significantly greater than that after fluticasone (1.3, p = 0.033), salmeterol (0.9, p < 0.001) and placebo (0.4, p < 0.001). Estimated differences at end point between treatment groups were 1.7 FSC vs. placebo, 0.7 FSC vs. fluticasone, 1.2 FSC vs. salmeterol, 1.0 fluticasone vs. placebo, and 0.5 salmeterol vs. placebo. The estimated difference between FSC and salmeterol or placebo exceeded the predefined criteria for clinical importance of 1 unit or more. In any case, there were no consistent differences among treatments for changes in CBSQ.

The TRISTAN study [17] reported improvements in breathlessness scores after treatment in favour of FSC vs. placebo, fluticasone and salmeterol [FSC mean: 1.47; fluticasone mean: 1.59 (p value vs. FSC = 0.006); salmeterol mean: 1.58 (p value vs. FSC = 0.010); placebo

Table 13.3 Long-term effect on symptoms of combination therapy in COPD

Study	Changes in explored symptoms
Hanania *et al.* [14]	Mean TDI scores for treatments with FSC (+1.7), salmeterol alone (+1.6; p = 0.043) and fluticasone alone (+1.7; p = 0.057) significantly greater than that with placebo (+1.0; p = 0.023). Estimated differences between treatment groups: 0.8 FSC vs. placebo, 0.1 FSC vs. fluticasone, 0.1 FSC vs. salmeterol, 0.7 fluticasone vs. placebo, and 0.7 salmeterol vs. placebo.
	Improvements in CBSQ with fluticasone (2.2) and FSC (2.1) significantly greater compared with placebo (1.4, p ≤ 0.017), but no significant differences among FSC and salmeterol or fluticasone.
Mahler *et al.* [15]	Mean TDI score for treatment with FSC (2.1) significantly greater than that after fluticasone (1.3, p = 0.033), salmeterol (0.9, p < 0.001) and placebo (0.4, p < 0.001). Estimated differences between treatment groups: 1.7 FSC vs. placebo, 0.7 FSC vs. fluticasone, 1.2 FSC vs. salmeterol, 1.0 fluticasone vs. placebo, and 0.5 salmeterol vs placebo.
	No consistent differences among treatments for changes in CBSQ.
Calverley *et al.* (TRISTAN study) [17]	Breathlessness significantly reduced by FSC vs. placebo (p = 0.0001), salmeterol (p = 0.006), and fluticasone (p = 0.010).
	Number of night-time awakenings per week significantly less in FCS group (2.31), compared with placebo (3.01, p = 0.006) and salmeterol (2.94, p = 0.011), but not with fluticasone (2.45, p = 0.591).
	Cough scores with FCS not significantly different compared with salmeterol (p = 0.639) and fluticasone (p = 0.34), but significantly different vs. placebo (FSC: 1.35 vs. placebo: 1.44, p = 0.018).
Szafranski *et al.* [18]	Decrease in total symptom scores after BFC (−1.61) significantly different compared with that after placebo (0.49, p < 0.001), budesonide (0.77, p < 0.001) and formoterol (1.20, p < 0.05). Symptom controlled days increased by 7% with BFC vs. placebo (p = 0.001), 1% with BFC vs. budesonide (p = ns) and 7% with formoterol vs. placebo (p < 0.001).
	Awakening free nights increased by 14% with BFC vs. placebo (p < 0.001), 10% with BFC vs. budesonide (p = 0.003) and 10% with formoterol vs. placebo (p = 0.001).
	Days free from shortness of breath increased by 12% with BFC vs. placebo (p < 0.001) and with BFC 9% vs. budesonide (p = 0.001).
Calverley *et al.* [19]	Total symptom score and individual symptom scores for shortness of breath, chest tightness and night-time awakenings significantly (p < 0.01) improved by BFC and formoterol vs. placebo. Night-time awakenings score significantly (p = 0.049) improved by budesonide vs. placebo.

mean: 1.66 (p value vs. FSC < 0.001)]. Also improvements in night time awakenings compared with salmeterol and placebo were reported [FSC mean number of nights per week: 2.31; salmeterol mean: 2.94 (p value vs. FSC = 0.011); placebo mean: 3.01 (p value vs. FSC = 0.006)]. However, the mean FSC score was not statistically significant compared with the fluticasone score (2.45, p = 0.591). Cough scores were not significantly different compared with salmeterol and fluticasone (p = 0.639 and 0.34, respectively), but there was a significant difference vs. placebo (FSC: 1.35 vs. placebo: 1.44, p = 0.018).

Szafranski *et al.* [18] reported a significant reduction in all symptom scores within the first week of treatment with BFC vs. budesonide, formoterol and placebo, which was sustained for 12 months for BFC vs. placebo, budesonide and, for formoterol, regarding the total score and awakenings. In particular, BFC led to a mean decrease of 1.61 in total symptom scores compared with a decrease of 0.49 with placebo treatment (p < 0.001), 0.77 with budesonide treatment (p < 0.001) and 1.20 with formoterol (p < 0.05). Symptom controlled days were increased with BFC by 7% vs. placebo (p = 0.001) and by 1% vs. budesonide (p = ns). No data on the comparison with formoterol were available, although there was a significant difference in favour of formoterol vs. placebo (7%, p < 0.001). Awakening free nights were increased by 14% with BFC compared with placebo (p < 0.001), that is equivalent to approximately one extra night per week, and by 10% with BFC vs. budesonide (p = 0.003). No data on the comparison with formoterol were available, although there was a significant difference in favour of formoterol vs. placebo (10%, p = 0.001). BFC led to a 12% increase in days free from shortness of breath vs. placebo (p < 0.001), that is equivalent to approximately one extra day per week, and 9% increase vs. budesonide (p = 0.001). There was no statistically significant difference observed vs. formoterol (2%, p = ns).

In the Calverley study [19], BFC and formoterol significantly (p < 0.01) improved the total symptom score and the individual symptom scores for shortness of breath, chest tightness and night-time awakenings compared with placebo. Budesonide also significantly (p = 0.049) improved the night-time awakenings score compared with placebo. None of the treatments significantly improved the cough score.

EVALUATION OF IMPACT ON ACUTE EXACERBATIONS

The impact on acute exacerbations of long-term treatments with combined therapy is shown in Table 13.4.

Hanania *et al.* [14] were unable to observe significant differences among treatment groups in terms of the numbers of exacerbations or the time to first exacerbation. However, this study was designed and powered to evaluate the treatment effect on FEV_1, which was the primary measure of efficacy, rather than to evaluate the rates of exacerbations.

In the Mahler study [15] there were no statistically significant differences between treatment groups in time to exacerbation (no data or p values reported). Moreover, this study reported no difference in the number of participants who exacerbated once (placebo: 8.8%; salmeterol: 5.6%; fluticasone: 10.1%; FSC: 8.5%, no p value presented).

Dal Negro *et al.* [16] observed a lower number of exacerbations after treatment with FSC (seven in six patients on FSC; 14 in six patients on salmeterol; 25 in six patients on placebo). The mean number of exacerbations/year dropped from 3.5 in the previous year to 1.2 in the FSC group (p < 0.001) and from 3.0 to 2.3 in the salmeterol group (p = ns), and rose from 3.2 to 4.2 in the placebo group (p = ns).

In the TRISTAN study [17], the rate of exacerbations fell by 25% in the combination group (p < 0.0001) and by 20% (p = 0.0027) and 19% (p = 0.0033) in the salmeterol and fluticasone groups, respectively, compared with placebo. In particular, there was a significant difference in the mean exacerbation rate per participant per year in favour of FSC when compared with placebo (FSC: 0.97 vs. placebo: 1.30; p < 0.0001). The treatment effect was more pronounced in patients with severe disease (i.e., a baseline FEV_1 <50% of predicted), who showed a 30% reduction with FSC compared with placebo, as against a 10% reduction in patients who had a baseline FEV_1 that was greater than 50% of that predicted. There was no significant difference when FSC was compared with salmeterol and fluticasone groups (salmeterol: 1.04, p = 0.345; and fluticasone: 1.05, p = 0.304). FSC reduced by 39% exacerbations requiring oral corticosteroids compared with placebo (0.46 vs. 0.76 exacerbations per year, p < 0.0001) but not compared with salmeterol and fluticasone (0.46 vs. 0.54 and 0.50,

Table 13.4 Long-term effect on exacerbations of combination therapy in COPD

Study	Changes in exacerbations
Mahler et al. [15]	No statistically significant differences between treatment groups in time to exacerbation.
	No difference in the number of participants who exacerbated once (placebo: 8.8%; salmeterol: 5.6%; fluticasone: 10.1%; FSC: 8.5%)
Dal Negro et al. [16]	Lower number of exacerbations after treatment with FSC.
	Mean number of exacerbations per year dropped from 3.5 in the previous year to 1.2 in the FSC group (p < 0.001) and from 3.0 to 2.3 in the salmeterol group (p = ns), and rose from 3.2 to 4.2 in the placebo group (p = ns).
Calverley et al. (TRISTAN study) [17]	Mean exacerbation/year significantly lower with FSC when compared with placebo (FSC: 0.97 vs. placebo: 1.30, p < 0.0001) with a more pronounced effect in patients with baseline FEV$_1$ <50% of predicted. No significant difference with FSC when compared with salmeterol (1.04, p = 0.345) and fluticasone (1.05, p = 0.304).
	Acute episodes of symptom exacerbation that required oral corticosteroids reduced by FSC (0.46 exacerbations per year) when compared with placebo (0.76 exacerbations per year, p < 0.0001) but not when compared with salmeterol (0.54 exacerbations per year, p = 0.12) and fluticasone (0.50 exacerbations per year, p = 0.45).
	No significant differences between active treatments with respect to their effect on the rate of episodes of symptom exacerbation, time to first exacerbation, or number of hospital admissions.
Szafranski et al. [18]	Reduction in the number of severe exacerbations by 24% in the BFC group vs. placebo (p = 0.035), by 23% vs. formoterol (p = 0.043) and 11% vs. budesonide (p = 0.385).
	Reduction in the number of oral steroid courses used in association with exacerbations in the BFC group vs. placebo (31%, p = 0.027) and vs. formoterol (28%, p = 0.039), and in the budesonide group vs. placebo (29%, p = 0.045).
	Reduction in the number of mild exacerbations by BFC when compared with placebo (62%, p < 0.001), budesonide (35%, p < 0.05) and formoterol (15%, p = 0.403).
Calverley et al. [19]	Time to first exacerbation and to first course of oral corticosteroids after randomisation significantly (p < 0.05 to p < 0.001) prolonged by BFC when compared with all other treatments.
	Reduction in exacerbation rate in the BFC group by 23.6% vs. placebo, by 25.5% vs. formoterol, and by 13.6% vs. budesonide.
	Reduction in the rate of oral corticosteroid courses in the BFC group by 44.7% vs. placebo, by 30.5% vs. formoterol, and by 28.2% vs. budesonide.

respectively, p value FSC vs. salmeterol and fluticasone, p = 0.12 and 0.45, respectively). Acute episodes of symptom exacerbation that required oral corticosteroids were reduced by 29% in the salmeterol group (p = 0.0003) and 34% in the fluticasone group (p = 0.0001) compared with placebo. There were no significant differences between active treatments with respect to their effect on the rate of episodes of symptom exacerbation, time to first exacerbation, or number of hospital admissions.

In the Szafranski study [18], mean exacerbation rates were 1.42, 1.59, 1.84 and 1.87 exacerbations per patient per year in the BFC, budesonide, formoterol and placebo treatment groups, respectively. The authors reported a reduction in the number of severe exacerbations by 24% in the BFC group vs. placebo (p = 0.035), by 23% vs. formoterol (p = 0.043) and 11% vs. budesonide (p = 0.385). This reflects a mean reduction in the average annual exacerbation rates of 0.42 (95% CI: 0.14–0.70), from 1.84 to 1.42 exacerbations per year. Budesonide produced a 15% reduction in severe exacerbations vs. placebo (p = 0.224). Compared with placebo, both BFC and budesonide reduced the number of oral steroid courses used in association with exacerbations (31%, p = 0.027 and 29%, p = 0.045, respectively, compared with 3% for formoterol vs. placebo, p = 0.853). BFC also significantly reduced the number of oral steroid courses compared with formoterol (28%, p = 0.039). Mild exacerbations were also reduced on BFC when compared with placebo (62%, p < 0.001), budesonide (35%, p < 0.05) and formoterol (15%, p = 0.403).

In the Calverley study [19], BFC prolonged time to first exacerbation compared with all other treatments (all, p < 0.05). Hazard rate analysis showed that the risk of having an exacerbation while being treated with BFC was reduced by 22.7, 29.5 and 28.5% vs. budesonide, formoterol and placebo, respectively. The exacerbation rate with BFC was reduced compared with placebo (23.6%) and formoterol (25.5%) but not with budesonide alone (13.6%). Neither budesonide nor formoterol affected either measure of exacerbation compared with placebo. BFC prolonged the time to first course of oral corticosteroids after randomisation; risk reductions were 32.7 and 33.8% vs. budesonide and formoterol, respectively (both p < 0.01), and 42.3% vs. placebo (p < 0.001). BFC also reduced the rate of oral corticosteroid courses by 28.2, 30.5 and 44.7% vs. budesonide, formoterol and placebo, respectively; budesonide alone reduced the number of oral corticosteroid courses compared with placebo but formoterol did not.

EVALUATION OF IMPACT ON QUALITY OF LIFE

Table 13.5 informs on the impact on quality of life of long-term treatments with combined therapy.

Hanania et al. [14] reported that treatment with FSC resulted in a clinically important increase from baseline in the mean overall Chronic Respiratory Disease Questionnaire (CRDQ) score (10.0), which was significantly greater compared with placebo (5.0; p = 0.006). The mean increases from baseline in the fluticasone and salmeterol groups were 10.4 and 6.4, respectively (fluticasone vs. placebo, p = 0.002).

Significant improvement in health status as measured by the CRDQ for those treated with FSC compared with placebo and fluticasone was observed in the Mahler study [15]. Mean change in CRDQ score from baseline was 10 in the FSC group, vs. 5 in the placebo group (p = 0.007), and vs. 4.8 in the fluticasone group (p = 0.017). The difference between FSC and salmeterol was not significant (mean change score in the salmeterol group was 8, p value vs. FSC not published).

In the TRISTAN study [17], mean absolute and change scores on the St. Georges Respiratory Questionnaire (SGRQ) were reported. There was a clinically significant improvement in health status in participants treated with FSC compared with baseline (−4.5 ± 12.9). This was statistically significant when compared with the change in placebo scores (−1.9, p = 0.008), and with the improvement in those treated with fluticasone (−2.5, p = 0.039). There were statistically significant differences between FSC and placebo and between FSC and fluticasone (FSC: 44.1 ± 0.5 vs. placebo: 46.3 ± 0.5 vs. fluticasone: 45.5 ± 0.4; FSC vs. placebo: p = 0.0003; FSC vs. fluticasone: p = 0.021). Absolute score vs. salmeterol was not significantly different (p = 0.071).

Szafranski et al. [18] reported a clinically significant improvement in health status as measured on the SGRQ in favour of BFC vs. placebo. Treatment with BFC led to a mean

Table 13.5 Long-term impact on health related-quality of life of combination therapy in COPD

Study	Changes in disease-specific measures
Hanania et al. [14]	Overall CRDQ score increase from baseline after FSC (10.0) significantly greater compared with placebo (5.0; p = 0.006) but not with salmeterol (10.4) and fluticasone (6.4).
Mahler et al. [15]	Overall CRDQ score increase from baseline after FSC (10.0) significantly greater compared with placebo (5.0, p = 0.007) and fluticasone (4.8, p = 0.017), but not with salmeterol (8.0).
Calverley et al. (TRISTAN study) [17]	SGRQ total score reduced by 4.5 after FSC. Differences vs. FSC at 12 months: placebo, −2.2, p = 0.0003; salmeterol, −1.1, p = 0.071; fluticasone, −1.4, p = 0.021.
Szafranski et al. [18]	SGRQ total score reduced by 3.9 after BFC, 1.9 after budesonide, 3.6 after formoterol, and 0.03 after placebo.
Calverley et al. [19]	SGRQ total score after BFC improved significantly (p ≤ 0.001) vs. placebo, but not vs. formoterol (p = 0.891) or budesonide (p = 0.120). Differences vs. placebo at 12 months: BFC, −7.5; budesonide, −3.0; formoterol, −4.1.

reduction of −5.4 in the BFC group vs. −2.3 in the placebo group (p = 0.048). BFC did not lead to statistically significant differences vs. formoterol or budesonide.

Inclusion of an optimised treatment phase in the Calverley study [19] justifies why at the end of the run-in period, SGRQ total scores had improved by a mean of 4.5 units (range 3.6–4.8). During the treatment period, the total scores fell further in the BFC group, representing an additional improvement beyond that achieved during run-in. Treatment with budesonide or formoterol allowed the initial improvement in HRQoL to be maintained, while HRQoL in the placebo group deteriorated to the pre run-in values. Thus, all active treatments improved the total score vs. placebo, with the greatest improvement occurring with BFC (differences at 12 months of −7.5, −3.0 and −4.1 vs. placebo for BFC, budesonide and formoterol, respectively).

COMPARISON BETWEEN ICS/LABA COMBINATION AND OTHER COMBINATIONS

Combinations of salmeterol 50 µg + fluticasone 250 µg or salmeterol 50 µg + fluticasone 500 µg twice daily, both from separate inhalers, were compared to a combination of salmeterol 50 µg + oral titrated theophylline twice daily in patients with well-controlled COPD [11]. A gradual increase in FEV_1 was observed with each of the three treatments. Maximum significant increases in FEV_1 over baseline values were observed after 3 months of therapy. They were as follows: salmeterol 50 µg + fluticasone 250 µg 0.188 l (95% CI: 0.089–0.287); salmeterol 50 µg + fluticasone 500 µg 0.239 l (95% CI: 0.183–0.296); and salmeterol 50 µg + titrated theophylline, 0.157 l (95% CI: 0.027–0.288). Salbutamol always caused a significant dose-dependent increase in FEV_1 (p < 0.001), although the 800-µg dose never induced further significant benefit when compared with the 400-µg dose. The mean difference between the highest salbutamol FEV_1 after salmeterol 50 µg + fluticasone 500 µg and that after salmeterol 50 µg + titrated theophylline twice daily was statistically significant (p < 0.05).

The efficacy in terms of improvement in symptoms and lung function of FSC vs. theophylline added to fluticasone in patients with COPD has recently been evaluated in 80 patients who were randomised to receive a 4-month treatment with fixed combination of FSC 500/50 µg twice daily or fluticasone 500 µg plus oral titrated theophylline twice daily [22]. Sixty-six patients completed the 4-month treatment period: 37 patients receiving FSC and 29 patients receiving fluticasone + theophylline. Patients were withdrawn for various reasons, the most common of which were poor compliance with the protocol, exacerbation and gastrointestinal events. A gradual increase in FEV_1 was observed with each treatment. Maximum significant increases in FEV_1 over baseline values that were observed after 4 months of treatment were as follows: FSC 0.1721 (95% CI: 0.084–0.260) and fluticasone + theophylline 0.1551 (95% CI: 0.054–0.256). FSC experienced significantly (p < 0.05) greater improvements in dyspnoea, and required significantly fewer supplemental salbutamol treatments than the fluticasone + theophylline group.

Results of a randomised, double-blind study of FSC 250/50 μg twice daily *via* Diskus vs. ipratropium/salbutamol 36/206 μg four times daily *via* MDI over 8 weeks, which enrolled 365 patients with symptomatic COPD patients defined as FEV_1/FVC of 0.7 or less and a FEV_1 of 40–70% of predicted normal values (baseline mean = 43.6%), and free of inhaled or oral corticosteroids for at least 30 days prior to randomisation, indicated that both combinations were well tolerated, but FSC significantly improved function and reduced symptoms [23]. In particular, both FSC and ipratropium bromide/salbutamol improved lung function, symptoms, and reduced supplemental salbutamol use compared with baseline. FSC was more effective than ipratropium bromide/salbutamol for improvement in morning pre-dose FEV_1, morning PEF, 6-hour FEV_1 AUC, TDI total score, daytime symptom score, night-time awakenings, sleep symptoms, and salbutamol-free nights (p < or = 0.013). Compared with day 1, at week 8 the FEV_1 AUC_{0-6h} significantly increased with FSC and significantly decreased with ipratropium bromide/salbutamol (p ≤ 0.003).

COMPARISON BETWEEN FSC AND BFC

Apparently, there is no substantial difference between FSC and BFC in patients with COPD when these combinations are prescribed at the dosages recommended for this pathology, at least after acute administration [24].

SYSTEMIC ADVERSE EFFECTS USING ICS/LABA COMBINATION IN THE MANAGEMENT OF COPD

Although there is clear evidence that the dose of ICSs can be reduced when combined with β_2-agonists, thus minimising the risk of side-effects [25], there is a real need to establish whether any side-effects induced by combination therapy with LABAs and ICSs are outweighed by the clinical advantages.

The combined use of fluticasone propionate and salmeterol in a single formulation provided additive benefit in the treatment of COPD but with comparable safety to the individual components used alone [14, 15, 17]. The safety profile of FSC treatment was consistent with that observed with the administration of salmeterol plus fluticasone, and was not different from that for the single components alone after a 12-week treatment period [11]. The overall adverse event profile of the combination therapy showed no new or unexpected adverse events. There was no evidence that combination treatment with FSC was associated with any increased risk of clinically relevant hypothalamic–pituitary–adrenal axis suppression (as assessed by cosyntropin stimulation testing) compared with fluticasone, salmeterol, or placebo. No unexpected cardiovascular effects, as assessed by Holter monitoring and routine electrocardiogram (ECG), were observed in those patients receiving FSC treatment compared with patients receiving salmeterol or placebo. In the Hanania study [14], drug-related adverse events that occurred at a frequency of ≥4% in any one treatment group were throat irritation, hoarseness/dysphonia, headaches, and candidiasis of the mouth and throat (incidence of candidiasis: placebo group, <1%; salmeterol group, 3%; fluticasone group, 6%; and FSC group, 9%). The number of patients who experienced adverse events resulting in withdrawal from the study was similar across treatment groups (range, 4–5%). At the selected sites where cosyntropin stimulation testing was performed, the incidence of abnormal cosyntropin stimulation values at end point was similar for the patients taking an ICS (i.e., fluticasone and

FSC, 9 patients) compared with those not taking an ICS (i.e., placebo and salmeterol, 6 patients). The incidence of clinically significant ECG abnormalities was comparable among treatment groups (placebo group, 3 patients; salmeterol group, no patients; fluticasone group, 1 patient; and FSC group, no patients). No treatment-related effects on vital signs, QTc, or cardiac rate were observed. Also in the Mahler study [15] a greater percentage of patients in the fluticasone and the FSC groups experienced candidiasis (mouth/throat) based on visual inspection compared with the placebo and salmeterol groups, as expected with the use of an ICS. However, there was no evidence that treatment with FSC was associated with any increased risk of clinically relevant hypothalamic–pituitary–adrenal axis suppression, as assessed by cosyntropin stimulation testing, compared with treatment with fluticasone, salmeterol, or placebo. The incidence of clinically significant electrocardiogram abnormalities was comparable among the treatment groups (4 patients in the placebo group, 4 patients in the fluticasone group, 2 patients in the salmeterol group, and 3 patients in the FSC group). No treatment-related effects on vital signs, QTc, or cardiac rate were observed. The incidence of ventricular ectopic events was similar in the placebo group compared with the active treatment groups at screening and at week 4. Only 5 patients experienced significant changes in Holter monitor results (1 patient each in the placebo, salmeterol, and FSC groups and 2 patients in the fluticasone group). In the TRISTAN study [17], all treatments were well tolerated, although the percentage of patients with oropharyngeal candidiasis was higher in groups receiving fluticasone-containing treatment (placebo 2%, salmeterol alone 2%, fluticasone alone 7%, salmeterol/fluticasone combination 8%). The majority of patients (96%) had serum cortisol within the reference range or not significantly changed from baseline. The incidence of skin bruising was low and comparable between treatment groups (placebo 6%, salmeterol alone 6%, fluticasone alone 7%, salmeterol/fluticasone combination 8%). ECG findings were unchanged by therapy.

BFC was also shown to be well tolerated and to have a safety profile similar to placebo and the single components in patients with moderate to severe COPD during 12 months of treatment in the Szafranski study [18]. Most adverse events were reported for respiratory system disorders, particularly COPD (17, 26, 13 and 19% in the BFC, placebo, budesonide alone and formoterol alone groups, respectively). No treatment-related patterns were discernible regarding death (n = 26) or serious adverse events (number of serious adverse events/1,000 treatment days: formoterol/budesonide, 0.8; placebo, 0.9; budesonide alone, 0.7; formoterol alone, 0.7). Discontinuations due to disease deterioration were highest in the placebo group (BFC, 10%; placebo, 21%; budesonide alone, 12%; formoterol alone, 14%), while the frequency of discontinuations due to other adverse events was similar in all groups (6–8%). No clinically important between-group differences were identified for laboratory or ECG measurements (including QTc prolongation). In the Calverley study [19], the most frequently reported adverse events were similar across the treatment groups. The number of serious adverse events related to COPD was 40, 40, 55 and 38 in the BFC, budesonide, formoterol and placebo groups, respectively.

POSITION OF ICS/LABA COMBINATION IN THE MANAGEMENT OF COPD

A formal meta-analysis of the different trials with ICS/LABA combinations is impossible because of substantial differences in sample size, effect size, research design, type of enrolled patients, primary efficacy outcomes (e.g., exacerbations or lung function), and duration of therapy across published studies. In such circumstances, it is difficult to determine if the differences between the study outcomes are due to chance, to inadequate study methods, or to systematic differences in the characteristics of the studies.

A recent Cochrane review [26] has concluded that compared with placebo, combination therapy led to clinically meaningful differences in quality of life, symptoms and exacerbations. However, there were conflicting results when the different combination therapies

Table 13.6 Definitions of COPD exacerbation used in combination therapy studies

Study	Definition
Hanania *et al.* [14]	Defined by treatment (moderate = exacerbations requiring treatment with antibiotics and/or corticosteroids; severe = exacerbations requiring hospitalisation)
Mahler *et al.* [15]	Defined by treatment (mild = increased use of salbutamol; moderate = use of either oral antibiotics and/or corticosteroids; severe = hospitalisation)
Dal Negro *et al.* [16]	Defined by treatment (mild = the condition requiring increased use of salbutamol prn by ≥ 2 occasions/24-hour period on two or more consecutive days compared with the baseline mean of last 7 days of run-in period; moderate = the condition requiring treatment with antibiotics and/or oral corticosteroids; severe = the condition requiring emergency hospital treatment and/or hospitalisation)
Calverley *et al.* (TRISTAN study) [17]	Worsening of COPD symptoms that required treatment with antibiotics, oral corticosteroids, or both
Szafranski *et al.* [18]	Severe = requirement for oral steroids and/or antibiotics and/or hospitalisation due to respiratory symptoms; mild = a day with ≥ 4 inhalations of reliever medication above the mean run-in use
Calverley *et al.* [19]	Event requiring medical intervention (oral antibiotics and/or corticosteroids or hospitalisation) due to respiratory symptoms

were compared with the single components alone. In particular, the results of the studies showed that BFC and FSC were effective and reduced the frequency of flare-ups compared with dummy medication to a level of three quarters of the previous rates, with one exacerbation prevented every 2 to 4 years in the participants in the clinical trials. When the combination treatment was compared with one of the component drugs given as single treatments, there was some meaningful benefit in QoL for BFC and FSC in comparison to the ICS component alone. BFC was better than its component LABA at reducing the frequency of flare-ups, but FSC did not show a significant advantage over LABA in one large study. FSC led to improvements in lung function compared with its component treatments given singly, and was better than ICS in reducing the need for rescue medication.

According to this Cochrane review [26], the conflicting findings between the results of the different studies may be accounted for by different study designs. In particular, definitions of exacerbation that have been used in the examined studies are rather different (Table 13.6). For example, in the Mahler study [15], exacerbation was defined by treatment (mild = increased use of salbutamol; moderate = use of either oral antibiotics and/or corticosteroids; severe = hospitalisation). In the Szafranski study [18], the definition of mild exacerbation was a day with ≥4 inhalations of reliever medication above the mean run-in use, whereas that of severe exacerbation was a requirement for oral steroids and/or antibiotics and/or hospitalisation due to respiratory symptoms. In the TRISTAN study [17], exacerbations were defined a priori as a worsening of COPD symptoms that required treatment with antibiotics, oral corticosteroids, or both. Episodes that required corticosteroid treatment or hospital admission were noted separately. Pauwels *et al.* [27] have correctly stressed that considerable heterogeneity in the aetiology and manifestation of COPD exacerbations makes identification and quantification of defining symptoms extremely difficult. However, with the emergence of a number of drugs designed or developed specifically to treat COPD and associated exacerbations, the absence of a uniform definition has become a significant issue. In fact, the choice of definition can significantly affect study outcomes, with varying criteria likely to result in different levels of demonstrated treatment success.

It is interesting to stress that patients enrolled in the TRISTAN study [17] had to have suffered from at least one episode of acute COPD symptom exacerbation per year in the previous 3 years, and at least one exacerbation in the year immediately before trial entry that required treatment with oral corticosteroids, antibiotics, or both. On the contrary, in the Szafranski study [18], patients had to have suffered from at least one severe COPD exacerbation within 2 ± 12 months before the first clinic visit. This fundamental difference indicates that the Szafranski study [18] enrolled patients with more severe disease or, at least, with a higher possibility of suffering from acute exacerbation. In fact, the mean pre-trial FEV_1 was 45% predicted in the TRISTAN study [17] and 36% predicted in the Szafranski study [18]. Moreover, the mean total exacerbation rate per patient per year under placebo was 1.30 in the TRISTAN study [17] and 1.9 in the Szafranski study [18]. Also in the Calverley study [19], the mean pre-trial FEV_1 was 36% predicted and the mean total exacerbation rate per patient per year under placebo was 1.80. As correctly highlighted by the authors of this paper [19], the more severe disease in the patients enrolled in BFC studies is the likely explanation for the greater number of episodes that they observed compared with other studies, a difference that increased the power of the study to detect an effect of treatment. It is also important to highlight that the authors of the three studies did not report the number of exacerbations in the year before the enrolment in the studies. This is a real lack of information because, as recently documented by Donaldson et al. [28], annual exacerbation frequency remains constant over time.

Rabe [29], in his editorial to the Calverley paper [19], affirmed that the data seem to indicate that patients experiencing more severe exacerbations benefit the most from combination therapy, whereas the relative effect of a LABA might be more pronounced in mild exacerbation. However, he also stressed the importance of definitions of exacerbations for clinical trials for having more solid conclusions.

In any case, it must be underlined that a treatment regimen with administration of an ICS and LABA in a single inhaler prolongs the time to a first COPD exacerbation, compared with treatment with the single components [19]. This finding is important because it indicates that following aggressive treatment of an acute exacerbation, therapy with an ICS/LABA combination may better control the disease than treatment with bronchodilator alone. In recent years, attention to the economic impact of treatment has become important in the choice and recommendations for health authorities worldwide. In view of the cost of an ICS/LABA combination, one could argue that this therapy should be reserved for patients who remain symptomatic in spite of optimised treatment with a LABA and/or an anticholinergic agent. This can be considered a correct approach because the price of drugs is only a part of the total cost of management of COPD [30]. In effect, the cost of each single exacerbation is very high, and there is a documentation that an ICS/LABA combination not only delays the onset of exacerbations, but also reduces their number [17–19].

Data from one-year studies have suggested that an ICS/LABA combination may reduce the rate of decline in FEV_1 over time compared with treatment with the single components [17–19]. Definitive conclusions would require a longer study period. However, this signal is exciting because it indicates the potential for the ICS/LABA combination to influence the natural history of COPD.

Another important finding is the early improvement in lung function in the ICS/LABA combination groups that is observed in the first day after starting treatment. This increase in lung function is further accentuated after 1-week's treatment compared with single components and maintained throughout the study period [14, 15, 17–19]. Rapid onset of bronchodilation is probably important both when starting and during treatment in providing immediate relief, potentially increasing confidence in the drug and aiding adherence to the treatment [18].

Hanania *et al.* [14] and Mahler *et al.* [15], who undertook a subgroup analysis according to reversibility of airway obstruction with salbutamol, reported that there was a modestly greater response to treatment in the reversible subgroup than in the non-reversible subgroup for pre- and post-dose FEV_1 with individual component therapy as well as combined therapy. This finding suggests that a treatment with an ICS/LABA combination must always be tried.

Airflow is traditionally used to assess both severity of COPD and response to treatment despite poor correlation with changes in symptoms, although any increase in expiratory airflow may contribute to improvements in clinical outcomes [15]. The converse, that symptomatic improvement may result when modest improvements occur in airflow, suggests that parameters other than airflow can affect the patient with COPD [31]. Dyspnoea is the most frequent complaint of patients with COPD requiring medical intervention and is the most prominent symptom limiting the activity of daily living. The comparison of the Hanania [14] and Mahler [15] studies, which were rather homogenous for sample size, research design, type of enrolled patients, primary efficacy outcomes, and durations of therapy, shows that FSC induced an improvement in pre-dose FEV_1 at the end of the studies that was similar (+165 ml in Hanania study [14] and +156 ml in Mahler study [15]). Nonetheless, when this combination was administered at the dosage of 250/50 µg twice daily, it was not possible to detect a significant modification in TDI scores compared to the single components and even placebo, whereas, at the dosage of 500/50 µg twice daily, estimated difference between FSC and salmeterol and between FSC and placebo exceeded the predefined criteria for clinical importance of 1 unit or more. This finding indicates that it is preferable to treat COPD patients with the dosage of 500/50 µg twice daily when the FSC is prescribed. This opinion contrasts with the fact that the US Food and Drug Administration (FDA) [32] has approved FSC 250/50 µg, but not 500/50 µg as new treatment of COPD because no additional improvement in lung function was observed in clinical trials with higher doses, and higher doses of ICSs may increase the risk of systemic effects.

A comparison of the Szafranski [18] and Carverley [19] studies, which were homogenous for sample size, research design, type of enrolled patients, primary efficacy outcomes, and durations of therapy as well, and used the same questionnaire, shows that the absolute changes in symptom score were similar. However, the Szafranski study [18] was alone in documenting a significant improvement in the total symptom score by combination therapy vs. all other comparators, whereas in the Calverley [19] study only the difference between BFC and placebo was significant.

This finding and the documentation that after an intensification regimen, administration of an ICS and LABA in a single inhaler prolongs the time to a first COPD exacerbation compared with treatment with the single components and the improvements in health status not only came on top of treatment optimisation and that these improvements were maintained over 12 months indicate that, before starting with a regular treatment with a ICS/LABA combination it may be better to optimise treatment with LABAs and oral corticosteroids. In any case, a steroid optimisation period of 2 weeks might not only help to differentiate between asthma and COPD; it will probably help to identify COPD patients who will undoubtedly benefit from combination therapy [29].

Because patients often modify their lifestyles to compensate for their dyspnoea, activity limitation associated with reduced expiratory airflow and other symptoms, it is important that treatment results in improvements in the patient's quality of life [14]. Health status generally slowly deteriorates in patients with COPD over time [33]. Nonetheless, health status was improved with both FSC and BFC relative to placebo, confirming the overall benefit of therapy to the patient. The additional effect of BFC on HRQoL compared with treatment with the single components observed in the Calverley [19] study is likely to reflect the lower number of exacerbations experienced by these patients, since HRQoL is known to be worse in frequent exacerbators [34]. In any case, the speed of change in health status was always less striking than in lung function tests.

The improvement in HRQoL may reflect the observation in all long-term studies [14–19] of a reduced need for reliever medication. On the other hand, greater reductions in the use of rescue salbutamol with active treatments compared with placebo further substantiate the clinical improvement in dyspnoea and in HRQoL.

Another important finding of all long-term studies [14–19] is the lack of significant difference between ICS/LABA combinations and comparators on the number of participants who withdrew due to adverse events other than COPD deterioration. Moreover, there is no evidence of an increase in adverse effects over and above that seen with the component medications alone.

CONCLUSION

Decisions in the management of COPD require consideration of multiple outcome measures. Although spirometry remains central in diagnosis and demonstration of efficacy, improvements in symptoms, HRQoL and prevention of exacerbations are of more concern to the patient and the medical profession and should be so also for health authorities. Recent advances in the treatment of patients who have COPD include the development of long-acting bronchodilators, and recognition of the benefits of ICS. In fact, treatment with long-acting inhaled bronchodilators and, in more severe disease, ICSs reduces symptoms and exacerbation frequency and improves health status [35].

We still do not know why combination therapy has improved efficacy in all levels of COPD severity. However, ICS/LABA combinations have a logical role in the treatment of severe-to-very severe COPD, offering the advantage of increased convenience and possibly improved compliance. In addition to improvements in lung function, symptom scores and HRQoL, the combination therapy reduces exacerbation rates, an outcome that contributes to favourable cost-effectiveness. Unquestionably, there are still unanswered questions [1, 26]. For example, combined therapy should be compared with separate administration of LABA and ICS in a double-dummy design study in large scale multi-centre studies, in order to assess whether combined therapy confers benefits over the simple addition of LABA to ICS treatment in separate inhalers. This should include an evaluation of patient compliance and preference. Moreover, a pharmacoeconomic analysis would be very helpful to assist purchasers of health care because we do not know if the higher medication cost of combination therapy with a LABA and ICS, compared with other treatments with single components, is really justified from a pharmacoeconomic point of view for COPD patients. Documentation of serious adverse events such as hospitalisation and intensive care support would be important. Additional studies could consider the effects of combined therapy compared with tiotropium, which may be able to reduce the rate of decline in FEV_1 over time [36, 37]. In addition, the effect of ICS, LABA and tiotropium administered separately and in combinations should be evaluated in long-term studies with different outcome parameters. Studies of the comparative effectiveness of fluticasone and budesonide and different regimens should be studied. Nonetheless, the data available strongly suggest that the fixed combination of ICS and LABAs in one inhaler is an efficacious, safe and practical approach for severe-to-very severe COPD patients.

REFERENCES

1. Cazzola M, Dahl R. Inhaled combination therapy with long acting β_2-agonists and corticosteroids in stable COPD. *Chest* 2004; 126:220–237.
2. Tse R, Marroquin BA, Dorscheid DR, *et al.* β-adrenergic agonists inhibit corticosteroid-induced apoptosis of airway epithelial cells. *Am J Physiol Lung Cell Mol Physiol* 2003; 285:L393–L404.
3. Soriano JB, Vestbo J, Pride NB, *et al.* Survival in COPD patients after regular use of fluticasone propionate and salmeterol in general practice. *Eur Respir J* 2002; 20:819–825.

4. Soriano JB, Kiri VA, Pride NB, *et al.* Inhaled corticosteroids with/without long-acting β-agonists reduce the risk of rehospitalization and death in COPD patients. *Am J Respir Med* 2003; 2:67–74.
5. Mak JC, Nishikawa M, Shirasaki H, *et al.* Protective effects of a glucocorticoid on downregulation of pulmonary β$_2$-adrenergic receptors *in vivo*. *J Clin Invest* 1995; 96:99–106.
6. Baraniuk JN, Ali M, Brody D, *et al.* Glucocorticosteroids induce β$_2$-adrenergic receptor function in human nasal mucosa. *Am J Respir Crit Care Med* 1997; 155:704–710.
7. Eickelberg O, Roth M, Lorx R, *et al.* Ligand-independent activation of the glucocorticoid receptor by β$_2$-adrenergic receptor agonists in primary human lung fibroblasts and vascular smooth muscle cells. *J Biol Chem* 1999; 274:1005–1010.
8. Pang L, Knox AJ. Synergistic inhibition by β$_2$-agonists and corticosteroids on tumor necrosis factor-α-induced interleukin-8 release from cultured human airway smooth-muscle cells. *Am J Respir Cell Mol Biol* 2000; 23:79–85.
9. Pang L, Knox AJ. Regulation of TNF-α-induced eotaxin release from cultured human airway smooth muscle cells by β$_2$-agonists and corticosteroids. *FASEB J* 2001; 15:261–269.
10. Korn SH, Jerre A, Brattsand R. Effects of formoterol and budesonide on GM-CSF and IL-8 secretion by triggered human bronchial epithelial cells. *Eur Respir J* 2001; 17:1070–1077.
11. Cazzola M, Di Lorenzo G, Di Perna F, *et al.* Additive effects of salmeterol and fluticasone or theophylline in COPD. *Chest* 2000; 118:1576–1581.
12. Cato AC, Nestl A, Mink S. Rapid actions of steroid receptors in cellular signaling pathways. *Sci STKE* 2002; (138):RE9.
13. Cazzola M, Santus P, Di Marco F, *et al.* Onset of action of formoterol/budesonide in single inhaler versus formoterol in patients with COPD. *Pulm Pharmacol Ther* 2004; 17:121–125.
14. Hanania NA, Darken P, Horstman D, *et al.* The efficacy and safety of fluticasone propionate (250 μg)/salmeterol (50 μg) combined in the Diskus inhaler for the treatment of COPD. *Chest* 2003; 124:834–843.
15. Mahler DA, Wire P, Horstman D, *et al.* Effectiveness of fluticasone propionate and salmeterol combination delivered *via* the Diskus device in the treatment of chronic obstructive pulmonary disease. *Am J Respir Crit Care Med* 2002; 166:1084–1091.
16. Dal Negro RW, Pomari C, Tognella S, *et al.* Salmeterol & fluticasone 50 μg/250 μg bid in combination provides a better long-term control than salmeterol 50 μg bid alone and placebo in COPD patients already treated with theophylline. *Pulm Pharmacol Ther* 2003; 16:241–246.
17. Calverley P, Pauwels R, Vestbo J, *et al.* Combined salmeterol and fluticasone in the treatment of chronic obstructive pulmonary disease: a randomised controlled trial. *Lancet* 2003; 361:449–456.
18. Szafranski W, Cukier A, Ramirez A, *et al.* Efficacy and safety of budesonide/formoterol in the management of chronic obstructive pulmonary disease. *Eur Respir J* 2003; 21:74–81.
19. Calverley PM, Boonsawat W, Cseke Z, *et al.* Maintenance therapy with budesonide and formoterol in chronic obstructive pulmonary disease. *Eur Respir J* 2003; 22:912–919.
20. American Thoracic Society/European Respiratory Society. Standards for the diagnosis and management of patients with COPD. Available at: http://www.thoracic.org. Accessed December 23, 2004.
21. Witek TJ Jr, Mahler DA. Meaningful effect size and patterns of response of the transition dyspnea index. *J Clin Epidemiol* 2003; 56:248–255.
22. Cazzola M, Noschese P, Centanni S, *et al.* Salmeterol/fluticasone propionate in a single inhaler device versus theophylline + fluticasone propionate in patients with COPD. *Pulm Pharmacol Ther* 2004; 17: 141–145.
23. Donohue JF, Kalberg C, Emmett A, *et al.* A short-term comparison of fluticasone propionate/salmeterol with ipratropium bromide/albuterol for the treatment of COPD. *Treat Respir Med* 2004; 3:173–181.
24. Cazzola M, Santus P, Di Marco F, *et al.* Combination therapy with salmeterol + fluticasone and formoterol + budesonide in patients with COPD. *Respir Med* 2003; 97:453–457.
25. Roth M, Johnson PR, Rudiger JJ, *et al.* Interaction between glucocorticoids and β$_2$ agonists on bronchial airway smooth muscle cells through synchronised cellular signalling. *Lancet* 2002; 360:1293–1299.
26. Nannini L, Cates CJ, Lasserson TJ, *et al.* Combined corticosteroid and long-acting β-agonist in one inhaler for chronic obstructive pulmonary disease. *Cochrane Database Syst Rev* 2004; (3):CD003794.
27. Pauwels R, Calverley P, Buist AS, *et al.* COPD exacerbations: the importance of a standard definition. *Respir Med* 2004; 98:99–107.
28. Donaldson GC, Seemungal TA, Patel IS, *et al.* Longitudinal changes in the nature, severity and frequency of COPD exacerbations. *Eur Respir J* 2003; 22:931–936.
29. Rabe K. Combination therapy for chronic obstructive pulmonary disease: one size fits all? *Eur Respir J* 2003; 22:874–875.

30. Cazzola M, Matera MG. Long-acting bronchodilators are the first choice option for the treatment of stable COPD. *Chest* 2004; 125:9–11.

31. Rennard SI, Anderson W, ZuWallack R, *et al*. Use of a long-acting inhaled β$_2$-adrenergic agonist, salmeterol xinafoate, in patients with chronic obstructive pulmonary disease. *Am J Respir Crit Care Med* 2001; 163:1087–1092.

32. FDAnews.com. Washington Drug Letter. FDA nod for pulmonary indication key to Advair. http://www.fdanews.com/pub/wdl/34_17/fda/3205–1.html.

33. Mahler DA, Tomlinson D, Olmstead EM, *et al*. Changes in dyspnea, health status, and lung function in chronic airway disease. *Am J Respir Crit Care Med* 1995; 151:61–65.

34. Seemungal TA, Donaldson GC, Paul EA, *et al*. Effect of exacerbation on quality of life in patients with chronic obstructive pulmonary disease. *Am J Respir Crit Care Med* 1998; 157:1418–1422.

35. Calverley PM, Walker P. Chronic obstructive pulmonary disease. *Lancet* 2003; 362:1053–1061.

36. Vincken W, van Noord JA, Greefhorst APM, *et al*. Improved health outcomes in patients with COPD during one year's treatment with tiotropium. *Eur Respir J* 2002; 19:209–216.

37. Casaburi R, Mahler DA, Jones PW, *et al*. A long term evaluation of once-daily inhaled tiotropium in chronic obstructive pulmonary disease. *Eur Respir J* 2002; 19:217–224.

14

Antioxidants and COPD

W. MacNee

ABSTRACT

An imbalance between oxidants and antioxidants or oxidative stress is considered to play a role in the pathogenesis of chronic obstructive pulmonary disease (COPD). There is considerable evidence that an increased oxidative burden occurs in the lungs of patients with COPD and this may be involved in many of the pathogenic processes in this condition. COPD is now recognised to have multiple systemic consequences, such as weight loss and skeletal muscle dysfunction and oxidative stress extending beyond the lungs may, through similar mechanisms as those in the lung, result in these systemic effects.

Strategies to repress local lung and systemic oxidative stress are therefore a logical therapeutic approach in COPD.

OXIDATIVE STRESS

Oxidative stress is said to occur when the balance between oxidants and antioxidants shifts in favour of oxidants, as a result of either an excess of oxidants and/or depletion of antioxidants. The lungs are continuously exposed to oxidants generated either endogenously (e.g., released from phagocytes) or exogenously (e.g., air pollutants or cigarette smoke). In addition, intracellular oxidants (e.g., from mitochondrial electron transport) are involved in cellular signalling pathways. The lungs are protected against this oxidative challenge by well-developed enzymatic and non-enzymatic antioxidant systems [1].

Smoking is the main aetiological factor in COPD. Cigarette smoke contains 10^{17} oxidant molecules per puff, and this, together with a large body of evidence demonstrating increased oxidative stress in smokers and in patients with COPD, has led to the proposal that an oxidant/antioxidant imbalance is important in the pathogenesis of this condition [2]. Oxidative stress not only produces direct injurious effects in the lungs, but also activates the molecular mechanisms that initiate lung inflammation [3], and may have a role in many of the processes in the complex pathological events which result in COPD.

Increasingly COPD is recognised not only to affect the lungs, but also to have significant systemic consequences, such as muscle dysfunction and weight loss [4]. Oxidative stress is also thought to play an important role in this aspect of the disease [5].

EVIDENCE OF OXIDATIVE STRESS IN THE LUNGS

Oxidative stress can be measured in several different ways: (1) direct measurements of the oxidative burden; (2) the responses to oxidative stress; or (3) the effect of oxidative stress on

William MacNee, MBChB, MD(Hons), FRCP (Glas), FRCP (Edin), Professor of Respiratory and Environmental Medicine, ELEGI Colt Laboratory, MRC Centre for Inflammation Research, University of Edinburgh Medical School, Edinburgh, UK.

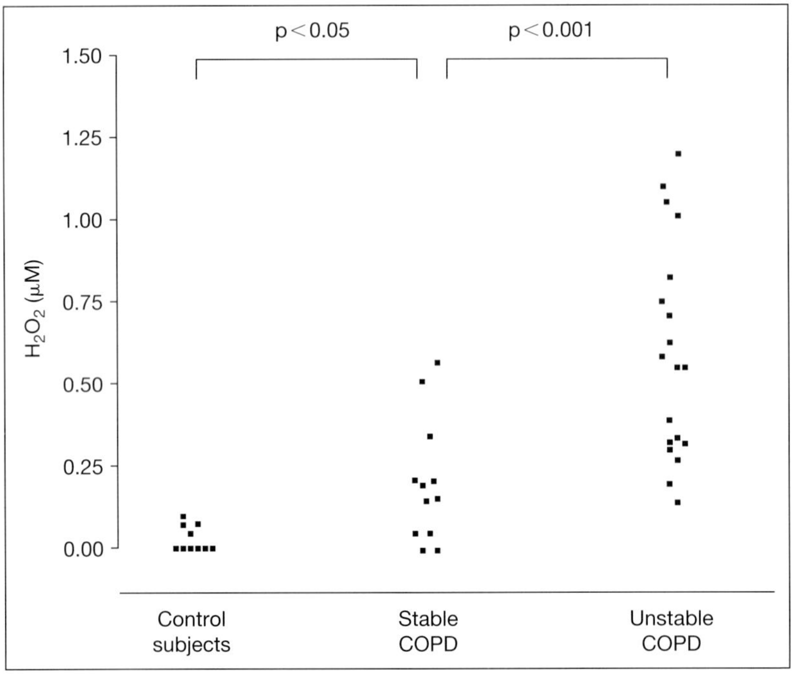

Figure 14.1   Individual data for hydrogen peroxide (H_2O_2) concentrations in breath condensate in control subjects and stable and unstable COPD. Modified from reference [7].

target molecules. Numerous studies which have assessed markers of oxidative stress using various techniques in exhaled breath, breath condensate, sputum, bronchoalveolar lavage and lung tissue have shown that oxidative stress is increased in the lungs of COPD patients compared with healthy subjects, but also compared with smokers with similar smoking history, but they have not developed COPD [2].

Direct measurements of the airspace oxidative burden, such as measurements of hydrogen peroxide in exhaled breath condensate, thought to derive from increased release of superoxide anion (O_2^-) by alveolar macrophages [6], show higher levels in smokers and patients with COPD than in ex-smokers with COPD or non-smokers [7, 8] (Figure 14.1). O_2^- anion and hydrogen peroxide (H_2O_2) are also derived from the xanthine/xanthine oxidase reaction, which shows increased activity in bronchoalveolar lavage fluid and in the plasma of smokers and in patients with COPD, compared with healthy smokers and non-smoking subjects [9, 10].

Nitric oxide (NO) has been used as a marker of airway inflammation and indirectly as a measure of oxidative stress. Increased levels of NO in exhaled breath occur in some [11–13], but not in other studies of patients with COPD [14, 15]. This may be due to the rapid reactivity of NO with O_2^- or with thiols which may alter NO levels in breath.

The levels of nitrosothiols have been shown to be higher in breath condensate in smokers and COPD patients compared to non-smoking subjects [16] (Figure 14.2). Peroxynitrite, formed by the reaction of NO with O_2^- can cause nitration of tyrosine to produce nitrotyrosine [17]. Nitrotyrosine levels are elevated in sputum leukocytes of COPD patients (Figure 14.2) and are negatively correlated with the forced expiratory volume in 1 second (FEV_1) [18].

Exhaled carbon monoxide (CO), as a measure of the response of haem oxygenase to oxidative stress, has been shown to be elevated in exhaled breath in CO compared with normal subjects [19].

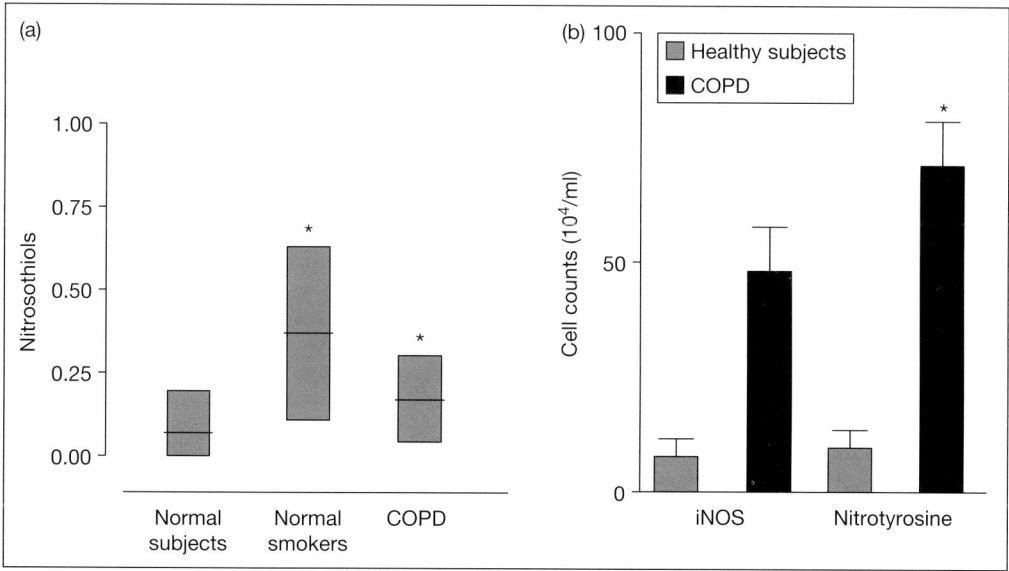

Figure 14.2   (a) Nitrosothiols, breath condensate in smokers and patients with COPD (modified from reference [16]). (b) Increased inducible nitric oxide (iNOS) and nitrotyrosine immunoreactivity in sputum leukocytes in COPD. Modified from reference [18].

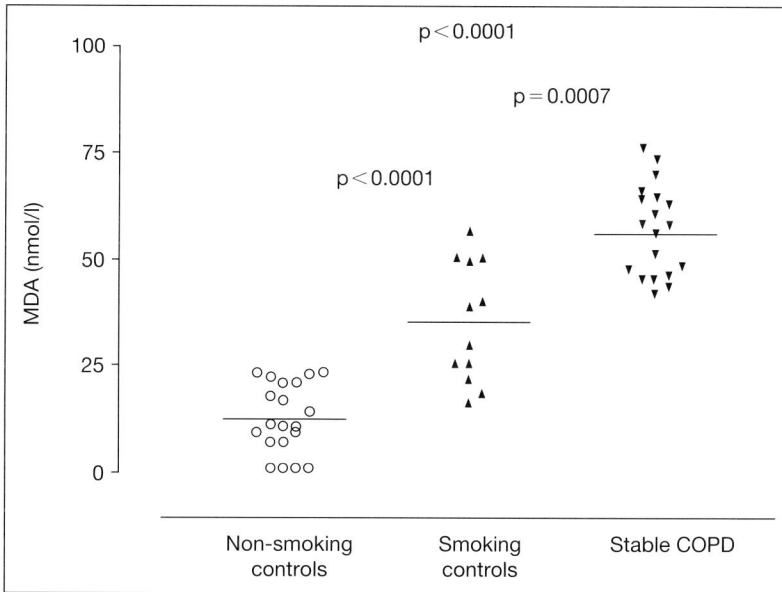

Figure 14.3   Malondialdehyde (MDA) levels in exhaled breath condensate are elevated in COPD patients. Modified from reference [21].

Lipid peroxidation products, such as thiobarbituric acid-reacting substances (TBARS) and malondialdehyde are elevated in sputum and breath condensate (Figure 14.3) in patients with COPD and are negatively correlated with the FEV_1 [20–22].

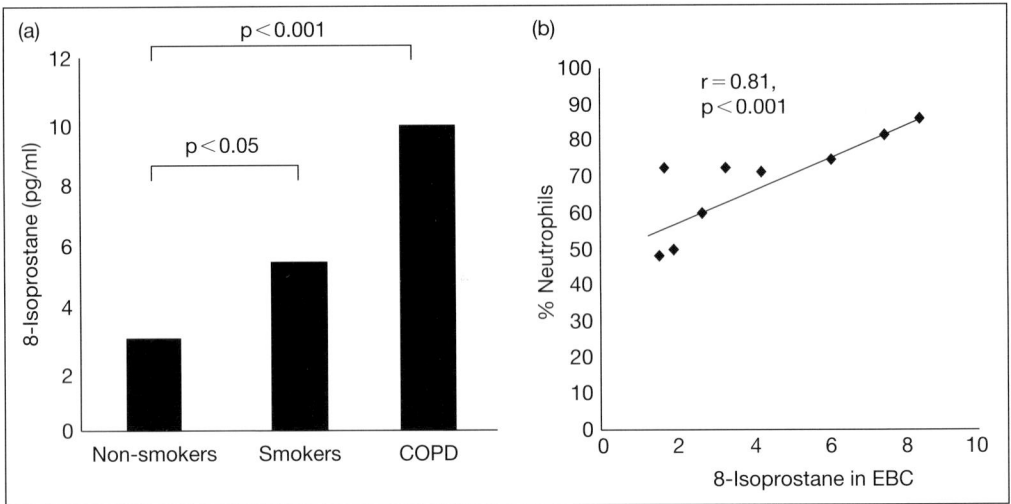

Figure 14.4 (a) Isoprostane levels in exhaled breath condensate in smokers with COPD. (b) Significant correlation between 8-isoprostane levels in exhaled breath condensate (EBC) and percent neutrophils in induced sputum. Modified from reference [24].

Isoprostanes, produced by reactive oxygen species (ROS)-mediated peroxidation of arachidonic acid are found in higher levels in breath condensate in patients with COPD, compared with normal subjects and smokers who have not developed the disease, and correlate with the degree of airways obstruction [23]. The levels of 8-isoprostane in breath condensate in COPD patients also show a positive correlation with the percentage neutrophils in induced sputum – suggesting that oxidative stress may be involved in the airway inflammation in COPD [24] (Figure 14.4). Increased levels of isoprostanes in plasma in smokers [25] and in urine in COPD patients [26] reflect increased systemic oxidative stress.

Hydrocarbon gases are by-products of ROS peroxidation of fatty acids [19]. Increased levels of exhaled breath ethane occur in COPD patients compared with control subjects, and the levels are negatively correlated with lung function [27].

Increased markers of oxidative stress are also present in lung cells in COPD patients. Increased nitrotyrosine, has been shown in sputum leukocytes in COPD patients compared with healthy subjects [18]. The lipid peroxidation product 4-hydroxynonenal reacts quickly with cellular proteins to form adducts, which are present in greater quantities in airway epithelial and endothelial cells in the lungs of COPD patients, compared with smokers with a similar smoking history who have not developed the disease (Figure 14.5) [28].

Thus the evidence of increased markers of oxidative stress in the airways and in lung tissue in COPD patients compared with normal subjects and smokers who have not developed the disease is now considerable. In addition many of these markers of oxidative stress correlate with the degree of airflow limitation in COPD, suggesting a role for oxidative stress in the decline in lung function in COPD.

SYSTEMIC OXIDATIVE STRESS

An increased systemic oxidative burden has been shown to occur in smokers. In COPD patients, peripheral blood neutrophils have been shown to release more ROS than in normal subjects and this is enhanced still further in exacerbations of the disease, associated with marked depletion of the plasma antioxidant capacity, indicating increased systemic

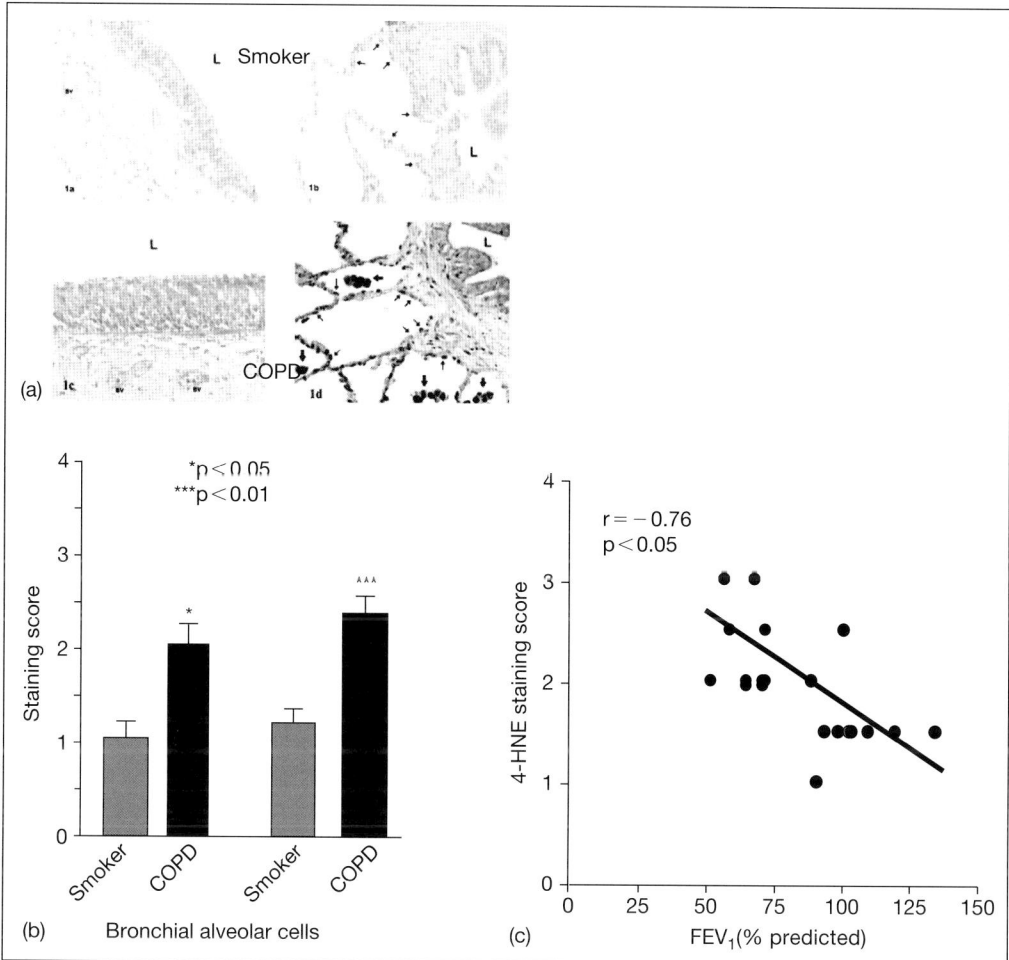

Figure 14.5 Immunostaining for lipid peroxidation product 4-hydroxynonenal adduct in the lungs of smokers with and without COPD. (a) Immunohistochemistry showing increased staining in both bronchial and alveolar epithelium in COPD patients who have the same smoking history as a group of smokers without COPD. (b) Staining score showing increased staining in COPD. (c) Correlation between 4-hydroxynonenal (4-HNE) staining score in the lungs and FEV_1 percent predicted. Modified from reference [28].

oxidative stress [29]. Products of lipid peroxidation are also increased in plasma in smokers with COPD, particularly during exacerbations [29]. Increased levels of nitrotyrosine have also been shown to occur in the plasma of COPD patients [17].

Exacerbations of COPD are known to result from increased levels of air pollutants, specifically particulate air pollution [30]. Particulate air pollution causes oxidative stress in the airways [31] and enhance inflammation by mechanisms involving redox-sensitive transcription factor activation, specifically NF-κB activation and decreased histone deacetylation and increased histone acetylation [3].

It is now recognised that COPD is not only a disease which affects the lungs, but also has important systemic consequences, such as cachexia of skeletal muscle function [32]. Evidence of similar mechanisms involving systemic oxidative stress and inflammation [33] may also be responsible for many of the systemic effects of COPD [32].

ANTIOXIDANTS IN COPD

A relationship between antioxidants, pulmonary function and the development of COPD has been shown in several population studies. The American Nutrition Examination Survey (NHANES) and the Dutch monitoring project for the risk factors for chronic diseases (MORGAN) have shown relationships between antioxidant dietary intake and airflow limitation. In NHANES (I) lower dietary intake of vitamin C was related to lower FEV_1 levels in a population survey [34]; data from the NHANES (II) showed an inverse relationship between both dietary and serum vitamin C and chronic respiratory symptoms [35]; and in NHANES (III) the levels of dietary vitamin C, vitamin E, selenium and β-carotene correlated positively with lung function [36]. Similarly, the MORGAN study also showed that a higher intake of vitamin C and β-carotene was associated with higher levels of the FEV_1, and this and other studies have shown associations between fruit intake and higher FEV_1 and lower symptoms in COPD patients [37–40].

As a response to oxidative stress induced by cigarette smoke, there appears to be up-regulation of protective antioxidant genes in the lungs. The antioxidant glutathione (GSH) is elevated in the epithelial lining fluid in chronic cigarette smokers, compared with non-smokers, an increase which does not occur during acute cigarette smoking [33]. The effects of chronic cigarette smoking can be mimicked by exposure of airspace epithelial cells to cigarette smoke condensate *in vitro*. This produces an initial decrease in intracellular GSH with a rebound increase after 24 h [41, 42]. This effect *in vivo* is mimicked by a similar change in GSH in rat lungs *in vivo* following exposure to cigarette smoke [42], associated with an increase in the oxidised form of GSH (GSSG). The increase in GSH following cigarette smoke exposure is due to transcriptional up-regulation of mRNA for γ-glutamylcysteine synthetase (γ-GCS), the rate limiting enzyme in GSH synthesis [42]. The mechanism of the up-regulation of γ-GCS mRNA is by the activation by cigarette smoke of the redox-sensitive transcription factor activator protein-1 (AP-1) [43, 44]. These events are likely to account for the increased GSH levels seen in epithelial lining fluid in chronic cigarette smokers, which acts as a protective mechanism. The injurious effects of cigarette smoke may occur repeatedly during and immediately after cigarette smoking when the lung is depleted of antioxidants including GSH. Animals exposed to whole cigarette smoke for up to 14 days also show increased expression of a number of antioxidant genes including manganese superoxide dismutase, metallothionein and GSH peroxidase [45].

OXIDATIVE STRESS AND THE PATHOGENESIS OF COPD

Although studies have shown that oxidative stress is increased in COPD and is related to the degree of airflow limitation, this does not indicate cause and effect, since oxidative stress may be an epiphenomenon related to the presence of inflammation [46]. There are as yet no longitudinal studies showing that the presence of enhanced oxidative stress relates neither to the decline in FEV_1 nor to the progression of the disease. However, there are many studies which indicate that oxidative stress is involved in many of the processes which are thought to be important in the pathogenesis of COPD.

It is thought that a relative 'deficiency' of antiproteases, such as $α_1$-antitrypsin, due to their inactivation by oxidants, creates a protease/antiprotease imbalance in the lungs, which forms the basis of the protease/antiprotease theory of the pathogenesis of emphysema [47, 48]. Although inactivation of $α_1$-antitrypsin by oxidants from cigarette smoke or oxidants released from inflammatory leukocytes has been shown *in vitro* [49, 50], the effect is less apparent *in vivo* [51]. However, a protease/antiprotease imbalance involving $α_1$-antitrypsin and elastase is an oversimplification, since other proteases and antiproteases are likely to have a role.

Oxidant-generating systems such as xanthine/xanthine oxidase have been shown to cause the release of mucus from airway epithelium [52]. Oxidants are also involved in the signalling pathways for the EGF receptor which has an important role in the release of mucus [53]. Oxidants such as H_2O_2 or HOCl in low concentrations (100 μM) have been shown to cause significant impairment of ciliary beating and even complete ciliary stasis [54]. Thus oxidant-mediated mucus hypersecretion and impaired mucociliary clearance may result in the accumulation of mucus in the airways contributing to airflow limitation.

Epithelial injury to the airway epithelium is an important early event following exposure to cigarette smoke as shown by an increase in airspace epithelial permeability. Increased epithelial permeability can be shown to result from cigarette smoke exposure both *in vitro* and *in vivo* [33, 55, 56] and is partially reversible by antioxidants. Extra- and intra-cellular GSH appears to be critical to the maintenance of epithelial integrity following exposure to cigarette smoke. Depletion of lung GSH alone can induce increased airspace epithelial permeability both *in vitro* and *in vivo* [56, 57]. Individual variability in antioxidant defences may be one factor in determining whether COPD develops after cigarette smoking.

There is now overwhelming evidence that COPD is associated with enhanced airway and airspace inflammation as shown in recent biopsy studies [58]. Oxidative stress may be a mechanism by which airspace inflammation is enhanced in COPD [59]. Oxidative stress may have a fundamental role enhancing inflammation through the up-regulation of redox-sensitive transcription factors such as NF-κB and AP-1 and also the ERK-junk and P38 MAP-Kinase signalling pathways. Cigarette smoke has been shown to activate all of these signalling mechanisms [3, 60, 61]. Genes for many inflammatory mediators are regulated by oxidant-sensitive transcription factors such as NF-κB [62, 63]. *In vitro* studies both in macrophage cell lines and alveolar and bronchial epithelial cells show that oxidants cause the release of inflammatory mediators such as IL-8, IL-1, and NO and that these events are associated with increased expression of the genes for these inflammatory mediators, and increased nuclear binding or activation of NF-κB [64, 65]. NF-κB has been shown to be activated and translocated to the nucleus in lung tissue in smokers and in patients with COPD compared with healthy subjects [60, 66]. NF-κB activation in lung tissue has been shown to correlate with the FEV_1 [67]. Linking of NF-κB to its consensus site in the nucleus leads to enhanced transcription of pro-inflammatory genes and hence inflammation, which itself will produce more oxidative stress, creating a vicious circle of enhanced inflammation resulting from the increased oxidative stress (Figure 14.6).

Animal models of smoke exposure show that neutrophil influx in the lungs is associated with increased IL-8 gene expression and protein release and with NF-κB activation [68, 69]. All of these events are associated with oxidative stress since they can be abrogated by antioxidant therapy (Figure 14.7) [68].

A further event induced by oxidative stress which may enhance the inflammation in the lungs is chromatin remodelling, which through activation of the core histones enables unwinding of DNA allowing access for transcription factors such as NF-κB and RNA polymerase to the transcriptional machinery, so enhancing gene expression. This process is known to be oxidant-sensitive and is controlled by histone acetyltransferases (HATs) which produce histone acetylation and histone deacetylases (HDACs) which reverse the process producing rewinding of DNA into a tight chromatin structure which leads to the suppression of gene transcription (Figure 14.8). Cigarette smoke exposure has been shown to decrease histone deacetylase 2 protein activity in the lungs of animals exposed to smoke [69] and in alveolar macrophages from smokers [70], which would add to enhanced gene transcription by preventing histone deacetylation (Figure 14.8).

A recent hypothesis in the pathogenesis of emphysema is that loss of lung cells in alveolar walls, both endothelial and epithelial cells, may occur in emphysema as a result of cell apoptosis [71]. Apoptosis has been shown to occur to a greater extent in emphysematous lungs than in non-smokers' lungs [72]. The process of endothelial apoptosis is thought to be under the influence of the VEGF R2 (KDR) receptor. Down-regulation of the VEGF receptor has been shown in animal models to produce emphysema [73] and down-regulation of VEGF

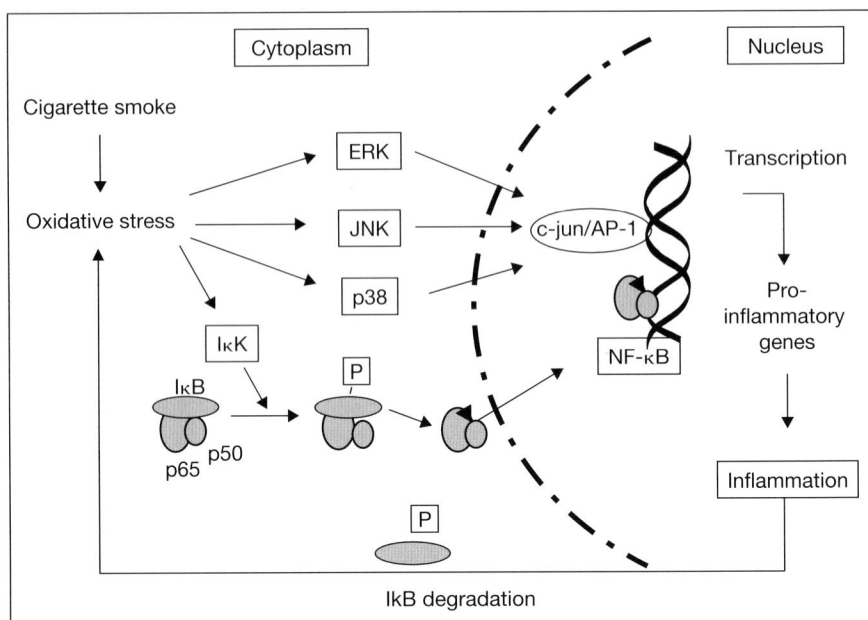

Figure 14.6 Activation of signal pathways by oxidative stress.

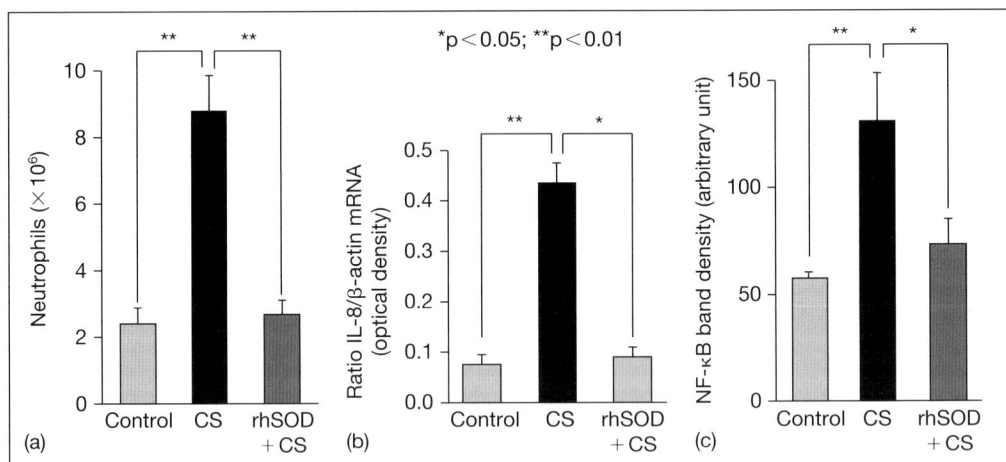

Figure 14.7 Effect of recombinant SOD (rhSOD) on cigarette smoke (CS)-induced neutrophil influx (a), IL-8 gene expression (b) and nuclear factor kappa B (NF-κB) nuclear binding (c) in guinea-pig lungs. Modified from reference [69].

R2 has been shown to occur in emphysematous human lungs [72]. Studies have also shown that the apoptosis/emphysema produced by VEGF inhibition in animal models is associated with increased markers of oxidative stress and is prevented by antioxidants [74], suggesting that oxidative stress is involved in this process.

Thus there is now considerable evidence of both local and systemic oxidative stress in COPD patients. There is also an increasing evidence that oxidative stress is involved in the

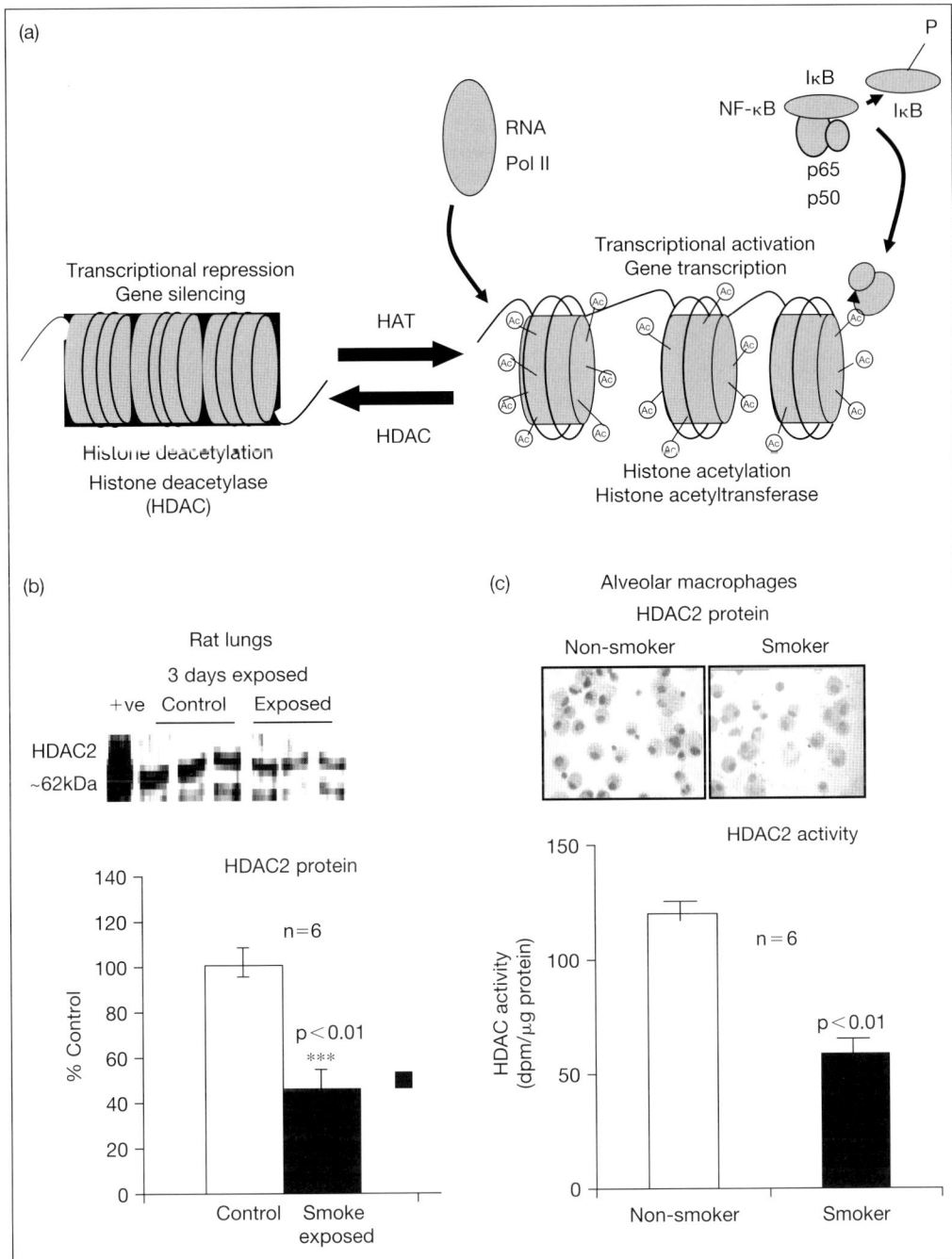

Figure 14.8 (a) Model of histone acetylation/deacetylation. (b) Decreased histone deacetylase 2 by Western blotting in rat lungs exposed to cigarette smoke (modified from reference [67]). (c) Decreased histone acetylase 2 protein (by immunohistochemistry) (top) and activity (bottom) in smokers' alveolar macrophages (modified from reference [71]).

pathogenesis of both local lung inflammation and in the injurious events and also the systemic events, such as skeletal muscle loss, which occurs in COPD [75].

ANTIOXIDANT THERAPY

Although there is now convincing evidence for an oxidant/antioxidant imbalance in COPD, proof of concept of the role of oxidative stress in the pathogenesis of COPD will come with studies of effective antioxidant therapy.

Various approaches have been tried to redress the oxidant/antioxidant imbalance. One approach is to give effective anti-inflammatory therapy to reduce lung inflammation, which will in turn decrease oxidative stress. Possible therapeutic options for this are drugs to prevent leukocyte influx into the lungs, either by interfering with the adhesion molecules necessary for migration, or preventing the release of inflammatory cytokines such as IL-8 or leukotriene B4 which result in neutrophil migration. It should also be possible to use agents to prevent the release of oxygen radicals from activated leukocytes or to quench those oxidants once they are formed, by enhancing the antioxidant screen in the lungs. Recent preliminary studies of the phosphodiesterase 4 inhibitor (PDE4) cilomilast have shown some therapeutic benefits in patients with COPD [76]. The mechanism by which such drugs act is by increasing cAMP which decreases neutrophil activation. In particular, the release of ROS by neutrophils may be decreased since increasing cAMP blocks the assembly of NADPH oxidase [77].

There are various options to enhance the lung antioxidant screen. One approach would be to use specific spin traps such as α-phenyl-N-tert-butyl nitrone to react directly with reactive oxygen and reactive nitrogen species at the site of inflammation. However, considerable work is needed to demonstrate the efficacy of such drugs *in vivo*. Inhibitors which have a double action, such as the inhibition of lipid peroxidation and quenching radicals, could be developed [78]. Another approach could be the molecular manipulation of antioxidant genes, such as GSH peroxidase or genes involved in the synthesis of GSH, such as γ-GCS or by developing molecules with activity similar to these antioxidant enzymes.

Recent animal studies have shown that recombinant SOD treatment can prevent the neutrophil influx into the airspaces and IL-8 release induced by cigarette smoking through a mechanism involving down-regulation of NF-κB [68] (Figure 14.7). This holds great promise if compounds can be developed with antioxidant enzyme properties which may be able to act as novel anti-inflammatory drugs by regulating the molecular events in lung inflammation.

A further approach would simply be to administer antioxidant therapy using antioxidants such as vitamins C and E. The results have been rather disappointing, although the antioxidant vitamin E has been shown to reduce oxidative stress in patients with COPD [79]. Attempts to supplement lung GSH have been made using GSH or its precursors [80]. GSH itself is not efficiently transported into most animal cells and an excess of GSH may be a source of the thiyl radical under conditions of oxidative stress [81]. Nebulised GSH has also been used therapeutically, but this has been shown to induce bronchial hyperreactivity [82].

The thiol cysteine is the rate-limiting amino acid in GSH synthesis [83]. Cysteine administration is not possible since it is oxidised to cysteine which is neurotoxic [83]. The cysteine-donating compound N-acetylcysteine (NAC) acts as a cellular precursor of GSH and is de-acetylated in the gut to cysteine following oral administration. It reduces disulphide bonds and has the potential to interact directly with oxidants. The use of NAC in an attempt to enhance GSH in patients with COPD has met with varying success [84, 85]. NAC given orally in low doses of 600 mg per day, to normal subjects, results in very low levels of NAC in the plasma for up to 2 h after administration [86]. After 5 days of NAC 600 mg three times daily, there was a significant increase in plasma GSH levels, however, there was no associated significant rise in BAL GSH or in lung tissue [87]. These data seem to imply that producing a sustained increase in lung GSH is difficult using NAC in subjects who are not already depleted of GSH.

Recent meta-analyses of the effects of NAC on exacerbations of COPD have shown positive effects [87], but this was not reflected in a recent randomised controlled trial of NAC in COPD patients, although there appeared to be some effects on exacerbations in a subgroup of patients who were not taking inhaled corticosteroids [88]. A study of N-isobutyrylcysteine, a derivative of NAC, also failed to reduce exacerbation rates in patients with COPD [89].

Nacystelyn (NAL) is a lysine salt of NAC. It is also a mucolytic and oxidant thiol compound which, in contrast to NAC which is acid, has a neutral pH. NAL can be aerosolised into the lung without causing significant side-effects [90]. Studies comparing the effects of NAL and NAC found that both drugs enhanced intracellular GSH in alveolar epithelial cells and inhibit H_2O_2 and O_2^- release from neutrophils harvested from peripheral blood from smokers and patients with COPD [89].

Molecular regulation of GSH synthesis by targeting γ-GCS has great promise as a means of treating oxidant-mediated injury in the lungs. Recent work by Manna *et al.* [91] has shown that recombinant γ-GCS in rat hepatoma cells completely protected against the TNF-α-induced activation of NF-κB, AP-1 and apoptosis/inflammatory process. Cellular GSH may be increased by increasing γ-GCS activity, which may be possible by gene transfer techniques, although this would be an expensive treatment that may not be considered for a condition such as COPD. However, knowledge of how γ-GCS is regulated may allow the development of other compounds that may act to enhance GSH.

REFERENCES

1. Halliwell B. Antioxidants in human health and disease. *Annu Rev Nutr* 1996; 16:33–50.
2. MacNee W. Oxidants/antioxidants and COPD. *Chest* 2000; 117(5 suppl 1):303S–317S.
3. Rahman I, MacNee W. Role of transcription factors in inflammatory lung diseases. *Thorax* 1998; 53(7):601–612.
4. Agusti AG. Systemic effects of chronic obstructive pulmonary disease. *Novartis Found Symp* 2001; 234:242–249.
5. Langen RC, Korn SH, Wouters EF. ROS in the local and systemic pathogenesis of COPD. *Free Radic Biol Med* 2003; 35(3):226–235.
6. Hoidal JR, Fox RB, LeMarbe PA, Perri R, Repine JE. Altered oxidative metabolic responses *in vitro* of alveolar macrophages from asymptomatic cigarette smokers. *Am Rev Respir Dis* 1981; 123(1):85–89.
7. Dekhuijzen PN, Aben KK, Dekker I, Aarts LP, Wielders PL, van Herwaarden CL *et al.* Increased exhalation of hydrogen peroxide in patients with stable and unstable chronic obstructive pulmonary disease. *Am J Respir Crit Care Med* 1996; 154(3 Pt 1):813–816.
8. Nowak D, Kasielski M, Pietras T, Bialasiewicz P, Antczak A. Cigarette smoking does not increase hydrogen peroxide levels in expired breath condensate of patients with stable COPD. *Monaldi Arch Chest Dis* 1998; 53(3):268–273.
9. Heunks LM, Vina J, van Herwaarden CL, Folgering HT, Gimeno A, Dekhuijzen PN. Xanthine oxidase is involved in exercise-induced oxidative stress in chronic obstructive pulmonary disease. *Am J Physiol* 1999; 277(6 Pt 2):R1697–R1704.
10. Pinamonti S, Muzzoli M, Chicca MC, Papi A, Ravenna F, Fabbri LM *et al.* Xanthine oxidase activity in bronchoalveolar lavage fluid from patients with chronic obstructive pulmonary disease. *Free Radic Biol Med* 1996; 21(2):147–155.
11. Delen FM, Sippel JM, Osborne ML, Law S, Thukkani N, Holden WE. Increased exhaled nitric oxide in chronic bronchitis: comparison with asthma and COPD. *Chest* 2000; 117(3):695–701.
12. Maziak W, Loukides S, Culpitt S, Sullivan P, Kharitonov SA, Barnes PJ. Exhaled nitric oxide in chronic obstructive pulmonary disease. *Am J Respir Crit Care Med* 1998; 157(3 Pt 1):998–1002.
13. Corradi M, Majori M, Cacciani GC, Consigli GF, de'Munari E, Pesci A. Increased exhaled nitric oxide in patients with stable chronic obstructive pulmonary disease. *Thorax* 1999; 54(7):572–575.
14. Rutgers SR, van der Mark TW, Coers W, Moshage H, Timens W, Kauffman HF *et al.* Markers of nitric oxide metabolism in sputum and exhaled air are not increased in chronic obstructive pulmonary disease. *Thorax* 1999; 54(7):576–580.
15. Clini E, Bianchi L, Pagani M, Ambrosino N. Endogenous nitric oxide in patients with stable COPD: correlates with severity of disease. *Thorax* 1998; 53(10):881–883.

16. Corradi M, Montuschi P, Donnelly LE, Pesci A, Kharitonov SA, Barnes PJ. Increased nitrosothiols in exhaled breath condensate in inflammatory airway diseases. *Am J Respir Crit Care Med* 2001; 163(4):854–858.

17. Petruzzelli S, Puntoni R, Mimotti P, Pulera N, Baliva F, Fornai E et al. Plasma 3-nitrotyrosine in cigarette smokers. *Am J Respir Crit Care Med* 1997; 156(6):1902–1907.

18. Ichinose M, Sugiura H, Yamagata S, Koarai A, Shirato K. Increase in reactive nitrogen species production in chronic obstructive pulmonary disease airways. *Am J Respir Crit Care Med* 2000; 162(2 Pt 1):701–706.

19. Paredi P, Kharitonov SA, Leak D, Ward S, Cramer D, Barnes PJ. Exhaled ethane, a marker of lipid peroxidation, is elevated in chronic obstructive pulmonary disease. *Am J Respir Crit Care Med* 2000; 162(2 Pt 1):369–373.

20. Nowak D, Kasielski M, Antczak A, Pietras T, Bialasiewicz P. Increased content of thiobarbituric acid-reactive substances and hydrogen peroxide in the expired breath condensate of patients with stable chronic obstructive pulmonary disease: no significant effect of cigarette smoking. *Respir Med* 1999; 93(6):389–396.

21. Tsukagoshi H, Shimizu Y, Iwamae S, Hisada T, Ishizuka T, Iizuka K et al. Evidence of oxidative stress in asthma and COPD: potential inhibitory effect of theophylline. *Respir Med* 2000; 94(6):584–588.

22. Corradi M, Rubinstein I, Andreoli R, Manini P, Caglieri A, Poli D et al. Aldehydes in exhaled breath condensate of patients with chronic obstructive pulmonary disease. *Am J Respir Crit Care Med* 2003; 167(10):1380–1386.

23. Montuschi P, Collins JV, Ciabattoni G, Lazzeri N, Corradi M, Kharitonov SA et al. Exhaled 8-isoprostane as an *in vivo* biomarker of lung oxidative stress in patients with COPD and healthy smokers. *Am J Respir Crit Care Med* 2000; 162(3 Pt 1):1175–1177.

24. Frangulyan R, Anderson D, Drost E, Hill A, MacNee W. Exhaled markers of inflammation in breath condensate in patients with bronchiectasis and COPD. *Thorax* 2003; 58(suppl III):S116.

25. Morrow JD, Frei B, Longmire AW, Gaziano JM, Lynch SM, Shyr Y et al. Increase in circulating products of lipid peroxidation (F2-isoprostanes) in smokers. Smoking as a cause of oxidative damage. *N Engl J Med* 1995; 332(18):1198–1203.

26. Pratico D, Basili S, Vieri M, Cordova C, Violi F, FitzGerald GA. Chronic obstructive pulmonary disease is associated with an increase in urinary levels of isoprostane F2alpha-III, an index of oxidant stress. *Am J Respir Crit Care Med* 1998; 158(6):1709–1714.

27. Habib MP, Clements NC, Garewal HS. Cigarette smoking and ethane exhalation in humans. *Am J Respir Crit Care Med* 1995; 151(5):1368–1372.

28. Rahman I, van Schadewijk AA, Crowther AJ, Hiemstra PS, Stolk J, MacNee W et al. 4-Hydroxy-2-nonenal, a specific lipid peroxidation product, is elevated in lungs of patients with chronic obstructive pulmonary disease. *Am J Respir Crit Care Med* 2002; 166(4):490–495.

29. Rahman I, Morrison D, Donaldson K, MacNee W. Systemic oxidative stress in asthma, COPD, and smokers. *Am J Respir Crit Care Med* 1996; 154(4 Pt 1):1055–1060.

30. MacNee W, Donaldson K. Environmental factors in COPD. In: Voelkel NF, MacNee W (eds) Chronic Obstructive Lung Disease. BC Decker, London, 2002, pp 145–160.

31. Donaldson K, Brown DM, Mitchell C, Dineva M, Beswick PH, Gilmour P et al. Free radical activity of PM10: iron-mediated generation of hydroxyl radicals. *Environ Health Perspect* 1997; 105 (suppl 5): 1285–1289.

32. Wouters EF, Creutzberg EC, Schols AM. Systemic effects in COPD. *Chest* 2002; 121(5 suppl):127S–130S.

33. Morrison D, Rahman I, Lannan S, MacNee W. Epithelial permeability, inflammation, and oxidant stress in the air spaces of smokers. *Am J Respir Crit Care Med* 1999; 159(2):473–479.

34. Schwartz J, Weiss ST. Relationship between dietary vitamin C intake and pulmonary function in the First National Health and Nutrition Examination Survey (NHANES I). *Am J Clin Nutr* 1994; 59(1):110–114.

35. Schwartz J, Weiss ST. Dietary factors and their relation to respiratory symptoms. The Second National Health and Nutrition Examination Survey. *Am J Epidemiol* 1990; 132(1):67–76.

36. Hu G, Cassano PA. Antioxidant nutrients and pulmonary function: the Third National Health and Nutrition Examination Survey (NHANES III). *Am J Epidemiol* 2000; 151(10):975–981.

37. Tabak C, Smit HA, Heederik D, Ocke MC, Kromhout D. Diet and chronic obstructive pulmonary disease: independent beneficial effects of fruits, whole grains, and alcohol (the MORGEN study). *Clin Exp Allergy* 2001; 31(5):747–755.

38. Miedema I, Feskens EJ, Heederik D, Kromhout D. Dietary determinants of long-term incidence of chronic nonspecific lung diseases. The Zutphen Study. *Am J Epidemiol* 1993; 138(1):37–45.

39. Strachan DP, Cox BD, Erzinclioglu SW, Walters DE, Whichelow MJ. Ventilatory function and winter fresh fruit consumption in a random sample of British adults. *Thorax* 1991; 46(9):624–629.

40. Tabak C, Feskens EJ, Heederik D, Kromhout D, Menotti A, Blackburn HW. Fruit and fish consumption: a possible explanation for population differences in COPD mortality (The Seven Countries Study). *Eur J Clin Nutr* 1998; 52(11):819–825.

41. Rahman I, Li XY, Donaldson K, Harrison DJ, MacNee W. Glutathione homeostasis in alveolar epithelial cells *in vitro* and lung *in vivo* under oxidative stress. *Am J Physiol* 1995; 269(3 Pt 1): L285–L292.

42. Rahman I, Smith CA, Lawson MF, Harrison DJ, MacNee W. Induction of gamma-glutamylcysteine synthetase by cigarette smoke is associated with AP-1 in human alveolar epithelial cells. *FEBS Lett* 1996; 396(1):21–25.

43. Rahman I, Antonicelli F, MacNee W. Molecular mechanism of the regulation of glutathione synthesis by tumor necrosis factor-alpha and dexamethasone in human alveolar epithelial cells. *J Biol Chem* 1999; 274(8):5088–5096.

44. Rahman I, Smith CA, Antonicelli F, MacNee W. Characterisation of gamma-glutamylcysteine synthetase-heavy subunit promoter: a critical role for AP-1. *FEBS Lett* 1998; 427(1):129–133.

45. Gilks CB, Price K, Wright JL, Churg A. Antioxidant gene expression in rat lung after exposure to cigarette smoke. *Am J Pathol* 1998; 152(1):269–278.

46. MacNee W. Oxidative stress and lung inflammation in airways disease. *Eur J Pharmacol* 2001; 429(1–3):195–207.

47. Janoff A, Carp H, Laurent P, Raju L. The role of oxidative processes in emphysema. *Am Rev Respir Dis* 1983; 127(2):S31–S38.

48. Stockley RA. Proteases and antiproteases. *Novartis Found Symp* 2001; 234:189–199.

49. Bieth JG. The antielastase screen of the lower respiratory tract. *Eur J Respir Dis Suppl* 1985; 139:57–61.

50. Evans MD, Pryor WA. Damage to human alpha-1-proteinase inhibitor by aqueous cigarette tar extracts and the formation of methionine sulfoxide. *Chem Res Toxicol* 1992; 5(5):654–660.

51. Abboud RT, Fera T, Richter A, Tabona MZ, Johal S. Acute effect of smoking on the functional activity of alpha1-protease inhibitor in bronchoalveolar lavage fluid. *Am Rev Respir Dis* 1985; 131(1):79–85.

52. Adler KB, Holden-Stauffer WJ, Repine JE. Oxygen metabolites stimulate release of high-molecular-weight glycoconjugates by cell and organ cultures of rodent respiratory epithelium *via* an arachidonic acid-dependent mechanism. *J Clin Invest* 1990; 85(1):75–85.

53. Nadel JA. Role of epidermal growth factor receptor activation in regulating mucin synthesis. *Respir Res* 2001; 2(2):85–89.

54. Feldman C, Anderson R, Kanthakumar K, Vargas A, Cole PJ, Wilson R. Oxidant-mediated ciliary dysfunction in human respiratory epithelium. *Free Radic Biol Med* 1994; 17(1):1–10.

55. Rusznak C, Mills PR, Devalia JL, Sapsford RJ, Davies RJ, Lozewicz S. Effect of cigarette smoke on the permeability and IL-1beta and sICAM-1 release from cultured human bronchial epithelial cells of never-smokers, smokers, and patients with chronic obstructive pulmonary disease. *Am J Respir Cell Mol Biol* 2000; 23(4):530–536.

56. Li XY, Donaldson K, Rahman I, MacNee W. An investigation of the role of glutathione in increased epithelial permeability induced by cigarette smoke *in vivo* and *in vitro*. *Am J Respir Crit Care Med* 1994; 149(6):1518–1525.

57. Li XY, Rahman I, Donaldson K, MacNee W. Mechanisms of cigarette smoke induced increased airspace permeability. *Thorax* 1996; 51(5):465–471.

58. Di Stefano A, Caramori G, Ricciardolo FL, Capelli A, Adcock IM, Donner CF. Cellular and molecular mechanisms in chronic obstructive pulmonary disease: an overview. *Clin Exp Allergy* 2004; 34(8):1156–1167.

59. Rahman I. Oxidative stress, transcription factors and chromatin remodelling in lung inflammation. *Biochem Pharmacol* 2002; 64(5–6):935–942.

60. Di Stefano A, Caramori G, Oates T, Capelli A, Lusuardi M, Gnemmi I *et al*. Increased expression of nuclear factor-kappaB in bronchial biopsies from smokers and patients with COPD. *Eur Respir J* 2002; 20(3):556–563.

61. MacNee W, Rahman I. Is oxidative stress central to the pathogenesis of chronic obstructive pulmonary disease? *Trends Mol Med* 2001; 7(2):55–62.

62. Janssen-Heininger YM, Macara I, Mossman BT. Cooperativity between oxidants and tumor necrosis factor in the activation of nuclear factor(NF)-kappaB: requirement of Ras/mitogen-activated protein kinases in the activation of NF-kappaB by oxidants. *Am J Respir Cell Mol Biol* 1999; 20(5):942–952.

63. Flohe L, Brigelius-Flohe R, Saliou C, Traber MG, Packer L. Redox regulation of NF-kappa B activation. *Free Radic Biol Med* 1997; 22(6):1115–1126.

64. Parmentier M, Hirani N, Rahman I, Donaldson K, MacNee W, Antonicelli F. Regulation of lipopolysaccharide-mediated interleukin-1beta release by N-acetylcysteine in THP-1 cells. *Eur Respir J* 2000; 16(5):933–939.

65. Jimenez LA, Thompson J, Brown DA, Rahman I, Antonicelli F, Duffin R *et al.* Activation of NF-kappaB by PM(10) occurs *via* an iron-mediated mechanism in the absence of IkappaB degradation. *Toxicol Appl Pharmacol* 2000; 166(2):101–110.

66. Szulakowski P, Drost E, Jimenez LA, Wickenden JA, Crowther AJ, Donaldson K *et al.* Role of histone acetylation in transcriptional regulation and promotion of inflammatory process in patients with chronic obstructive pulmonary disease. *Am J Respir Crit Care Med* 2004; 169:A275.

67. Crowther AJ, Rahman I, Antonicelli F, Jimenez LA, Salter D, MacNee W. Oxidative stress and transcription factors AP-1 and NF-B in human lung tissue. *Am J Respir Crit Care Med* 1999; 159:A816.

68. Nishikawa M, Kakemizu N, Ito T, Kudo M, Kaneko T, Suzuki M *et al.* Superoxide mediates cigarette smoke-induced infiltration of neutrophils into the airways through nuclear factor-kappaB activation and IL-8 mRNA expression in guinea-pigs *in vivo*. *Am J Respir Cell Mol Biol* 1999; 20(2): 189–198.

69. Marwick JA, Kirkham P, Stevenson CS, Danahay H, Giddings J, Butler K *et al.* Cigarette smoke alters chromatin remodelling and induces pro-inflammatory genes in rat lungs. *Am J Respir Cell Mol Biol* 2004; 31:633–642.

70. Ito K, Lim S, Caramori G, Chung KF, Barnes PJ, Adcock IM. Cigarette smoking reduces histone deacetylase 2 expression, enhances cytokine expression, and inhibits glucocorticoid actions in alveolar macrophages. *FASEB J* 2001; 15(6):1110–1112.

71. Tuder RM, Petrache I, Elias JA, Voelkel NF, Henson PM. Apoptosis and emphysema: the missing link. *Am J Respir Cell Mol Biol* 2003; 28(5):551–554.

72. Kasahara Y, Tuder RM, Cool CD, Lynch DA, Flores SC, Voelkel NF. Endothelial cell death and decreased expression of vascular endothelial growth factor and vascular endothelial growth factor receptor 2 in emphysema. *Am J Respir Crit Care Med* 2001; 163(3 Pt 1):737–744.

73. Kasahara Y, Tuder RM, Taraseviciene-Stewart L, Le Cras TD, Abman S, Hirth PK *et al.* Inhibition of VEGF receptors causes lung cell apoptosis and emphysema. *J Clin Invest* 2000; 106(11):1311–1319.

74. Tuder RM, Zhen L, Cho CY, Taraseviciene-Stewart L, Kasahara Y, Salvemini D *et al.* Oxidative stress and apoptosis interact and cause emphysema due to vascular endothelial growth factor receptor blockade. *Am J Respir Cell Mol Biol* 2003; 29(1):88–97.

75. Agusti A, Morla M, Sauleda J, Saus C, Busquets X. NF-kappaB activation and iNOS upregulation in skeletal muscle of patients with COPD and low body weight. *Thorax* 2004; 59(6):483–487.

76. Compton CH, Gubb J, Cedar E, Nieman RB, Amit O, Brambila C *et al.* SB 207499, a second generation oral PDE4 inhibitor, first demonstration of efficacy in patients with COPD. *Eur Respir J* 1999; 14:281S.

77. Torphy TJ. Phosphodiesterase isozymes: molecular targets for novel antiasthma agents. *Am J Respir Crit Care Med* 1998; 157(2):351–370.

78. Chabrier PE, Auguet M, Spinnewyn B, Auvin S, Cornet S, Demerle-Pallardy C *et al.* BN 80933, a dual inhibitor of neuronal nitric oxide synthase and lipid peroxidation: a promising neuroprotective strategy. *Proc Natl Acad Sci USA* 1999; 96(19):10824–10829.

79. Steinberg FM, Chait A. Antioxidant vitamin supplementation and lipid peroxidation in smokers. *Am J Clin Nutr* 1998; 68(2):319–327.

80. MacNee W, Bridgeman MM, Marsden M, Drost E, Lannan S, Selby C *et al.* The effects of N-acetylcysteine and glutathione on smoke-induced changes in lung phagocytes and epithelial cells. *Am J Med* 1991; 91(3C):60S–66S.

81. Ross D, Norbeck K, Moldeus P. The generation and subsequent fate of glutathionyl radicals in biological systems. *J Biol Chem* 1985; 260(28):15028–15032.

82. Marrades RM, Roca J, Barbera JA, de Jover L, MacNee W, Rodriguez-Roisin R. Nebulized glutathione induces bronchoconstriction in patients with mild asthma. *Am J Respir Crit Care Med* 1997; 156(2 Pt 1):425–430.

83. Meister A, Anderson ME. Glutathione. *Annu Rev Biochem* 1983; 52:711–760.

84. Bridgeman MM, Marsden M, MacNee W, Flenley DC, Ryle AP. Cysteine and glutathione concentrations in plasma and bronchoalveolar lavage fluid after treatment with N-acetylcysteine. *Thorax* 1991; 46(1): 39–42.

85. Bridgeman MM, Marsden M, Selby C, Morrison D, MacNee W. Effect of N-acetyl cysteine on the concentrations of thiols in plasma, bronchoalveolar lavage fluid, and lung tissue. *Thorax* 1994; 49(7): 670–675.

86. Drost EM, Selby C, Lannan S, Lowe GD, MacNee W. Changes in neutrophil deformability following *in vitro* smoke exposure: mechanism and protection. *Am J Respir Cell Mol Biol* 1992; 6(3):287–295.

87. Stey C, Steurer J, Bachmann S, Medici TC, Tramer MR. The effect of oral N-acetylcysteine in chronic bronchitis: a quantitative systematic review. *Eur Respir J* 2000; 16(2):253–262.

88. Decramer M, Dekhuijzen PN, Troosters T, van Herwaarden C, Rutten-van Molken M, van Schayck CP *et al*. The Bronchitis Randomized On NAC Cost-Utility Study (BRONCUS): hypothesis and design. BRONCUS-trial Committee. *Eur Respir J* 2001; 17(3):329–336.

89. Gillissen A, Jaworska M, Orth M, Coffiner M, Maes P, App EM *et al*. Nacystelyn, a novel lysine salt of N-acetylcysteine, to augment cellular antioxidant defence *in vitro*. *Respir Med* 1997; 91(3):159–168.

90. Nagy AM, Vanderbist F, Parij N, Maes P, Fondu P, Neve J. Effect of the mucoactive drug nacystelyn on the respiratory burst of human blood polymorphonuclear neutrophils. *Pulm Pharmacol Ther* 1997; 10(5–6):287–292.

91. Manna SK, Kuo MT, Aggarwal BB. Overexpression of gamma-glutamylcysteine synthetase suppresses tumor necrosis factor-induced apoptosis and activation of nuclear transcription factor-kappa B and activator protein-1. *Oncogene* 1999; 18(30):4371–4382.

15

Antiprotease therapy

T. D. Tetley

INTRODUCTION

The hypothesis that an increased protease burden in the lung was the biochemical basis of emphysema emerged in the early 1960s. This followed the observation that (a) a deficiency of α-1 antitrypsin (AAT; also called α-1 proteinase inhibitor, the major serum inhibitor of neutrophil elastase) is associated with early development of emphysema [1] and (b) papain, a proteinase with high elastinolytic activity, induced emphysema when instilled intratracheally into experimental animals [2]. An important component of chronic obstructive pulmonary disease, notably emphysema, is the loss of elastic recoil due to loss of elastin, and an abnormal repair leading to abnormal elastic tissue structure, suggesting that increased elastinolytic proteinases are responsible. The evidence to support this hypothesis is substantial, although it is highly unlikely that a single protease is responsible.

The most likely source of increased protease burden is the inflammatory cells; macrophages, neutrophils, lymphocytes, mast cells and eosinophils have all been found to be increased in the lungs of those affected [3, 4]. However, the numbers and profile of the cellular response vary depending on the level of the respiratory tract that is affected, the degree of disease and the presence of exacerbations, as well as smoking habits and history. In addition, each type of inflammatory cell occupies specific compartments of the lung and may preferentially exist in the airspaces, the epithelium, subepithelium, within smooth muscle, respiratory parenchyma or secretory glands [4]. All these cells are capable of releasing proteolytic enzymes into the extracellular environment and ultimately any tissue damage will depend on the site of action and efficacy of the endogenous antiprotease screen. Clearly, such factors will have a significant effect on the pathological process and clinical consequences.

Since COPD is largely a disease of smokers, and most smokers have inflamed lungs, but only approximately 15% develop clinically significant COPD, it is likely that, in those affected, the inflammatory cells release significantly greater quantities of deleterious enzymes, or alternatively that the antiprotease screen is overwhelmed, or both. Another contributory factor may be that repair mechanisms may be inadequate, or abnormal. Thus, together with the inflammatory cells that are recruited to the lung, there are other sources of proteases, which include resident epithelial cells and parenchymal cells such as fibroblasts, myofibroblasts and smooth muscle cells, that release proteases during normal and abnormal cell turnover and repair. Cigarette smoke-induced injury to resident cells may trigger

Teresa D. Tetley, BSc, PhD, Reader in Lung Cell Biology, National Heart & Lung Institute, Imperial College, London, UK.

increased tissue remodelling, part of which includes release of matrix metalloproteinases (MMPs) and probably cysteine proteinases to deal with damaged connective tissue and enable repair.

NEUTROPHIL-DERIVED PROTEASES

Neutrophils contain high concentrations (mM) of potent serine proteinases, neutrophil elastase, proteinase-3, and cathepsin G [5]. Because these enzymes are pre-packaged and stored in azurophil (primary) granules in their active form, on cellular activation, they can be rapidly released and form powerful, pericellular pockets of proteinase activity. Two MMPs, MMP8 (neutrophil collagenase) and MMP9 (gelatinase B) are stored in secondary and tertiary granules. Neutrophil elastase is commonly measured as a marker of neutrophil load and activation in the lungs of COPD subjects. Extracellular neutrophil elastase is elevated in lung secretions from those with bronchitis, during infection and exacerbation of COPD and in preclinical and clinically significant emphysema [5, 6]. Sputum from COPD subjects contains high extracellular neutrophil elastase and MMP9, particularly during exacerbations. In addition, neutrophil-derived MMP9 (i.e., lipocalin-bound) is elevated in bronchoalveolar lavage from patients with emphysema [7]. It is interesting that, although neutrophils are elevated in the peripheral parenchyma during emphysema, their numbers decrease in proportion to the degree of airspace enlargement [8], unless there is a full-blown disease, for example, requiring transplantation, when inflammatory cells reach many times the control numbers [9]. Serine proteinases can affect many processes (Figure 15.1). Neutrophil elastase is a potent enzyme that is a secretagogue, is ciliostatic, can activate complement, stimulates interleukin (IL)-8 and TGF-α synthesis and can proteolytically activate and inactivate cytokines and chemokines. In addition, it can amplify proteolytic potential

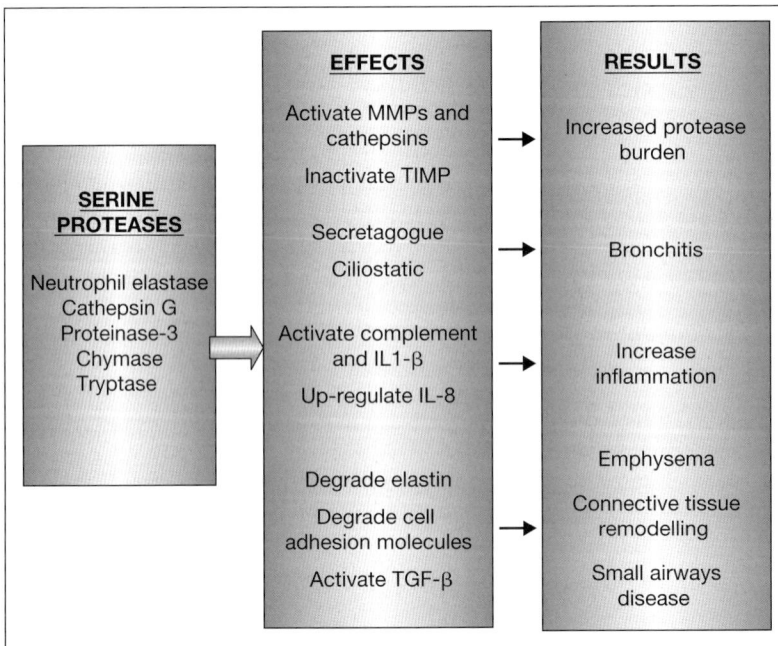

Figure 15.1 Pro-inflammatory effects of serine proteases and role in COPD.

by activating latent MMPs and inactivating their inhibitors [10] as well as processing cathepsins (Figure 15.1).

MACROPHAGE-DERIVED PROTEASES

Macrophages store enzymes within lysosomes and can up- and down-regulate protease synthesis in response to endogenous and external stimuli. Macrophages synthesise and release a number of MMPs, including MMP1 (collagenase), MMP2 (gelatinase A), MMP9 (gelatinase B), MMP12 (macrophage metalloelastase) and MMP14 (membrane-bound type 1) [10, 12]. MMP1 and MMP9 mRNA expression and protein secretion by macrophages from subjects with emphysema are increased [7, 13]. The presence of elevated MMP1 and MMP9 in macrophages from subjects with emphysema was confirmed by immunohistochemistry of human lung tissue [14]. *In vitro* release of MMP9 by macrophages from COPD subjects is elevated above those without COPD, particularly in response to cigarette smoke extract [15, 16]. In addition to MMP1 and MMP9, there is evidence showing that macrophages from COPD subjects contain elevated MMP2 and 14 [17], while studies of MMP12 knockout mice suggest that macrophage metalloproteinase could also be significant in the development of human emphysema [18]. MMPs are important in inflammation. They degrade connective tissue, generating chemotactic fragments. They inactivate AAT whilst activating other MMPs, thus amplifying protease activity. They also activate/inactivate cytokines and chemokines (Figure 15.2).

Macrophages also synthesise cysteine proteinases, including cathepsins B, H, K, L and S, which are stored in the lysosomes [19]. It is not yet clear whether cathepsin K is present in mature alveolar macrophages, although it is present in intravascular macrophages. Cathepsins K, L and S have potent elastinolytic activity at acid pH and may be important in acidic microenvironments, while cathepsin S retains a significant amount of its activity

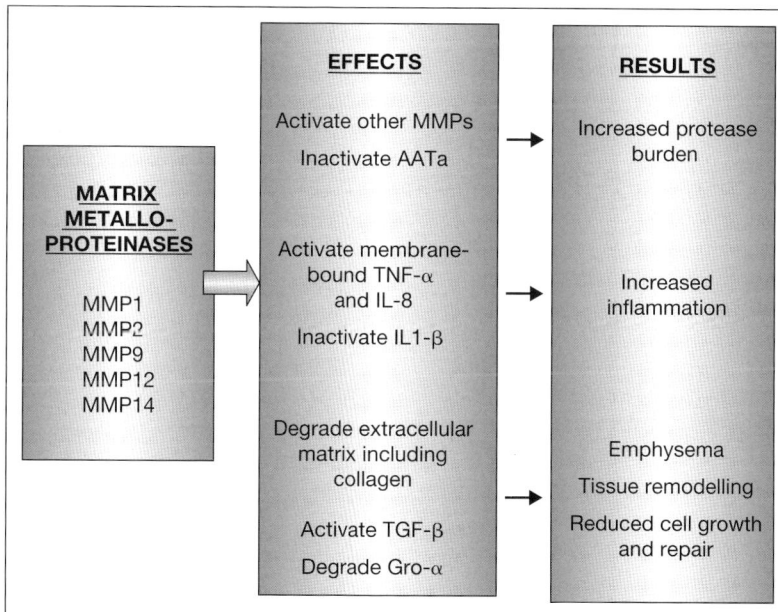

Figure 15.2 Pro-inflammatory effects of matrix metalloproteinases and role in COPD.

at neutral pH. Cysteine proteinase activity and cathepsin L release by pulmonary macrophages from cigarette smokers is elevated [20, 21]. Recent investigations of lung resection tissue showed that the mRNA expression for cathepsin S and B was high in alveolar macrophages and correlated with each other, as well as correlating with smoking [22]. Furthermore, cathepsin B expression was related to the degree of airflow obstruction. Overexpression of IFN-γ by transgenic mice causes emphysema [23], suggested to be due to up-regulation of cathepsins, notably cathepsin S, which in turn induces cathepsin B and K; macrophages may be one source of cathepsins in these studies. In addition to MMPs and cathepsins, macrophages contain receptors for neutrophil elastase, and may act as a reserve, contributing to retention of neutrophil elastase in the lungs of COPD patients [24]. Cathepsins process proteases and other cathepsins. They can also break down connective tissue and inactivate inhibitors of serine proteinases (Figure 15.3).

OTHER SOURCES OF INCREASED PROTEASE ACTIVITY

CD8 and CD4 T cells are markedly elevated in the subepithelial region throughout the respiratory tract of patients with severe COPD and emphysema, and are also increased in the airspaces [4]. Although it is the increase in CD8 T cells and CD8/CD4 T-cell ratio that is currently attracting the most attention, these cells contain cathepsin S and other cathepsins for intracellular protein processing. In addition, cytotoxic T cells exhibit membrane-bound cathepsin B (and possibly other cysteine proteinases) to facilitate migration [25]. Elevated mast cell numbers have been described in some studies of COPD; these cells contain high levels of tryptase and chymase, release of which may contribute to the disease process. They also release cathepsins C and L. Examination of lung tissue sections following immunostaining or *in situ* hybridisation studies highlights the presence of proteolytic enzymes in other cell types, for example MMP1, MMP2 and MMP14, which are increased in alveolar epithelial type II cells in emphysematous tissue [14, 17] while MMP1 and 2 are increased in bronchial epithelial cells in tissues from subjects with COPD. MMP9 and other proteinases increase during epithelial cell repair and regeneration [26]. Examination of normal human lung tissue confirms cathepsin H, L and S in macrophages, and identifies cathepsin K and L in bronchial epithelial cells and cathepsin H in alveolar type II cells [19]. Bronchial epithelial cells secrete cathepsin B *in vitro* [11]. Fibroblasts release cathepsins B and K, while

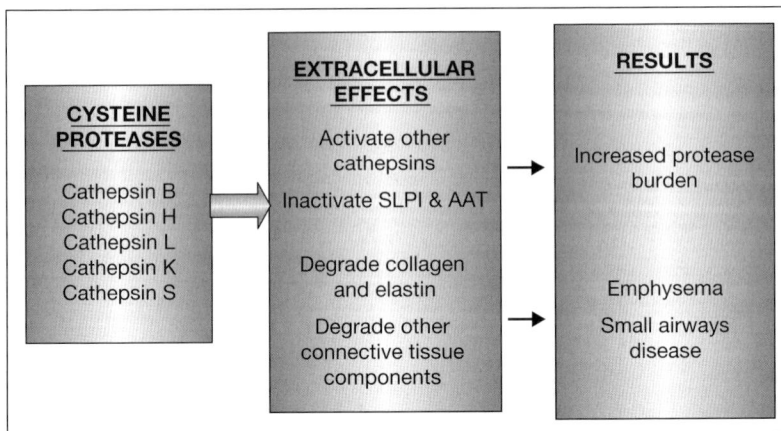

Figure 15.3   Pro-inflammatory effects of cysteine proteases, cathepsins, and role in COPD.

Table 15.1 Examples of protease inhibitors that may have therapeutic potential and that are currently used to investigate the role of proteases in COPD

Protease class	Endogenous lung inhibitors	Examples of possible therapeutic and developmental inhibitors
Serine proteases	α-1 antitrypsin (AAT) Secretory leukoprotease inhibitor (SLPI) Elafin	Proteins: AAT; rAAT rSLPI; 1/2SLPI
		Other protein-based inhibitors: EPI-HNE-4, PAI-1 mutant
		Synthetic, low MWt inhibitors: Acyl-enzyme inhibitors Transition-state inhibitors
Matrix metalloproteinases	TIMPs 1–4	Synthetic, low MWt inhibitors: BMS-27529 (periostat) RS-113456 RS-132908 CP-471,474
Cysteine proteases	Cystatin C	Some specific cysteine protease (cathepsin) inhibitors: Inhibitor-polymer conjugates for cathepsin K
		Peptide aldehyde derivatives e.g., 2-Phe-Tyr(Obut)-COCHO for cathepsin L
		1,2,4-thiadiazole heterocyclic compounds for cathepsin B

smooth muscle cells release cathepsins K and S [see 19]. Cathepsins B and L are elevated in lung secretions from subjects with emphysema and COPD, suggesting release from epithelial cells and/or macrophages and possibly interstitial cells [11, 21]. Clearly, there is significant potential for parenchymal cell proteinases to contribute to the increased proteolytic load in the pathogenesis of COPD.

SERINE PROTEASES

Thus, at least three classes of proteolytic enzymes may contribute to the aetiology of COPD - serine proteinases, MMPs and cysteine proteinases. The neutrophil-derived serine proteinases neutrophil elastase, cathepsin G and proteinase-3 (all approximately 30 kD), have broad substrate specificity and all have a conserved juxtaposition of histidine, aspartate and serine amino acid at the reactive site. A charge relay system transfers an electron from the carboxyl moiety of the histidine residue through aspartate to the oxygen on the serine residue, which results in a nucleophile that splits the amino acid carbonyl group of the substrate. Mast cell tryptase exists at high concentrations in mast cell granulesis. It is tetrameric and access of the substrate to the central pore reactive site limits substrate specificity [27], although it also acts *via* a catalytic histidine-aspartate-serine triad. Its unique, narrow substrate specificity is believed to be related to initiating a series of inflammatory events through limited proteolysis, rather than digesting proteins and it cannot be easily accessed by proteinase inhibitors; there is no endogenous inhibitor of human mast cell tryptase. Mast cell chymase degrades the extracellular matrix and activates TGF-β1 and IL-1β, as well as activating MMP1 which in turn cleaves type I collagen (Figure 15.1) [28].

ENDOGENOUS SERINE PROTEASE INHIBITORS

The best known endogenous inhibitors of these serine proteinases are AAT, secretory leukocyte proteinase inhibitor (SLPI) and elafin. AAT ($\sim$54 kD) is a serpin (SERine Proteinase INhibitor) synthesised in the liver and released into the circulation [29], but is also synthesised at low levels by lung cells and can be up-regulated by cytokines, which may be an important source during neutrophilic inflammation. It is an irreversible inhibitor of neutrophil elastase, cathepsin G and proteinase 3, binding covalently at a 1:1 molar ratio. It can also inhibit mast cell chymase. A glutamic acid-to-lysine substitution at amino acid 342 (Z AAT) causes AAT accumulation in the liver. Polymerisation of Z AAT is believed to account for this, as well as reduced functional activity of both circulating, and pulmonary, Z AAT [30, 31]. SLPI ($\sim$12 kD) and elafin ($\sim$6 kD; also called elastase-specific inhibitor skin-derived anti-leukoproteinase) form the anti-leukoproteinase family [32]; both these proteins are acid stable, unlike AAT. SLPI is a potent, reversible inhibitor of neutrophil elastase and can also inhibit cathepsin G, trypsin, chymase and chymotrypsin, although its ability to inhibit mast cell tryptase is arguable [27]. SLPI is synthesised constitutively by pulmonary epithelial cells as well as alveolar macrophages and neutrophils. It forms a significant proportion of the serine proteinase inhibitory capacity of large airway secretions, reflecting release from bronchial and glandular epithelial cells [32]. Although contributing less of the total anti-proteinase activity in the distal airway, SLPI is synthesised by Clara cells and alveolar epithelial type II cells and is present in the bronchoalveolar lavage [33, 34]. Elafin ($\sim$6 kD) is synthesised by the same pulmonary epithelial cells that synthesise SLPI; it inhibits neutrophil elastase and proteinase-3. Usually present at relatively low levels, elafin is synthesised in response to inflammatory mediators such as cytokines, for example, tumour necrosis factor (TNF) and IL-1β [32, 34], as well as lipopolysaccharide and, interestingly, is up-regulated by neutrophil elastase itself [35], which may be a feedback mechanism. SLPI is usually present at higher concentrations than elafin, but is also up-regulated by the same mediators.

α-1 ANTITRYPSIN AUGMENTATION THERAPY

Early investigation of antiprotease treatment using intravenous serum-derived AAT in AAT-deficient subjects showed that it was possible and practical to increase pulmonary (bronchoalveolar lavage) AAT levels above the critical threshold [36]. This has been confirmed in a number of later studies [37]. Two studies of the effect of IV treatment with 60 mg/kg AAT at weekly intervals on decline in FEV_1 in patients with severe AAT deficiency and reduced FEV_1 [37–39] showed a reduction in the rate of decline in FEV_1 in subjects who had an initial FEV_1 between 30% and 65% predicted. Intravenous AAT also resulted in a reduction in sputum elastase activity and LTB4 following a 4-week trial [40], illustrating the anti-inflammatory potential of AAT, and suggesting that inhalation might be an effective alternative route of delivery. These and other similar studies suggest that intravenous AAT augmentation therapy may be beneficial, particularly in AAT-deficient subjects [reviewed by Stoller et al.; 37]. However, intravenous AAT treatment is expensive and time consuming. Other problems relate to the availability of sufficient quantities and safety (e.g., pathological prion or viral contamination) of plasma-derived AAT. Recombinant AAT can be generated in quantity and at high purity and would, therefore, be a good substitute, and likely to be effective by inhalation.

LOW-MOLECULAR-WEIGHT PROTEASE INHIBITOR THERAPY

As SLPI is a relatively smaller protein than AAT, delivery either by inhalation or intravenously will result in rapid transudation into tissues and fluids. However, the half-life of SLPI is also rapid (12 h), but a twice-daily intravenous dose should be adequate. In patients with cystic fibrosis, neutrophil numbers and elastase activity in lung secretions decreased following inhalation of SLPI [41]. Neutrophil elastase-induced brochoconstriction in guinea-pigs is inhibited by intravenous recombinant, ½ SLPI [containing the neutrophil elastase inhibitory domain; 42]. Furthermore, SLPI stimulated expression of anti-inflammatory cytokines, IL-10 and transforming growth factor-β (TGF-β), by LPS-stimulated macrophages *in vitro* [43]. As elafin, like SLPI, is also a small protein, it will readily access tissues. Again, there are relatively few experimental studies of the efficacy of this inhibitor in lung disease. Neutrophil elastase-induced acute lung injury in hamsters could be inhibited by pre-elafin (also a member of the Trappin family, Trappin-2) but not by elafin [44]. The efficacy of elafin has not been tested in man. A potentially important aspect of treatment with SLPI and elafin is their role in antimicrobial defence, as they also exhibit properties of defensins [45]. Because SLPI and elafin are reversible inhibitors it may be that dual therapy with AAT might prove more effective, since release of enzyme previously bound to, and inactivated by, SLPI or elafin, in the absence of sufficient AAT, may not be cleared and may just prolong its activity within the lung [33]. In this respect, the efficacy of fusion proteins that combine the activity of both types of inhibitor, i.e., SLPI and AAT, are currently being investigated.

ENGINEERED PROTEINS

DX-890 (EPI-HNE-4) is a recombinant protein of an active region of human inter-α-trypsin inhibitor, which has potent irreversible activity against neutrophil elastase. It is not susceptible to oxidative inactivation and is active at acid pH. It protects rats from lung injury following intratracheal instillation of neutrophil elastase or the soluble phase of cystic fibrosis sputum (i.e., containing serine proteinase activity [46]). It is currently being investigated for cystic fibrosis therapy, and may be effective for emphysema [47]. Very recently, a mutant form of plasminogen activator inhibitor type-1 has been shown in an *in vivo* model of pulmonary inflammation to be more effective against neutrophil elastase and cathepsin G than the endogenous inhibitors [48]. This approach offers an alternative strategy, although it might prove expensive to produce and administer such drugs.

SYNTHETIC SERINE PROTEASE INHIBITORS

There are a number of compounds designed to inhibit neutrophil elastase. The most promising are acyl-enzyme inibitors and transition-state inhibitors. These have been the subject of a recent review [49]. Both types of inhibitor form a stable complex with neutrophil elastase to prevent its activity. Sivelestat (ONO-5046), an acyl-enzyme inhibitor, is very successful in reversing the effects of a number of pro-inflammatory agents (LPS, LTB4, ozone) in animal models and may be useful in Man in acute lung injury [50]. However, because it has to be administered intravenously, it is not likely to be used for chronic conditions such as COPD. Another acyl-enzyme inhibitor, which is showing promise for use in COPD, midesteine (MR-889), has low oral toxicity and inhibits mucus production and is currently being evaluated to treat COPD [51]. Amongst the transition-state inhibitors, ONO-6818 is promising. In animal models of pulmonary inflammation and emphysema (i.e., LPS and neutrophil elastase exposure), oral ONO-6818 is very effective [52]. Because it is effective orally, it has potential for use in chronic disease such as emphysema and COPD. In an animal model of cigarette smoke-induced emphysema, ZD0892 neutrophil elastase inhibitor inhibited inflammatory chemokine and cytokine levels and reduced the degree of airspace enlargement [53]. Mast cell chymase inhibitors include NK3201 and BCEAB, which have been shown to be effective in animal models of cardiovascular disease, but not yet in animal models of COPD and emphysema [28].

MATRIX METALLOPROTEINASES

The MMPs are a large, growing family of structurally related proteases that degrade extra-cellular matrices. Their common name reflects their ability to degrade extracellular matrix components at neutral pH. They depend on divalent metal ions, Zn^{2+} and Ca^{2+}, for their activity. They have a conserved zinc-binding motif, HExxHxxGxxH, and a C-terminal methionine residue within a 1,4-met-turn, whose side chain provides a hydrophobic region that protects the zinc-binding site [see Belvisi and Bottomly; 54]. The glutamic acid next to the N-terminal histidine acts as a nucleophile in association with water to cleave the peptide substrate. Thus, the catalytic zinc atom binds to the carbonyl group of the sessile peptide bond to trigger hydrolysis. In the latent pro-MMP molecule, a conserved cysteine-switch motif, C-terminal to the zinc-binding site, co-ordinates with the zinc ion, preventing the access of water and conferring latency as long as the pro-region of the MMP remains intact.

MMPs are secreted as inactive zymogens, and are activated extracellularly, for example, by proteolytic cleavage of the pro-peptide. All the MMPs have a prepro-peptide, which precedes the catalytic domain [55]. With the exception of MMP3, this is followed by a hemo-pexin-like domain. MMP2 and 9 also contain three fibronectin-like sequences N-terminal to the catalytic domain, which enhance enzyme–substrate interactions. Some membrane-bound MT-MMPs contain a transmembrane region N-terminal to the hemopexin-like domain, consisting of a sequence of hydrophobic amino acids that anchors the protein at the cell surface. Other MT-MMPs bind to the cell surface *via* a sequence that binds to glycophosphatidyl inositol. The membrane-bound MT-MMPs have the potential to be catalytically active on secretion. Because of the structural heterogeneity of MMPs (they vary in size from 30 to 100 kD), once released into the extracellular environment, or membrane-bound and functional in the pericellular zone, and activated, MMPs can degrade most extracellular connective tissues and are important during development of normal tissue as well as remodelling damaged tissue [10, 12]. Synthesis, storage and secretion of MMPs is strictly regulated in response to the tissue environment, and expression is controlled by factors such as cytokines, endotoxin, phagocytosis and growth factors. Extracellular-MMPs can control the activity of cytokines, for example, by the proteolytic activation of TGF-β, membrane-bound TNF-α, and IL-8 and degradative inactivation of IL-1β. They also activate other MMPs (e.g., MMP14 activates MMP2) and they can inactivate proteinase inhibitors such as AAT. Thus, they can influence many processes of importance in COPD (Figure 15.2) [10, 12, 54].

TISSUE INHIBITORS OF MATRIX METALLOPROTEINASES

The tissue inhibitors of matrix metalloproteinases are the endogenous inhibitors of MMPs. Four have been described, TIMP1, 2, 3 and 4. They range in size from 21–29 kD and inhibit MMPs on a 1:1 molar ratio. They are usually secreted alongside MMPs and are believed to confer strict control over MMP activity. TIMP1 release by alveolar macrophages from COPD subjects is reduced at the same time that MMP9 is increased [15], and similarly, the ratio of TIMP1 to MMP9 has been reported to be reduced in sputum from COPD subjects [56]. This suggests that reduced TIMP may also contribute to COPD, together with increased MMP activity. However, unlike AAT, the use of natural or recombinant TIMP to augment the anti-MMP screen has not been thoroughly investigated.

Most research has concentrated on developing low-molecular-weight, synthetic inhibitors of MMPs. These inhibitors are designed to target the reactive zinc molecule and the substrate recognition site of the enzyme. Although several MMP inhibitors are being evaluated to treat cancer, rheumatoid arthritis and periodontal disease, there have been no clinical trials of COPD. Unfortunately, a number of potent inhibitors have either proven to be ineffective and/or toxic in clinical trials for cancer and rheumatoid arthritis (e.g., Marimastat [BB-256], Prinomastat [AG3340]), while others are still on trial (e.g., Periostat, BMS-27529). The failure of synthetic MMP inhibitors on trial in other inflammatory diseases discourages their use in COPD. However, synthetic MMP inhibitors (e.g., RS-113456, RS-132908) have been used very successfully in the smoking mouse model of emphysema [55, 57], which has previously been demonstrated to involve MMP12 [macrophage metalloelastase; 18], where they markedly reduce or halt the degree of cigarette smoke-induced emphysema, even when administered after the onset of alveolar enlargement [55]. CP-471, 474, a broad spectrum synthetic MMP inhibitor, successfully reduced the degree of emphysema in a guinea-pig model [58]. These studies in experimental animals support the concept that MMPs are important in the development of emphysema and that inhibition of MMP activity in the lungs of COPD subjects is a viable future therapeutic strategy.

CYSTEINE PROTEASES – CATHEPSINS

Cathepsins have received much attention for their role in cancer, osteoporosis and rheumatoid arthritis. Cathepsins are proteinases that are located in lysosomes and exist in an acidic environment within the lysosome. They vary in size between 21 and 30 kD. They are synthesised as inactive pro-enzymes and are activated on release of the pro-peptide. This generally occurs as a result of proteolytic cleavage by other cathepsins [19]. Their optimal activity is at acid pH and they lose activity at neutral and alkaline pH. However, cathepsin S and, to some extent, cathepsin K retain some activity at neutral pH, which disappears over time. Cathepsins include enzymes from different classes. Thus, while cathepsin G is a serine proteinase, cathepsins B, H, K, L and S are thiol proteinases [19, 59]. The active site consists of a series of 5–7 amino acid residues. The specificity of action is defined by the second substrate binding pocket (S2) which, for most lysosomal cysteine proteinases, accepts hydrophobic amino acids such as phenylalanine and leucine, although cathepsin B also accepts arginine. Cathepsin K is remarkable in that it accepts proline at the S2 subsite. This means that it can degrade collagen types I and II in the proline-rich helical region, which is normally resistant to proteolysis and which also means that it is able to degrade collagen independently of other proteinases [60]. In contrast, degradation of collagen by MMPs takes place in co-operation with cathepsin L-like proteases. Since cathepsins K, L and S can degrade elastin, possibly within protected acidic niches, but also at neutral pH (e.g., cathepsin S and K), release of cathepsins into the extracellular environment is likely to trigger connective tissue turnover. Cathepsin K is one of the most potent elastinolytic enzymes, and cathepsin L and S have very high activity at optimal pH. Intratracheal instillation of cathepsin B causes emphysema in hamsters [61]. Overexpression of IFN-γ and IL-13 in mice results in emphysema and up-regulation of MMP12 and a number of cathepsins [23, 62]. Use of E64, a cysteine protease inhibitor, abrogated the condition supporting a role for cathepsins in the development of emphysema. Furthermore, cathepsins with elastinolytic activity (cathepsins B, L and S) are capable of rapidly degrading SLPI, even with a 400 molar excess of SLPI [63], while cathepsin L degrades AAT [64], thus enhancing activity of the serine proteinases (Figure 15.3). Inhibition of cathepsins, particularly those with elastinolytic activity, is likely to prove beneficial in emphysema and COPD.

CYSTATIN C

Cystatins are the endogenous inhibitors of cathepsins. Intracellular cystatins A and B control the very high cathepsin concentrations found in lysosomes (1 mM), and cystatins C, D and F, as well as serpins and α-2 macroglobulin, control extracellular activity [19, 59]. Cystatin C (~13.5 kD) is widely distributed in the body, a very potent inhibitor and the most ubiquitous inhibitor of extracellular cysteine proteinases in the lung. The inhibitory activity of cystatins is reversible and involves hydrophobic interactions between the binding region of cystatin and the binding pockets of the enzyme. The Arg, Leu and Val at positions 8, 9 and 10 in the N-terminal region of cystatin C, are believed to be important in the inhibitory process [59]. Cystatin C has not been extensively studied in emphysema and COPD, partly because the relevance of cysteine proteinases to these conditions is only just becoming clear. In one study, cystatin C was found to be increased in bronchoalveolar lavage from subjects with subclinical emphysema [65], while release of cystatin C by human macrophages was coincident with the release of cathepsin B [11].

SYNTHETIC CYSTEINE PROTEINASE (CATHEPSIN) INHIBITORS

As mentioned earlier, most of the research into cathepsins, and hence therapy, has centred on cancer, rheumatoid arthritis and bone disease. The challenge has been to develop potent, but selective inhibitors because of the wide tissue distribution of these enzymes and possibility of side-effects. There are no studies of cysteine protease (cathepsin) inhibitors in COPD.

An inhibitor commonly used in laboratory studies is an oxyrane-inhibitor, E-64, (2S, 3S-trans-epoxysuccinyl-L-leucyl-agmatine), which was originally isolated from cultures of *Aspergillus japonicus*; it is a very strong, irreversible inhibitor of cysteine proteinases [66]. This inhibitor works in animal models of emphysema and against cathepsins released from human alveolar macrophages [17, 23, 62]. Due to the lack of specificity of many cysteine proteinase inhibitors, the objective is to develop drugs that are selective and potent. Thus, a series of novel cathepsin inhibitors are currently being developed. These include very selective bioavailable ketoamides for cathepsin K [67]. Cathepsin K-inhibitor-polymer conjugates, which allow for specific targeting of the inhibitor [68], are potent, selective oral inhibitors which are being developed because of the lack of specificity of other synthetic cathepsin inhibitors. A peptide aldehyde derivative, Z-Phe-Tyr(OBut)-COCHO, is a recently described, very specific, potent inhibitor of cathepsin L [69]. A novel class of specific synthetic inhibitors of cathepsin B are based on 1,2,4-thiadiazole heterocycle as the thiol-trapping pharmacophore [70]. Many other cysteine protease (cathepsin) inhibitors are currently in development, but there are few laboratory or human studies relating to COPD.

CONCLUSION

Antiprotease therapy is not currently in routine use for the treatment of emphysema and COPD. This is despite accumulating evidence that the protease burden is increased and contributes to the disease process. Investigation of the efficacy of proteinase inhibitors in COPD is complicated by the chronic and slow progress of the disease, and the problems associated with detecting therapeutic benefits, which take years to establish [37]. While AAT deficiency is an obvious reason for AAT augmentation therapy, the exact mechanisms of cigarette smoke-induced COPD in patients with normal levels of AAT are not certain. In addition, continued exposure to cigarette smoke may affect therapy due to oxidative inactivation or other effects on the therapeutic compounds. Some early investigations of anti-neutrophil elastase therapy in Man were not successful. However, it seems likely that the multitude of cellular sources of proteases being released into different compartments of the lung may have masked the effect of an inhibitor of one class of enzyme. As the research over the last thirty years has shown, many classes of enzyme are involved, forming a potent protease cocktail that amplifies inflammation (Figures 15.1, 15.2 and 15.3). New strategies for antiprotease therapy should probably consider targeting the specific site of action with inhibitors of more than one class of protease.

REFERENCES

1. Laurell CB, Eriksson S. The electrophoretic alpha 1-globulin pattern of serum in alpha 1-antitrypsin deficiency. *Scan J Clin Lab Invest* 1963; 15:132–140.
2. Gross P, Pfitzer EA, Tolker E, Babyak MA, Kaschak M. Experimental emphysema: its production with papain in normal and silicotic rats. *Arch Environ Health* 1965; 11:50–58.
3. Saetta M, Turato G, Maestrelli P, Mapp CE, Fabbri LM. Cellular and structural bases of chronic obstructive pulmonary disease. *Am J Respir Crit Care Med* 2001; 163:1304–1309.
4. Turato G, Zuin R, Saetta M. Pathogenesis and pathology of COPD. *Respiration* 2001; 68:117–128.
5. Stockley RA. Neutrophils and the pathogenesis of COPD. *Chest* 2002; 121(suppl 5):S151–S155.
6. Barnes PJ. New concepts in chronic obstructive pulmonary disease. *Annu Rev Med* 2003; 54:113–129.
7. Finlay GA, Russell KJ, McMahon KJ, D'arcy EM, Masterson JB, FitzGerald MX, O'Connor CM. Elevated levels of matrix metalloproteinases in bronchoalveolar lavage fluid of emphysematous patients. *Thorax* 1997; 52:502–506.
8. Niewoehner DE, Kleinerman J, Rice DB. Pathologic changes in the peripheral airways of young cigarette smokers. *N Engl J Med* 1974; 291:755–758.
9. Retamales I, Elliott WM, Meshi B, Coxson HO, Pare PD, Sciurba FC *et al.* Amplification of inflammation in emphysema and its association with latent adenoviral infection. *Am J Respir Crit Care Med* 2001; 164:469–473.
10. Tetley TD. Macrophages and the pathogenesis of COPD. *Chest* 2002; 121 (suppl 5):S156–S159.
11. Burnett D, Abrahamson M, Devalia JL, Sapsford RJ, Davies RJ, Buttle DJ. Synthesis and secretion of procathepsin B and cystatin C by human bronchial epithelial cells *in vitro:* modulation of cathepsin B activity by neutrophil elastase. *Arch Biochem Biophys* 1995; 317:305–310.
12. Shapiro SD. Proteinases in chronic obstructive pulmonary disease. *Biochem Soc Trans* 2002; 30:98–102.
13. Finlay GA, O'Driscoll LR, Russell KJ, D'arcy EM, Masterson JB, FitzGerald MX, O'Connor CM. Matrix metalloproteinase expression and production by alveolar macrophages in emphysema. *Am J Respir Crit Care Med* 1997; 156:240–247.
14. Segura-Valdez L, Pardo A, Gaxiola M, Uhal BD, Becerril C, Selman M. Upregulation of gelatinases A and B, collagenases 1 and 2, and increased parenchymal cell death in COPD. *Chest* 2000; 117:684–694.
15. Russell RE, Thorley A, Culpitt SV, Dodd S, Donnelly LE, Demattos C *et al.* Alveolar macrophage-mediated elastolysis: roles of matrix metalloproteinases, cysteine, and serine proteases. *Am J Physiol Lung Cell Mol Physiol* 2002; 283:L867–L873.
16. Russell RE, Culpitt SV, DeMatos C, Donnelly L, Smith M, Wiggins J, Barnes PJ. Release and activity of matrix metalloproteinase-9 and tissue inhibitor of metalloproteinase-1 by alveolar macrophages from patients with chronic obstructive pulmonary disease. *Am J Respir Cell Mol Biol* 2002; 26:602–609.
17. Ohnishi K, Takagi M, Kurokawa Y, Satomi S, Konttinen YT. Matrix metalloproteinase-mediated extracellular matrix protein degradation in human pulmonary emphysema. *Lab Invest* 1998; 78:1077–1087.
18. Hautamaki RD, Kobayashi DK, Senior RM, Shapiro SD. Requirement for macrophage elastase for cigarette smoke-induced emphysema in mice. *Science* 1997; 277:2002–2004.
19. Buhling F, Waldburg N, Reisenauer A, Heimburg A, Golpon H, Welte T. Lysosomal cysteine proteases in the lung: role in protein processing and immunoregulation. *Eur Respir J* 2004; 23:620–628.
20. Reilly JJ, Jr., Mason RW, Chen P, Joseph LJ, Sukhatme VP, Yee R, Chapman HA, Jr. Synthesis and processing of cathepsin L, an elastase, by human alveolar macrophages. *Biochem J* 1989; 257:493–498.
21. Takahashi H, Ishidoh K, Muno D, Ohwada A, Nukiwa T, Kominami E, Kira S. Cathepsin L activity is increased in alveolar macrophages and bronchoalveolar lavage fluid of smokers. *Am Rev Respir Dis* 1993; 147:1562–1568.
22. Crothers K, Zheng T, Cheng GS, Chen G, Chupp G, Elias JA, Homer RJ. Elevated expression of cathepsin S and B in lung tissue of current smokers. *Am J Respir Crit Care Med* 2004; 169;A835.
23. Wang Z, Zheng T, Zhu Z, Homer RJ, Riese RJ, Chapman HA *et al.* Interferon gamma induction of pulmonary emphysema in the adult murine lung. *J Exp Med* 2000; 192:1587–1600.
24. Campbell EJ, Wald MS. Fate of human neutrophil elastase following receptor-mediated endocytosis by human alveolar macrophages. Implications for connective tissue injury. *J Lab Clin Med* 1983; 101:527–536.

25. Layton GT, Harris SJ, Bland FA, Lee SR, Fearn S, Kaleta J et al. Therapeutic effects of cysteine protease inhibition in allergic lung inflammation: inhibition of allergen-specific T lymphocyte migration. *Inflamm Res* 2001; 50:400–408.

26. Buckley S, Driscoll B, Shi W, Anderson K, Warburton D. Migration and gelatinases in cultured fetal, adult, and hyperoxic alveolar epithelial cells. *Am J Physiol Lung Cell Mol Physiol* 2001; 281:L427–L434.

27. Sommerhoff CP. Mast cell tryptases and airway remodeling. *Am J Respir Crit Care Med* 2001; 164:S52–S58.

28. Doggrell SA, Wanstall JC. Vascular chymase: pathophysiological role and therapeutic potential of inhibition. *Cardiovasc Res* 2004; 61:653–662.

29. Lomas DA, Parfrey H. Alpha1- pathophysiology. 4: molecular pathophysiology *Thorax* 2004; 59:529–535.

30. Mulgrew AT, Taggart CC, Lawless MW, Greene CM, Brantly ML, O'Neill SJ, McElvaney NG. Z alpha1-antitrypsin polymerizes in the lung and acts as a neutrophil chemoattractant. *Chest* 2004; 125:1952–1957.

31. Lomas DA, Mahadeva R. Alpha1-antitrypsin polymerization and the serpinopathies: pathobiology and prospects for therapy. *J Clin Invest* 2002; 110:1585–1590.

32. Sallenave JM. Antimicrobial activity of antiproteinases. *Biochem Soc Trans* 2002; 30:111–115.

33. Bingle L, Tetley TD. Secretory leukoprotease inhibitor: partnering alpha 1-proteinase inhibitor to combat pulmonary inflammation. *Thorax* 1996; 51:1273–1274.

34. Bingle L, Tetley TD, Bingle CD. Cytokine-mediated induction of the human elafin gene in pulmonary epithelial cells is regulated by nuclear factor-kappaB. *Am J Respir Cell Mol Biol* 2001; 25:84–91.

35. Reid PT, Marsden ME, Cunningham GA, Haslett C, Sallenave JM. Human neutrophil elastase regulates the expression and secretion of elafin (elastase-specific inhibitor) in type II alveolar epithelial cells. *FEBS Lett* 1999; 457:33–37.

36. Wewers MD, Casolaro MA, Sellers SE, Swayze SC, McPhaul KM, Wittes JT, Crystal RG. Replacement therapy for alpha 1-antitrypsin deficiency associated with emphysema. *N Engl J Med* 1987; 316:1055–1062.

37. Stoller JK, Fallat R, Schluchter MD, O'Brien RG, Connor JT, Gross N et al. Augmentation therapy with alpha1-antitrypsin: patterns of use and adverse events. *Chest* 2003; 123:1425–1434.

38. Seersholm N, Wencker M, Banik N, Viskum K, Dirksen A, Kok-Jensen A, Konietzko N. Does alpha1-antitrypsin augmentation therapy slow the annual decline in FEV1 in patients with severe hereditary alpha1-antitrypsin deficiency? Wissenschaftliche Arbeitsgemeinschaft zur Therapie von Lungenerkrankungen (WATL) alpha1-AT study group. *Eur Respir J* 1997; 10:2260–2263.

39. Wencker M, Banik N, Buhl R, Seidel R, Konietzko N. Long-term treatment of alpha1-antitrypsin deficiency-related pulmonary emphysema with human alpha1-antitrypsin. Wissenschaftliche Arbeitsgemeinschaft zur Therapie von Lungenerkrankungen (WATL)-alpha1-AT-study group. *Eur Respir J* 1998; 11:428–433.

40. Stockley RA, Bayley DL, Unsal I, Dowson LJ. The effect of augmentation therapy on bronchial inflammation in alpha1-antitrypsin deficiency. *Am J Respir Crit Care Med* 2002; 165:1494–1498.

41. Vogelmeier C, Gillissen A, Buhl R. Use of secretory leukoprotease inhibitor to augment lung antineutrophil elastase activity. *Chest* 1996; 110(suppl 6):S261–S266.

42. Suzuki T, Wang W, Lin JT, Shirato K, Mitsuhashi H, Inoue H. Aerosolized human neutrophil elastase induces airway constriction and hyperresponsiveness with protection by intravenous pretreatment with half-length secretory leukoprotease inhibitor. *Am J Respir Crit Care Med* 1996; 153:1405–1411.

43. Sano C, Shimizu T, Sato K, Kawauchi H, Tomioka H. Effects of secretory leucocyte protease inhibitor on the production of the anti-inflammatory cytokines, IL-10 and transforming growth factor-beta (TGF-beta), by lipopolysaccharide-stimulated macrophages. *Clin Exp Immunol* 2000; 121:77–85.

44. Vachon E, Bourbonnais Y, Bingle CD, Rowe SJ, Janelle MF, Tremblay GM. Anti-inflammatory effect of pre-elafin in lipopolysaccharide-induced acute lung inflammation. *Biol Chem* 2002; 383:1249–1256.

45. Hiemstra PS. Novel roles of protease inhibitors in infection and inflammation. *Biochem Soc Trans* 2002; 30:116–120.

46. Delacourt C, Herigault S, Delclaux C, Poncin A, Levame M, Harf A et al. Protection against acute lung injury by intravenous or intratracheal pretreatment with EPI-HNE-4, a new potent neutrophil elastase inhibitor. *Am J Respir Cell Mol Biol* 2002; 26:290–297.

47. Grimbert D, Vecellio L, Delepine P, Attucci S, Boissinot E, Poncin A et al. Characteristics of EPI-hNE4 aerosol: a new elastase inhibitor for treatment of cystic fibrosis. *J Aerosol Med* 2003; 16:121–129.

48. Stefansson S, Yepes M, Gorlatova N, Day DE, Moore EG, Zabaleta A et al. Mutants of plasminogen activator inhibitor-1 designed to inhibit neutrophil elastase and cathepsin G are more effective in vivo than their endogenous inhibitors. J Biol Chem 2004; 279:29981–29987.

49. Ohbayashi H. Novel neutrophil elastase inhibitors as a treatment for neutrophil-predominant inflammatory lung diseases. Drugs 2002; 5:910–923.

50. Zeiher BG, Matsuoka S, Kawabata K, Repine JE. Neutrophil elastase and acute lung injury: prospects for sivelestat and other neutrophil elastase inhibitors as therapeutics. Crit Care Med 2002; 30(suppl 5):S281–S287.

51. Luisetti M, Sturan C, Sella D, Madonini E, Galavotti V, Bruno G et al. MR889, a neutrophil elastase inhibitor, in patients with chronic obstructive pulmonary disease: a double-blind, randomized, placebo-controlled clinical trial. Eur Respir J 1996; 9:1482–1486.

52. Kuraki I, Ishibashi M, Takayama M, Shiraishi M, Yoshida M. A novel oral neutrophil elastase inhibitor (ONO-6818) inhibits human neutrophil elastase-induced emphysema in rats. Am J Respir Crit Care Med 2002; 166:496–500.

53. Wright JL, Farmer SG, Churg A. Synthetic serine elastase inhibitor reduces cigarette smoke-induced emphysema in guinea-pigs. Am J Respir Crit Care Med 2002; 166:954–960.

54. Belvisi MG, Bottomley KM. The role of matrix metalloproteinases (MMPs) in the pathophysiology of chronic obstructive pulmonary disease (COPD): a therapeutic role for inhibitors of MMPs? Inflamm Res 2003; 52:95–100.

55. Shapiro SD, Tong SE, Van Wart HE, Martin RL. Marophage Metalloelastase Inhibitors. In: Barnes PJ, Harse TT (eds) New Drugs for Asthma, Allergy and COPD. Karger, Basel, 2001, pp 177–180.

56. Beeh KM, Kornmann O, Buhl R, Culpitt SV, Giembycz MA, Barnes PJ. Neutrophil chemotactic activity of sputum from patients with COPD: role of interleukin 8 and leukotriene B4. Chest 2003; 123:1240–1247.

57. Churg A, Dai J, Zay K, Karsan A, Hendricks R, Yee C et al. Alpha-1-antitrypsin and a broad spectrum metalloprotease inhibitor, RS113456, have similar acute anti-inflammatory effects. Lab Invest 2001; 81:1119–1131.

58. Selman M, Cisneros-Lira J, Gaxiola M, Ramirez R, Kudlacz EM, Mitchell PG, Pardo A. Matrix metalloproteinases inhibition attenuates tobacco smoke-induced emphysema in guinea-pigs. Chest 2003; 123:1633–1641.

59. Grzonka Z, Jankowska E, Kasprzykowski F, Kasprzykowska R, Lankiewicz L, Wiczk W et al. Structural studies of cysteine proteases and their inhibitors. Acta Biochem Pol 2001; 48:1–20.

60. Garnero P, Borel O, Byrjalsen I, Ferreras M, Drake FH, McQueney MS et al. The collagenolytic activity of cathepsin K is unique among mammalian proteinases. J Biol Chem 1998; 273:32347–32352.

61. Lesser M, Padilla ML, Cardozo C. Induction of emphysema in hamsters by intratracheal instillation of cathepsin B. Am Rev Respir Dis 1992; 145:661–668.

62. Zheng T, Zhu Z, Wang Z, Homer RJ, Ma B, Riese RJ, Jr. et al. Inducible targeting of IL-13 to the adult lung causes matrix metalloproteinase- and cathepsin-dependent emphysema. J Clin Invest 2000; 106:1081–1093.

63. Taggart CC, Lowe GJ, Greene CM, Mulgrew AT, O'Neill SJ, Levine RL, McElvaney NG. Cathepsin B, L, and S cleave and inactivate secretory leucoprotease inhibitor. J Biol Chem 2001; 276:33345–33352.

64. Johnson DA, Barrett AJ, Mason RW. Cathepsin L inactivates alpha 1-proteinase inhibitor by cleavage in the reactive site region. J Biol Chem 1986; 261:14748–14751.

65. Takeyabu K, Betsuyaku T, Nishimura M, Yoshioka A, Tanino M, Miyamoto K, Kawakami Y. Cysteine proteinases and cystatin C in bronchoalveolar lavage fluid from subjects with subclinical emphysema. Eur Respir J 1998; 12:1033–1039.

66. Matsumoto K, Mizoue K, Kitamura K, Tse WC, Huber CP, Ishida T. Structural basis of inhibition of cysteine proteases by E-64 and its derivatives. Biopolymers 1999; 51:99–107.

67. Tavares FX, Boncek V, Deaton DN, Hassell AM, Long ST, Miller AB et al. Design of potent, selective, and orally bioavailable inhibitors of cysteine protease cathepsin K. J Med Chem 2004; 47:588–599.

68. Wang D, Li W, Pechar M, Kopeckova P, Bromme D, Kopecek J. Cathepsin K inhibitor-polymer conjugates: potential drugs for the treatment of osteoporosis and rheumatoid arthritis. Int J Pharm 2004; 277:73–79.

69. Lynas JF, Hawthorne SJ, Walker B. Development of peptidyl alpha-keto-beta-aldehydes as new inhibitors of cathepsin L–comparisons of potency and selectivity profiles with cathepsin B. Bioorg Med Chem Lett 2000; 10:1771–1773.

70. Leung-Toung R, Wodzinska J, Li W, Lowrie J, Kukreja R, Desilets D et al. 1,2,4-thiadiazole: a novel Cathepsin B inhibitor. Bioorg Med Chem 2003; 11:5529–5537.

16

Mucoactive drugs

L. Allegra

MUCOCILIARY CLEARANCE IN CHRONIC BRONCHIAL DISEASES

The precise interaction between airflow obstruction, reduced mucociliary clearance, smoking, hypersecretion and infection, and their individual and interactive importance to respiratory morbidity and subsequent mortality in separate conditions remains at best debatable and at worst a mystery. Detailed research into sputum over the past two decades has greatly increased our depth and breadth of knowledge. Let us hope that continuing studies in this field will lead, perhaps through adaptation of the quantity or quality of respiratory mucus, to new and more successful therapeutic strategies.

MUCOCILIARY DYSFUNCTION

The accumulation of mucus in the conducting airways is thought to result from epithelial hypersecretion combined with a defect in ciliary function. Both component functions of mucociliary interaction have been shown to be already impaired in simple cigarette smokers with neither pathological signs and symptoms nor functional abnormalities. Of course, defective mucociliary function is recognised as the marker of several pathological respiratory conditions, the majority of the studies having been dedicated to chronic bronchitis, both simple and obstructive.

CHRONIC BRONCHITIS

Histologically characterised by bronchial inflammation and secretory cell hyperplasia and hypertrophy (with increased Reid index), chronic bronchitis (for which cigarette smoking remains the main etiological agent) is associated with a reduction in mucociliary clearance, hypersecretion, and 'abnormal mucus'. This has a typical epithelial glycoprotein content (with characteristic features of buoyant density and chemical constitution – large molecular weight), which together with a predominantly glycolipid component, disturbs the viscoelastic properties of the respiratory tract secretions [1–3]. Elastase activity is also raised [4]. Persistent mucus accumulation and airway obstruction (in concert with recurrent infection in the later stages of the disease) eventually lead to severe airflow limitation and chronic respiratory failure. Chronic bronchitis is defined clinically as 'chronic productive cough' with a duration time of >3 months/year for at least 2 consecutive years. This definition implies an abnormality in the production and clearance of lower airway secretion,

Luigi Allegra, MD, Professor, Respiratory diseases, University of Milan; Director, Cardiorespiratory Department, IRCCS, Policlinico Hospital, Milan,Italy.

which is common to both the clinical presentations of the disease, the 'simple chronic bronchitis' as well as the 'obstructive' one (COPD), the latter being characterised by clinical and spirographic signs and symptoms of obstruction in addition to cough and phlegm. Cigarette smoking is the single most common cause of chronic bronchitis, and therefore it is not surprising that the actions of cigarette smoke on the mucociliary apparatus of the airways has been the subject of intense investigation. There is general agreement that cigarette smoke has detrimental effects on mucociliary function, and some of the mechanisms responsible for the cigarette smoke and chronic-bronchitis-associated mucociliary dysfunction have been elucidated.

Another important question, however, is whether the presence of excessive mucus in the airways of patients with chronic bronchitis limits airflow. Epidemiological data are conflicting. In patients with chronic obstructive lung disease, survival has been reported to be inversely related to forced expiratory volume in 1 s (FEV$_1$) whether or not productive cough is present [5]. Likewise, a long-term study has found that death rates in chronic obstructive lung disease are not significantly related to initial sputum production [6]. On the other hand, a 22-year mortality survey of >1,000 men has shown not only that the severity of airflow obstruction (e.g. FEV$_1$/FVC) is correlated with mortality, but also that chronic phlegm production is significantly associated with mortality [7].

In Europe and America it is widely accepted that the important primary cause of hypersecretion is smoking cigarettes, particularly those with a high tar content [8]. Other exogenous factors that may contribute to the hypersecretion (and further bronchopulmonary damages characterising chronic bronchitis) include metropolitan (and micro-environmental) air pollution, occupational dust exposure (including exposure to asbestos and other carcinogenic airborne particles), domestic pollution, for example, from poor ventilation, gas fires in urban areas and cooking fuels in rural communities, passive smoking, climatic factors, childhood factors such as repetitive bronchial infections, hereditary factors linked, for example, with protease-antiprotease imbalance, demographic factors, social classes, promiscuity and malnutrition.

So, smoking, hypersecretion and chronic bronchitis (simple or obstructive) are strongly associated. This is explained at a microscopic level, at least in part, by the description of the Reid index, describing the diameter of submucosal glands as a proportion of the gland to bronchial wall thickness [9]. Chronic hypersecretion is also found in other pulmonary diseases such as cystic fibrosis, α-1-antitrypsin deficiency, hypogammaglobulinaemia and asthma, even in those with asthma who have never smoked [10, 11].

The role of infection in the progression of lung disease is unclear. It as been known for 30 years that the bronchial tree may not be sterile in conditions of hypersecretion [12, 13]. Initially it was believed that infection precipitated further airway damage. Although some studies seem to have supported this [14], others have not shown any general correlation between frequency of infection and the rate of decline of FEV$_1$ in the presence of hypersecretion and mild airways obstruction [6, 15, 16]. However, where added immunological or physiological factors are present (such as in cystic fibrosis, bronchiectasis, hypogammaglobulinaemia or severe airways obstruction), frequency of infection does seem to be related to deterioration in FEV$_1$ [5, 11, 15, 17] in the mild to moderate COPD patients, although it has been demonstrated to be responsible for progressive steps of deterioration in the severe phases of the disease, those characterised by FEV$_1$ <35% pred. [18].

PRIMARY CILIARY ABNORMALITIES

Respiratory mucus accumulation and resultant airway obstruction are clearly exemplified in cases of primary ciliary dyskinesia, for example, in syndromes such as Kartagener's (bronchiectases, sinusitis and *situs viscerum inversus*) and Young's (obstructive azoospermia with normal spermatogenesis, sinusitis and alteration of pancreatic secretions). These are two of a group of autosomal recessively inherited disorders characterised by a primary defect in mucociliary transport. In the former, many ciliary structural defects have been identified; in Young's syndrome the reason for the mucociliary impairment is believed to be abnormal mucus. Mucus accumulation is the consequence, and airways obstruction leads to recurrent pulmonary infections.

BRONCHIECTASIS

This is defined as 'a permanent, irreversible, more or less circumscribed dilatation of the bronchial lumen'. Permanent dilatation of the bronchial tree can also occur in chronic bronchitis; however, this is of a lesser degree and is more diffused. These two diseases are almost always associated. Pure bronchiectases are rather rare and represent a simple anatomical alteration. Due to the presence of chronic inflammation, they become a precisely defined clinical reality that sometimes has been defined as 'bronchiectatic chronic bronchitis'. Persistent dry cough, at times accompanied by modest episodes of hemoptysis, is the only symptom of non-infective bronchiectases. However, there is almost always an abundant emission of more or less purulent sputum, which becomes mucopurulent (never serous) during phases of remission.

BRONCHIAL ASTHMA

In bronchial asthma, besides other reasons of bronchoconstriction such as airways hyper-reactivity, bronchospasm, inflammation and oedema of the mucosa, respiratory mucus also demonstrates peculiar glycoprotein patterns and glycolipid predominance, with resultant alteration in physical properties and quali-quantitative changes in rheological properties which contribute to the flow limitation along the airways. The pH within the respiratory mucus tends to be lower than normal, affecting mast cell degranulation. Evidence suggests that mucociliary clearance impairment is mirrored by a deteriorating clinical state, with mucus clogging in association with bronchospasm and an easier than normal tendency to overinfections.

CYSTIC FIBROSIS

Hypersecretion, abnormal mucus (with peculiar epithelial glycoprotein and glycolipid content), reduced mucociliary clearance, and increased elastase activity are associated with chronic respiratory tract colonisation and infection, especially with *Staphylococcus aureus* and *Pseudomonas aeruginosa*. Eventually, bronchiectasis results. The primary cause still remains unknown, although abnormalities of epithelial permeability and associated bio-electrical alterations are common features of the disease.

MUCOACTIVE NATURAL PRINCIPLES IN THE HISTORY

INTRODUCTION

The history of mucoactive therapy is more relevant than the history of most drugs for several reasons:
(a) Many therapeutic principles in current use have been employed for thousands of years.
(b) The popularity of some agents, in numerous unrelated cultures, suggests that they may offer benefits that cannot readily be detected by methods of evaluation of simple and diffuse utilization. A number of traditional drugs have provided the source for developing new agents that have been successfully introduced into current respiratory therapy.
(c) The traditional confusion between expectorants, antitussives, demulcents, pectorals and other agents that affect the respiratory tract points to the need to make a finer distinction in the assessment of the effects of mucokinetic agents.

(d) The recognition that many traditional agents have a multiplicity of therapeutic applications is reciprocated in contemporary discoveries that current agents, such as N-acetyl-L-cysteine (NAC), also have multiple effects (at higher than normal doses showing potent antioxidant and antidotal properties in addition to their basic mucokinetic actions).

(e) The lessons of history are applicable to today's examination of drugs, and the same wide-ranging scope of enquiry needs to be directed at some mucoactive agents that find a place in the pharmacopoeias of today.

MEDITERRANEAN AND WESTERN DRUGS

Most of the drugs currently available throughout the world for the treatment of pulmonary disorders characterised by abnormal mucus are derivatives of ancient medications, many of which are known to have been in use for over 5,000 years. In every geographic area, people have experimented with plants, minerals and animal products, and have gradually come to find certain derivatives to be helpful and safe in treating disorders such as bronchitis, asthma and milder respiratory infections. The number of natural drugs that have been accepted by differents societies is immense, and the supposed indications for specific agents can differ enormously. It would seem that those respiratory drugs that are discovered independently by different people might offer true benefits, but unfortunately this is not necessarily so. Western drug therapy had its origins in Mediterranean and surrounding civilizations. Oriental medicine arose independently in China and India, and many remedies remain indigenous to these countries. Thus, the historical origin of agents can best be analysed by examining these two broad cultural groups separately.

Mesopotamian drugs

Sumerians, Akkadians, Babylonians and Assyrians left evidence of a systematised knowledge of drug therapy [19–21]. For example, the Assyrians used over 500 drugs; one chest remedy included Ammi, the plant group from which cromones were subsequently derived. Many of the Mesopotamian cultures, for example, used mandrake, a plant with anticholinergic properties that continued to be invested with magical powers for thousands of years. Other Assyrian remedies for treating lung diseases remain in use even today [22]. The Akkadians used spices and resins, and appeared to favour sulphur, and extracts of balsamic plants [20]. The favoured drugs of the Mesopotamian cultures had a profound influence on the neighbouring Egyptians and Greeks.

Egyptian drugs

The ancient Egyptians used drugs in ceremonial and decorative fashion as well as for therapy. They developed the use of cosmetics, fragrances, perfumes and incenses, further extended by the Egyptians' sophisticated commitment to preserving dead bodies through embalming.

The word perfume is derived from the Latin *per fumum* (through smoke), and indicated that perfumes and incenses had similar constituents [23].

Other antibacterial agents used in Egypt included onion and garlic, as well as a resin mixture found in the mummy of Meneptah, son of Ramses II, that had a pleasant odour 'like Friar's balsam' [20]. All of these agents were incorporated in oral medications, in chest plasters or in fumigations/incenses for inhalation, each form of administration being recognised as useful in the treatment of respiratory disorders. As an example, the famous Ebers' *Papyrus* dating from 1600 B.C. recommended the following formula for bronchial diseases: figs, grapes, sycamore fruit, frankincense, cumin, juniper, wine, goose grease and sweet beer [22].

'Biblical' drugs

Cautious use of medications was recommended and relatively few drugs were described in the Bible; most of these came from Egyptian sources [22, 24, 25]. But overall, it is reasonable to conclude that the Bible, with its limited drug repertoire, provided a pharmacopoeia that appeals mainly to the respiratory specialist.

Greek and Roman drugs

The excesses of the Mesopotamian and Egyptian cultures and the cautious use of medications in the Biblical era provided a historical basis for the philosophical Greeks to select a balanced approach to pharmacology and therapy. Moreover, the Greeks developed a framework of scientific reasoning to try to formalise rational explanations for the physiological and pharmacological interactions in the body. Names of famous doctors and medical school leaders begin to be linked to new medical theories and discoveries, namely Empedocles (504–433 B.C.), Hippocrates (about 460–370 B.C.) and Aristotle's pupil Theophrastus (327–287 B.C.). The majority of their respiratory drugs were similar to those of the Egyptians [26]. Some treatments were more invasive (intratracheal instillations) and inhalations with balsam or fumigation with vapours of hyssop (which was primarily used as an emetic) were often suggested [27]. Thus, cinnamon, radish, garlic, honey, and flax were good for coughs, particularly 'old' ones, while 'comfrey doth rid up noisome stuff from ye lungs', mandrake 'doth expel upward phlegm', and lesser celandine 'purge all things out of the thorax'. Even more abstruse is the suggestion that leek is suitable 'for all griefs in the thorax', while pepper is advised for 'all ye passions about the thorax'. Many agents were used for coughs nonspecifically, such as honey and pine extract (used equally uncritically today!). Almond oil, rhubarb, scilla and many other agents were recommended for asthma. Of particular interest is the advice to treat lung diseases by inhaling the smoke from burning sweetflag, terebintha (turpentine) or coltsfoot, which would 'break impostumes (abscesses) in the thorax' [28].

Some centuries later Dioscorides, a Greek doctor who was particularly famous in his adoptive land, Rome, produced a brilliant textbook in Latin, *De Materia Medica* (78 A.D.). Another famed (Roman) authority who wrote extensively in the first century A.D. was Celsus. The works of Dioscorides and Celsus were reflected in the writings of Galen in the 2nd century A.D. These authorities were destined to influence therapeutics for the next 1,500 years, and many of their remedies are still popular today. Thus, Celsus' favourite agents such as thymol, storax, turpentine, hyssop and elecampane persist as expectorants in current pharmacopoeias [22].

The only Europeans who developed a more extensive herbal knowledge than the Greeks and Romans were the Anglo-Saxon herbalists. These healers, or leeches, became familiar with at least 500 medical plants, and the 'Leech Book of Bald' that appeared in the first half of the 10th century showed a wider range of therapeutic knowledge than any other contemporaries, including physicians of the Salerno School. The Salerno School was emerging in Italy at that time and its doctors were inclined to dedicate their interests more to the effects of the inhalatory administration of smoke or vapours obtained from plants and mineral products than to the natural principles contained in them. This form of inhalational therapy was then popularised in Europe by them [29]. Thus, Bernard the Provincial gave antimony vapours for cough and galbanum for suffocation, while Archimathoeus advised arsenical fumigations for chronic bronchial catarrh [21]. Many of the traditional folk medications that are currently used in Britain date back to the leeches of a millennium ago [30].

Arabic drugs

The waning of the Greek and Roman cultures left an intellectual void into which the emergent Moorish culture eventually exploded with a vigorous new dedication to science. Although many Arabic writers and their students in conquered lands made contributions to medicine, much of their pharmacology was directly based on the work of Dioscorides. Thus, the

pharmaceutical manuscripts of Abulcasis in the 10th century [31] and the books on pharmacy and *materia medica* of Al-Biruni in the 11th century [32] were filed with quotations from
Dioscorides and Galen. These writers extolled spices and advised using incenses, inhalations, poultices, syrups and oral preparations of numerous drugs for respiratory disease. The
great Persian clinician of the 10th century, Avicenna, in his influential Canon of Medicine,
added little more, although he nevertheless described about 758 compounds [22, 33], with an
emphasis on holistic therapy rather than drugs. The Arabs did introduce several new drugs,
including camphor, and developed syrups for treating respiratory afflictions [34].

The most important book on respiratory therapeutics during the Moorish era was that of
Maimonides, whose famous 'Treatise on Asthma' appeared in the 12th century [35, 36].
Among the foods, spices and herbal drugs, an extract of tea (today's theophylline) was
recommended to be used in asthma. Of major importance was Maimonides' exhortation
that chicken soup (flavoured with spices such as ginger, cloves, coriander and spikenard) be
employed for aiding in the coughing up of phlegm. Very curiously, in the late 1970s, a paper
on improvement of pathologic mucociliary clearance in humans, thanks to the ingestion of
chicken soup, was published after 'peer review' by the group of Marvin A. Sackner [37],
American Thoracic Society President at the time, and got an enormous number (thousands!)
of requests for reprints, resulting in one of the biggest successes of scientific respiratory literature ever (Sackner, personal communication).

Evolution of modern drugs in Europe and the New World

Following the conquest of the Moors, in the 15th century, centres of medical progress developed in Italy, England, France, Germany, Holland and other countries in Europe. The discovery of the New World resulted in the introduction of new drugs. Although the Spanish
colonists destroyed all writings of the Native Americans, about 1,200 Mexican plants, representing the enormous herbal knowledge of the native cultures, gradually became known
to European physicians and herbalists [34]. The 'Aztec Herbal of Mexico' was published in
Europe in 1552, and by 1649 in 'History of the Plants of new Spain'', about 3,000 plants were
described [38]. The Mexican drugs that were used for respiratory diseases included some
well-known agents as well as many obscure ones. In 1447, the first European pharmacopoeia
was published in Germany, but the initial influential account of therapeutics was
the London Pharmacopoeia of 1616 [22]. Its extension, Salmon's brilliant 'New London
Dispensatory of 1678, continued to describe similar drugs including ancient medicines such
as oxymel and hyssop, which he agreed were good for expelling phlegm [39]. His lack of
discrimination demonstrated that there had been little true progress since the time of
Dioscorides. In 1654, Nicholas Culpepper died at the age of 49 after publishing one of the
most influential herbals, which is still readily available to the public today [40].

ORIENTAL DRUGS

Extensive lists of drugs have been assembled over the years by many Oriental cultures. The
most impressive is the wide-ranging and thoughtful assemblage of agents that has grown
consistently in China over the course of the last 5,000 years. Although most of the agents are
quite unfamiliar to contemporary Westerners, a surprising number are similar to those used
in Europe several hundred years ago. However, analysis of the early histories of the two
cultures suggests that most basic discoveries were made independently, although cross-
fertilization has occurred, especially during the past nineteenth century. Liquorice, for
example, is a drug that has been used by Oriental and Western cultures independently, and
its reputation as an expectorant persists. It is important to recognise that many of our current respiratory drugs were direct descendants of old, established Oriental agents, and there
could possibly be further developments of new drugs from Chinese, Indian or other Asiatic

folk medicines [41]. Since the Asiatic cultures have given close attention to diseases accompanied by abnormal phlegm, it is reasonable to expect that traditional Oriental pharmacopoeias may be worth examining for suitable new mucokinetic agents [42].

Chinese drugs

The Chinese have had a continuing interest in herbal medications for thousands of years [43, 44]. A favoured ancient remedy for respiratory disorders was *ma huang*, which is the source of ephedrine. This is obtained from the bush *Ephedra sinensis*.

The initial Chinese Book of Herbs (*Pen Ts'ao*) was attributed to the legendary Red Emperor, Shen Nung, who lived around 3500 B.C. [43]. The book listed 365 drugs. The Great Pharmacopoeia' of Li Shih-chen, the *Pen-ts'ao Kang-mu*, published in 1596 A.D. and available in greatly modified form in English [45], forms the backbone of contemporary practice in Chinese herbalism, although there are currently around 5,000 plants recognised in China as medicinal ones, with 1,000 being in common use [46]. Complex theoretical bases underlie combinations of dozens of drugs in a typical formula. This explains some of the difficulties that investigators presently encounter in trying to evaluate the effects of traditional Chinese pulmonary formulations for treating abnormal mucus.

Indian drugs

Drugs in Indian traditional practice have arisen from more extraneous sources than those in Chinese traditional medicine. The earliest evidence of systematised Indian medicine reveals that it relied much less on magic than did contemporaneous Egyptian and other Middle Eastern systems. *Ayurveda*, the 'science of life', became a separate practice of medicine with little reliance on magic. Many Ayurvedic drugs are relatively obscure, and translation of their names from the Sanskrit, Hindi or other languages of India is difficult [47]. Moreover, the Indians incorporated Chinese drugs into their therapies, and in the 13th century Persian influences brought in the Greek-Roman system that had been modified by the Arabs [48]. Subsequently, the European colonisers of the 16th century introduced their medical practice into India, thus extending the complex Indian pharmacopoeia much further.

Other Asiatic drugs

The medicinal plants of Pakistan, Sri Lanka, Indonesia, Malaysia and Philippines include many unique agents that are alleged to have expectorant properties [49], drugs that are not used in China or India. However, since most agents are used for many diseases, and their pulmonary indication is often vague, it is unlikely that any major mucokinetic drug will readily emerge from this vast potential source. Most of the common expectorants of the West are prescribed in Asia, but many of the scores of Indian expectorant drugs are not used elsewhere [50]. It is possible that a few drugs from India and surrounding countries may eventually yield new agents that will be introduced into Western mucoactive therapy.

AGENTS THAT ACT ON BRONCHIAL MUCUS AND MUCOSA

CLASSIFICATION BY FUNCTION

A first approach to the problem of bringing order to the different agents on a functional basis (Table 16.1) is to start with a group termed *primary agents*: those drugs with direct effects on the production of secretions or on changes in their composition, resulting in improved movement of mucus through the respiratory tree or increased effectiveness of mucociliary clearance. The other group, *secondary agents*, do not have a specific action on mucus, but produce a general benefit on airway structure and function, secondary to correction of the pathophysiological mechanisms that result in abnormal secretion. However, since many

Table 16.1 Classification of mucoactive drugs showing primary and secondary agents acting on bronchial secretions (modified from 51)

Primary agents		
Agents affecting mucus production	Hydrating agents	Water Salt solutions
	Mucoregulators	Carbocysteine Bromhexine Sobrerol
	Bronchorrheics	Balsams Pinenes Terpenes
	Broncho-mucotropics Expectorants	Iodides Guaifphenesin Ipecacuanha Sodium, potassium and ammonium salts
Agents affecting mucus structure	Diluents	Water Salt solutions
	Mucospissics	Tetracyclines and other antibiotics Glucocorticosteroids Anticholinergic agents
	Mucolytics	Cysteine and derivatives Acetylcysteine (NAC) Erdosteine α-Mercaptopropionylglycine 2-Mercaptoethanesulfonate Enzymes Urea Ascorbic acid Hypertonic salt solutions Sulphurous spring water
Agents affecting mucociliary clearance	Ciliary excitants	Cholinergic agents Adrenergic agents Others
	Detergents or surfactants or wetting agents	Ambroxol Tyloxapol Sodium bicarbonate Ethyl alcohol
Secondary agents		
Bronchodilators		Sympathomimetics Methylxanthines and antiphosphodiesterases Anticholinergics Antileukotrienes
Anti-inflammatory		Corticosteroids Decongestants
Anti-infective agents		Antibiotics Antiviral agents
Antiallergic drugs		Antihistamines Cromones Mast cell stabilisers
Respiratory or cough stimulants		Hypertonic aerosols Airway irritants Analeptics

agents have overlapping effects, it is simpler to classify specific drugs according to their major actions, and to describe the importance of their secondary effects [51].

Another approach to classify drugs that act on bronchial secretions arises from the same observation as above, that there is first a dichotomy between drugs with *direct action* and drugs with *indirect action* on mucus. In this case, the term direct action often indicates an effect resulting in the rupture of the molecular bonds of mucoprotein. Thus, this class can be defined as the class of agents that break the polymeric structure of mucus, so that they always act specifically on mucus rather than causing a general improvement of airway conditions. Table 16.2 lists the different types of action of this heterogeneous group of substances on different parameters such as mucin biochemistry, mucus secretion, adhesiveness of the gel layer, modification of the sol layer and gastric vagal reflex. It is readily appreciated that traditional agents, such as water, hypotonic salt solutions, iodide, balsams and guaiphenesin, can have more than one mechanism of action. They should therefore be placed in several classes, according to their apparent main action. This observation could be extended to newer agents, whose overall effect on the bronchial mucus system is achieved through complex alterations, resulting in volume changes and mucus clearance. These multiple differing variables are closely interlinked. In this classification, we have not included the huge number of different proprietary or traditional combinations of mucoactive drugs that are compounded with each other or with other drugs, including historical substances whose use can no longer be scientifically justified [51].

Among the large number of substances reported to have mucoactive effects, some are not used in clinical practice, but are only intended for studies *in vitro*.

GLOSSARY OF TERMS USED IN BRONCHIAL MUCOLOGY

The above classifications are based on 'terminology' accumulated over recent years to explain with a single word the action of a drug on mucus according to its function. Different investigators and clinicians tend to give individual meanings according to their personal experience and interpretation. So, over the years, the birth of new therapeutic agents has resulted in new terms being coined to try to explain their activity. Year after year, the terminology has continued to evolve considerably, reflecting the different backgrounds and points of view of the experts. Since many of them seek to explain the same property with only minor differences, confusion can arise. The specific terms are defined in the glossary section of Table 16.3, which provides an explanation of the most frequent terminology regarding drugs that act on mucus [51].

DRUGS BREAKING MUCUS POLYMERIC STRUCTURE

MUCOLYTIC MOLECULES PROVIDED WITH SULPHYDRYL GROUPS (THIOLS)

Cysteine and its derivatives

Cysteine is an amino acid (not an essential one); it is a derivative of alanine, synthesised from methionine and serine through a trans-sulphuration process. Most of the sulphur in our diet is obtained from ingesting proteins that contain cysteine or methionine. Cysteine is found as a constituent of animal proteins, including glutathione, and is a major component in tissue such as those of hoofs, hair and skin. Industrially, it can be manufactured by hydrolysing the proteins from sources such as the feathers, hair or skins of various animals.

In 1963, Sheffner [52] published his extraordinary finding on the mucolytic properties of L-cysteine and its derivatives. He did not explain the rationale for examining cysteine, but recorded the fact that during a search for a therapeutic mucolytic agent, the properties of cysteine were carefully evaluated. It was apparent that the sulphydryl or thiol group (-SH) of cysteine was essential for conferring mucolytic properties, and that most congeners with

Table 16.2 Classification of mucoactive drugs according to direct or indirect effects on bronchial secretions (modified from 51)

Direct action	Drugs breaking mucus polymers	Thiols	Cysteine Methylcysteine Ethylcysteine Acetylcysteine (NAC) Erdosteine a-mercaptopropionylglycine (thiopronine) 2-mercaptoethane sulfonate (mesna)
		Enzymes	Trypsin, α-chymotrypsin, streptodornase, streptokinase, serratiopeptidase, sfericase, onoprose, DNA-ase
		Other agents	Urea Ascorbic acid Hypertonic salt solutions Inorganic iodides Sulphurous spring water[2]
Indirect action	Drugs modifying mucin biochemistry and mucus secretion		S-carboxymethylcysteine Letosteine Stepronine[1], thiopronine Sobrerol Iodoethylene glycerol (domiodol) Iodopropylidene glycerol
	Drugs modifying adhesivity of gel layer		Bromhexine Ambroxol Tyloxapol[2] Propylene glycol[2] Sodium ethasulphate[2] Sodium bicarbonate[2]
	Drugs modifying sol layer and hydratation		Water[2] Sodium salts[2] Potassium salts[2]
	Volatile inhalants and balsams		Pinenes Terpenes Methenes Phenol derivatives
	Drugs stimulating gastropulmonary reflex		Ammonium chloride Sodium citrate Guaiphenesin Ipecacuanha
	Drugs modifying bronchial gland activity		Adrenergic agents Cholinergic agents Corticosteroids Antihistamines Antileukotrienes
	Muco spissic drugs		Antibiotics Diuretics Others

Not all drugs reported are in clinical use
[1]Stepronine is a prodrug for thiopronine
[2]Topically administered

Table 16.3 Glossary of terms used in mucology, referred for: (A) drug activity and (B) mucus characteristics (modified from 51)

Term	Definition
(A) Bronchomucotropic	Acts directly on bronchial glands to augment their output of mucoid secretion
Bronchorrheic	Acts by non-specific irritation or hyperosmolality to increase the transepithelial secretion of water
Ciliary excitant	Increases rate and/or effectiveness of ciliary beating
Detergent	Reduces adhesiveness of secretions to mucosal surface by surface-active effect
Diluent	Dilutes the respiratory secretions by simple addition of water
Expectorant	Acts reflexively on bronchial glands to increase their output of mucoid secretion
Fluidifier	Term used to describe drug causing increased mucus mobility through several mechanisms
Hydrating agent	Causes water to be incorporated into the structure of respiratory secretions
Liquifier	Same as mucolytic
Mucoactive	Term to indicate all drugs having a beneficial effect on respiratory secretions without specific regard to the mechanism of action
Mucolytic	Breaks up glycoproteins, other protein, DNA and macromolecules into smaller components
Mucokinetic	Term used to describe all drugs that improve mobilisation and clearance of abnormal respiratory secretions
Mucomodifying	Same as mucoactive
Mucoregulator	Causes the synthesis of normal biochemical components of mucus
Mucosecretolytic	Same as fluidifier
Mucospissic	Causes thickening of abnormally hypoviscous mucus
Secretolytic	Same as fluidifier
Surfactant agent	Stimulates type II alveolar cell secretion of surface active phospholipids
Tensioactive	Reduces the surface tension of a liquid
Wetting agent	Same as detergent
(B) Adhesiveness	The phenomenon of holding materials together by surface attachment (interfacial forces)
Consistency	Resistance offered by a material to deformation
Elasticity	Property of a material to deform reversibly and to recover original asset and shape immediately upon release of the stress
Pourability	Capacity of a fluid to adhere to the walls of a container and flow under gravity
Spinability	Ability of bronchial mucus to be drawn into threads when stretched
Stickiness	Same as adhesiveness
Tixotropy	Reversible decrease of apparent viscosity with time when a constant shear rate is applied
Viscosity	Property of a material to flow, with the rate of flow being function of the stress
Yield stress	Minimal shear stress necessary to apply to a substance for it to flow

a similar effect on mucus possess a mercapto grouping (-CH$_2$SH). Thiol agents that are sensitive to autoxidation, such as cysteine, have considerable mucolytic action, whereas very stable compounds have little activity. Sheffner found that, during the breakdown of mucoprotein, the disulphide bridges interconnecting the protein molecules are ruptured by an interchange reaction with the free sulphydrilic grouping of cysteine.

Many chemicals with a free sulfhydryl group (cysteine derivatives, NAC and dithiothritol) reduced the viscosity of sputum *in vitro* and are also used regularly in laboratories for such a property. It is noteworthy that reduced glutathione, which is synthesised in the body from cysteine, is an effective mucolytic [52, 53]. It was also recognised that one of the most suitable congeners of L-cysteine for therapeutic use was NAC, since it has less taste and odour, and is much less toxic than L-cysteine. It is also more stable and forms highly soluble disulphide oxidation products.

Acetylcysteine (N-acetyl-L-cysteine: NAC)

The excellent *mucolytic activity* of NAC has been well known since the 1960s, such effects having been demonstrated both *in vitro* and *in vivo*. The NAC molecule includes a thiolic group, i.e. a free -SH group, capable of substituting and opening the -S-S- link between two cysteine groups belonging to the complex mucin molecule. This medicament induces a decrease in the number of intra- and intermolecular links, causing a rupture of the mucus polymeric structure (i.e. a depolymerisation), an event that reduces mucus viscosity and facilitates its expulsion. Its excellent oral and injective tolerability (at doses much higher than usual) permits the long-term use of the drug in these modes of administration. The only problem could lie in the episodes of bronchospasm which have been described, but only in cases of aerosol administration.

In recent years, NAC has been used all over the world in several experimental and clinical research studies, most of which have focussed on its *antioxidant activity*, which has become progressively more evident from the 1980s, giving an already out-of-patent drug a 'second youth' and renewed interest from various fields of clinical research such as pneumology, cardiology, nephrology, infectious diseases, radiology etc. The antioxidant action has a dual mechanism: (a) NAC acts as a direct donor of hydrogen radicals (due to the free -SH group) with consequent reduction of all extracellular reactive oxygen species (ROS), (b) NAC undergoes intracellular deacetylation with production of L-cysteine, an indispensable amino acid for the synthesis of glutathione and the consequent increase of the reserve of such a molecule in cells and plasma, where it exerts the most powerful antioxidant action. Since the clinical needs of mucolytic activity have been previously discussed, it is perhaps useful to present here some data on the conditions where the antioxidant properties of NAC are of importance.

In *chronic bronchitis*, the high number of publications has permitted three independent meta-analyses, all performed between 2000 and 2001 [54–56], demonstrating the efficacy of NAC in preventing winter exacerbations, with the further consideration that, due to the low cost of the drug, this expenditure is largely offset by reduced hospital fees. A recent Dutch study [57] has shown a dose-dependent reduction of hospitalisation risk following long-lasting therapy with NAC, probably due to a double protective effect; mucolytic as well as antioxidant. The dose-dependency of the antioxidant action in COPD has already been observed in a double-blind Italian study [58], the results being more evident with an oral daily dose (1,200 mg) which is double the most commonly used oral daily doses proven to be mucolytic (600 mg).

An interesting original observation has resulted from a very recent European polycentric study (acronym: Ifigenia) on *idiopathic cystic fibrosis* where one-year administration of a still higher daily dose (1,800 mg) in addition to the usual therapy (corticosteroid + azathioprine) reduces the decline in vital capacity (VC) by 9% and in diffusion capacity by 24%, NAC thus being one of the few drugs able to slow the evolution of the disease. This effect, of course, is not attributable to its mucolytic properties but more to its antioxidant ones [59].

Finally a polycentric double-blind Italian study (acronym: Nacis) has shown a significant reduction in the frequency and severity of *influenza* symptoms in non-vaccinated elderly persons and patients suffering from chronic diseases, effects which have been attributed to the NAC acting to reduce the high production of free radicals in these diseases [60].

The fact that the oral daily 'antioxidant' dose results from two or three times 'mucolytic' dose (1,200–1,800 vs 600 mg), is confirmed by the return to normal of the erythrocyte morphology, which is profoundly altered in COPD patients, together with a significant decrease of H_2O_2 and increase in total thiols in these cells, effects that are obtained by the long-term administration of such high NAC doses [61, 62].

Finally, other effects of high or very high doses of NAC have been documented that are independent of its mucolytic activity, having been attributed to its action against ROS: these include protection from nephrotoxicity due to contrast means, reduction of vascular risk in dialysed patients, dimensional reduction of the damage following myocardial infarction, mortality reduction in AIDS, protection from the effects of intoxication by paracetamol and poisoning due to the mushroom *Amanita phalloides*, protection against atomic radiation, severe renal failure developing in transplanted liver patients, rejection and veno-occlusive liver disease in patients submitted to bone marrow transplant and from haemorrhagic cystitis induced by cyclophosphamide [63].

In the most severe of the above-mentioned cases, the oral or infused daily dosages can be as much as 6–10 g up on the 40 g/day administered by enema to cystic fibrosis patients undergoing terminal ileum subocclusion [64].

Erdosteine (N-carboxymethylthioacetyl-omocysteine thiolactone)

Erdosteine is one of the most recently proposed mucoactive drugs [65] and is already available in several countries. It contains two sulphur atoms; one in an aliphatic chain, the other in a heterocyclic ring. It is a prodrug; after ingestion it is metabolised, producing an active metabolite (Met I) which has an unblocked -SH group; this metabolite (but not the prodrug) can thus be classified under the group of mucolytic thiols. The drug has proven to be well-tolerated and efficacious in the treatment of patients suffering from airway diseases characterised by tracheobronchial mucus hypersecretion with rheological changes due to alterations in mucus visco-elasticity. In addition, the Met I of erdosteine, in concentrations compatible with its therapeutic use, shows inhibitory activity on bacterial (Gram+ as well as Gram−) adhesion in humans [66]. It also has antioxidant activity, thus acting as a scavenger of oxidant radicals [67]. The administration of erdosteine increases glutathione intracellular levels. Recently, its capacity to control neutrophil elastase has also been demonstrated (Braga, personal communication).

Mesna (sodium 2-mercaptoethane sulphonate)

Together with NAC, this is one of the most widely clinically employed and studied products both in children and adults needing mucolytic activity. This thiolic agent has a clear-cut mucolytic activity leading to a reduced mucus viscosity.

Sulphurous spring water

Aerosols of sulphydritic molecules characteristic of the hot spring waters of several spas, mainly in continental Europe and Japan, are a 'classic' remedy used for centuries by millions of patients suffering from bronchial or nasal secretory chronic disturbances of an inflammatory nature. The mechanism of action is similar to that of thiolic agents. The high degree of safety of such aerosols is also due to the fact that they are administered under medical conditions in adequately equipped resorts.

ENZYMES

Proteases

Mucoprotein and deoxyribonucleic acid are the major components of mucus contributing to its viscosity. A reduction in size of these complex molecules to smaller components results in a marked decrease in viscosity. Various enzymes can be included among the agents known to cause rupture of the molecules. A number of proteolytic enzymes produced by animal organs such as the pancreas, or by bacteria, are considered to have therapeutic properties. Relatively few from plant sources have proved to be useful; among these are papain, bromelain and ficin. Their mucolytic effects have been extensively studied, and enzymes grew in popularity as topical therapeutic agents during the 1950s and 1960s. Subsequently, more effective and less expensive agents with lower toxicity, such as NAC, have almost completely replaced enzymes as mucokinetic agents.

Enzymes are organic catalysts, which usually exist as water-soluble colloids; they are readily affected by temperature, pH of the medium and various heavy metal ions. All enzymes are proteins, and they depend for their action upon the presence of non-protein co-enzymes, some of which are vitamins.

In different countries, a certain number of molecules with enzymatic properties have been used therapeutically in humans, or submitted to clinical trials: these include proteases such as trypsin (also under nebulised form), chymotrypsin, streptokinase, streptodornase, serratiopeptidase, sphericase, onoprose and, more recently, DNA-ase (deoxyribonuclease).

For several reasons, this group of agents appears to be of secondary importance when compared with more widely employed drugs such as NAC, mainly as a result of a relative lack of potency and/or safety, difficult handling and high costs.

DNA-ase (deoxyribonuclease)

In more recent years, great hopes have been placed on this enzyme, for a number of reasons: it was the first mucoactive agent obtained by genetic engineering, the first studied and produced in the USA by American scientists and the first with a specific substrate of nuclear that has been origin, a characteristic that has been investigated in depth. However, high resources and huge multicentric studies were eventually followed by the withdrawal of the product from the market due to its disproportionately high cost, and perhaps to its poor ease of handling and relatively high toxicity.

HYPERTONIC SOLUTIONS, UREA, AND ASCORBIC ACID

Hypertonic salt solutions

Physiological response to hypertonic solutions

Body fluids normally have an osmotic pressure corresponding to that of a 0.9% solution of sodium chloride. Thus, 'normal' saline solution will exist in equilibrium with blood and with moist mucous membranes, without any net interchange of fluid occurring between them. Fluid solutions that demonstrate this property could be called normal, iso-osmotic or iso-tonic. In the case of solutions of sodium chloride, or saline, 0.9% is considered isotonic. When a hypertonic solution is brought into contact with a mucosal surface, water will be withdrawn from the tissue until the osmotic pressure of the solution becomes isotonic; the additional volume of fluid may cause blockage of small airways. In contrast, a hypotonic solution will have its water content absorbed into the tissues until it achieves isotonicity [68]. When hypertonic solutions of sodium chloride are instilled or nebulised into the respiratory tree, the initial response will be the transference of water from the tissues across the epithelial membrane to dilute the saline [69]. Once this becomes hypotonic, the diluted saline, whose volume will be increased, is either removed by the mucociliary escalator or by coughing. The ability of hypertonic saline solution to withdraw fluid from the respiratory tract epithelium has been recognised for many years. This action is a bronchorrheic effect, and it has led to the use of aerosol administration of light hyperosmolar solutions for the induction of expectoration in patients who have no spontaneous sputum production. Such bronchorrheic stimuli have proven to be invaluable in securing cytological or microbiological specimens.

Urea

In 1966, Waldron-Edward and Skoryna reported that several amides, of which urea (carbamide) was the most suitable, had mucolytic properties. The action of 'mucolytic amides' on mucoproteins appears to be a non-specific denaturing one, resulting in large molecules being disrupted to form smaller and less viscous components [70]. In further studies, however, urea proved not to be of value in treating respiratory tract mucus. No controlled clinical trials on urea or other amides have been reported since 1971 [71] and clinical interest in them has subsequently faded.

Ascorbic acid

There is some evidence that ascorbic acid has mild antihistaminic properties, and that it may have slight bronchodilator qualities [72–75]. However, the effects are insufficient to be of clinical relevance, and thus the drug cannot compete with established antihistamines and bronchodilators. In the early 1960s, Palmer [76] reported that uncontrolled studies suggested that aerosolisation of ascorbic acid in combination with sodium percarbonate and copper sulphate had a mucolytic action in bronchitic patients. This was attributed to depolymerisation of mucoprotein macromolecules by the organic reducing agent (ascorbic acid) undergoing active oxidation. In spite of these promising results, no further interest has been shown in the potential mucokinetic value of ascorbic acid alone or in Asc-Oxreaction mixture [77]. Current thinking is that the hypertonicity of the mixture may have a non-specific effect that cannot be ascribed to the chemical reaction. Any further clinical studies on ascorbic acid would have to carefully control the tonicity of the solution, and since outcomes of such studies with hypertonic salt solutions often lead to equivocal results, it is unlikely that ascorbic acid alone or in chemical mixtures will prove to have any clinical value.

DRUGS MODIFYING MUCIN BIOCHEMISTRY AND MUCUS SECRETION

CARBOCYSTEINE (CARBOXYMETHYLCYSTEINE) AND CARBOCYSTEINE-LYSINE (CARBOXYMETHYLCYSTEINE LYSINE SALT)

Mechanism of action

This substance is proposed for the treatment of acute and chronic infections of the upper airways in cases of obstruction with stagnation of secretions resulting from alterations of their physico-chemical properties. Oral administration of carbocysteine induces an increase in the production of sialomucins and a reduction in the fucomucins: sialomucins ratio.

Carbocysteine was prepared in the 1930s during research into the protective nature of glutathione and cysteine as poison antidotes. Interest in its mucolytic activity began in the 1960s and it is now widely used in the treatment of respiratory disorders [78]. Havez *et al* [79] showed that cysteine has two different groups of derivatives: the first is characterised by a free thiol group; the second by a blocked thiol group. Carbocysteine is undoubtedly the most representative molecule of cysteine derivatives with a blocked thiol group. It does not act as a reducing agent on bronchial mucus, but induces biochemical mucus modifications. Like other mucomodifying drugs, carbocysteine is capable of affecting various parameters such as mucus production and composition as well as specific histological aspects of the tracheobronchial mucosa. Louisot and Meister [80] showed that carbocysteine is able to activate microsomic pulmonary sialyltransferase. The result of such an induction of sialyltransferase activity is the incorporation of neuraminic acid on desalinised glycopeptides of bronchial origin. This type of action explains the increase in sialomucins in the tracheobronchial secretions induced by the drug. In 1974, the protective role of carbocysteine on mucociliary clearance was studied by us in sheep [81]. After 5 days of exposure to ozone, placebo-treated animals showed a marked reduction of their mucociliary transport speed (-33%), while in the carbocysteine group this decrease was significantly less pronounced (−9%). Three days after the last exposure, mucociliary transport speed reached the baseline value in the carbocysteine group, whereas no improvement was observed in the placebo group (−31%). These data confirm once more the protective role of carbocysteine against respiratory tract damage induced by air pollution. These experimental observations have been confirmed in humans, since the drug induces improved mucociliary transport [82].

Clinical Pharmacology
Different studies show an increase in secretory IgA production after carbocysteine administration. Havez and Degand [79, 83] showed modifications of mucus glycoproteins after carbocysteine. In patients with chronic bronchitis, fucomucins are higher than sialomucins and sulphomucins: this fact negatively influences the rheological properties of secretions. In humans, after a 10-day treatment with relatively high doses of carbocysteine, sialomucins increase while fucomucin significantly decrease.

In vivo clinical studies
The results mentioned above are compatible not only with the mode of action of carbocysteine but in general with the existence of different subpopulations of chronic bronchitics, in relation to mucus characteristics. In spite of this, carbocysteine seems to improve the clinical condition of such patients. According to Puchelle *et al* [84], it is possible to claim that carbocysteine not only has mucolytic properties but also mucoregulating ones. Carbocysteine has been, furthermore, successfully studied in some ENT pathological conditions, namely secretory otitis media, other acute or chronic otitis, glue ear and chronic sinusitis.

Safety
Gastric problems, which have occasionally been linked with the long-term use of high doses of carbocysteine, have been prevented by the more recent lysinated preparation of carbocysteine, which provides gastric protection.

LETOSTEINE (CARBOXYTHIAZOLIDINILETHYL-2-MERCAPTOETHYLACETIC ACID)

This substance is proposed, from the clinical point of view, for its effect on mucoactivity of the mucoregulatory type and also (with a somehow inappropriate extension) for the treatment of acute and chronic infections of the upper airways in cases of obstruction due to stagnation of secretions resulting from alterations in their physico-chemical properties. Letosteine does not interfere with the mechanisms of expectoration, whose regular function is essential and has to be preserved after fluidification of the bronchial secretions.

In humans, experiments on the drug's properties have clarified its modality of action: it tends to interfere with the different pathogenic mechanisms responsible for the modification of the 'secretory function' at the level of the bronchial mucosa.

The molecule is a cyclic derivative of cysteine with a blocked thiolic group. As in other molecules characterised by such blocked groups, it favours the synthesis of mucins with polyanionic character, rich in N-acetylneuraminic acid, a phenomenon attributed to sialyltransferase activation. This enzyme, by regulating the attack of the glycidic side chains to the central proteic axis of the mucus fibres, contributes to the synthesis of sialomucins, thus restoring a correct balance between the various glycoproteic fractions so as to produce mucus with viscoelasticity characteristics typical of the normal range [85, 86], particularly with regard to 'viscosity' [87]. The increase in sialomucin level induced by the drug contributes to the inactivation of mucosal inflammatory mediators such as kinins [87]. The increase of IgA induced by letosteine has been attributed to this antikinin action of sialomucins, with a beneficial effect on the deficiency in secretory IgA (IgAs) that partially reflects the dysfunctional status of the bronchial mucosa [87, 88].

Stepronine (2-α-thenoilthiopropionylglycine lysine salt)

Stepronine exerts its mucoactivity through two mechanisms: (i) inducing changes in the rheological characteristics of already-produced secretion and (ii) reducing the production of new secretions [89]. Stepronine interacts by means of its sulfhydryl group (-SH), which appears after metabolisation, with the sulphydrilic bridges of the mucoproteins, producing an exchange that causes S-S bonds to break [90]. In addition, it promotes the synthesis of sialomucins by activating sialyltransferase, thus modifying the structure and hydration of the mucus [91]. This reducing action is, therefore, carried out directly in the secretions, thus modifying the rheological characteristics of the bronchial mucus. Due to the aforementioned action, and since in the original structure the -SH group is not free ('covered'), the drug is listed in this list of mucoregulators and not in that of thiols (that are characterised by free -SH groups). Therefore, stepronine carries out a fluidifying action that improves pathological mucociliary clearance and encourages the removal of mucus hypersecretions from the airways. Besides the modification of the physical characteristics of the bronchial mucus, stepronine lysinate also acts favourably on mucociliary clearance in its complex, integrating its mucolytic action with the activation of ciliary movements. Moreover, by virtue of the bond between the -SH group and thenoyl group, stepronine does not damage gastric mucosal secretion with its mucolytic action while transiting through the stomach [92]. In particular, in a double-blind crossover trial in patients affected by chronic rhino-bronchial obstruction, stepronine administered *via* aerosol and compared with placebo was proven effective. The results showed significantly improved nasal resistance to air flow during treatment with stepronine together with a significant increase in the functional test results.

A number of clinical studies carried out using stepronine have pointed out the safety of the molecule; in particular, its safety profile (especially its good gastric safety) was studied in an open nationwide Italian trial [93].This may be attributed to the structural characteristic of the bond between the -SH group and the thenoyl group, which protects the gastric mucosa from being attacked [89].

Thiopronine (α-mercapto-propionyl-glycine)

This sulphuric compound has also been used in the past for its mucolytic properties. Its high efficacy has been demonstrated *ex vivo* on rheological mucus properties, and *in vivo* on the consequent increase in tracheal mucus velocity.

Sobrerol [1-methyl-4(2-hydroxy-isopropyl]-cyclohexyl-1,2-en-6)]

Physical properties of mucus

Using a forced oscillation technique, a dynamic test to measure viscoelasticity, a statistically significant reduction in both viscosity and elasticity was observed (unpublished observations). The effect of sobrerol was also evaluated on another rheological parameter frequently altered in chronic bronchitis: spinnability, i.e. the capacity of mucus to form threads. A significant improvement in this parameter (increased value) was observed after 7 days of treatment with sobrerol.

Mucus production

Treatment with sobrerol has been shown to increase the volume of expectoration for 2–3 days. Following this initial peak, the volume of expectoration tends to decrease constantly.

Mucociliary clearance

An example of the modification of mucociliary clearance by sobrerol is offered by the experimental model of asthmatic attacks after *Ascaris suum* sensitisation in sheep: a challenge with such an allergen induces the impairment of mucociliary function. A 5-day pre-treatment with sobrerol was able to selectively prevent this reduction without affecting other aspects of the response to the challenge (i.e. bronchoconstrictive responses) [94].

Tracheal mucus velocity

This is one of the most probative tests to study the activity of mucomodifying drugs on mucociliary clearance. In chronic bronchitics, sobrerol increases tracheal mucus velocity (TMV) measured with 99 mTc albumin microspheres in a crossover design [95] or with Teflon particles in a design *versus* placebo [96]. Another indirect method for measuring this effect consists of placing the secretions of chronic bronchitis patients before and after sobrerol treatment on a preparation of frog's palate. A marked increase of clearance induced by sobrerol was also shown with this technique [97].

Cough

Sobrerol is able to improve cough during airway infections [98, 99]. During sobrerol treatment, the production of bronchial mucus with improved rheological characteristics makes cough more productive, gradually removing the stimuli for coughing. Auscultatory patterns appear to be improved in these patients and a similar trend was observed for dyspnoea.

In chronic bronchitis

Some airway obstruction may be caused by excessive production of viscous and inelastic mucus. Improving mucus characteristics may, therefore, determine abnormalities of respiratory function. Several studies addressed this point and interesting results were obtained for some respiratory indices [96, 100, 101]. The variability of patients, in terms of disease severity, often seems to obscure these trends. Using a more suitable technique (marked particle distribution), it has been shown that sobrerol favours the clearance of some airways (especially the most disadvantaged) and that the distribution of particles in the dependent zones is increased.

The effects of a long-term treatment (3 months) with sobrerol have been studied *versus* placebo [102]: over 600 patients were recruited and the drug's effects on winter exacerbations of chronic bronchitis were monitored. A constant improvement of expiratory indices such as FEV_1 and residual volume (RV) was reported during the 3 months of therapy with sobrerol. In addition, sobrerol reduced the number of exacerbations evaluated both historically (previous year) and during treatment, where the percentage of patients with exacerbations and number of episodes during the 3 months were significantly lower in the sobrerol group in comparison with the placebo group.

Safety

Sobrerol has been shown to be particularly safe and without important side-effects. In fact, in all of the studies carried out, including controlled trials, no side-effects requiring a specific pharmacological intervention were seen; in a few cases only, administration was interrupted. Sobrerol has been marketed since 1970, in Japan, Switzerland and Italy (where, together with NAC, it has been a category leader for decades). During these years of wide clinical use, no severe side-effect associated with drug administration was seen, further supporting the safety of the drug.

IODIDES

Iodides are a favourite ingredient of anticough mixtures and have been used to treat asthma for more than 100 years [103]. However, some patients receiving inorganic iodine preparations experienced an offensive taste, gastric irritation and other adverse reactions. Organic iodides were therefore synthesised and introduced into clinical practice. These are more stable in storage and their taste and tolerability are much better.

Inorganic iodides

There has been a long and consistent belief that iodide is beneficial in lung diseases, although clinical proof has been relatively unsatisfactory. Nevertheless, many current textbooks continue to recommend the utilizsation of iodides if abnormal sputum is a problem. In contrast, numerous authorities advise that iodides should not be used because their indisputable toxicity outweighs their disputable effectiveness. This is true for inorganic iodide preparations such as iodine, calcium iodide, hydriodic acid and iodoniacin, but not for organic ones.

Organic iodides

Domiodol (4-hydroxymethyl-2-iodomethyl-1,3-dioxolane)

Several mechanisms of action have been postulated as contributing to the activity of iodides on the respiratory mucosa [69, 104]: stimulation of bronchial glands to secrete a low-viscosity, watery mucus; stimulation of the gastro-pulmonary vagal reflex (particularly by the inorganic preparations); direct mucolytic effect ('lyotropic' effect), or modification by the iodides on partially organised, inspissated mucus lying within the chronically infected respiratory tract.

Domiodol proved to be active in patients with various bronchopulmonary diseases. It rapidly improved objective signs and symptoms: the daily quantity of sputum, sputum viscosity, expectoration difficulty and dyspnoea. Domiodol is a well-tolerated drug. Three clinical trials were specifically designed to evaluate the safety of domiodol, with particular reference to thyroid function and gastric tolerability. This iodide did not affect gland function and had no unfavourable effects on the mucus protecting the gastric mucosa.

Iodopropylidene glycerol (IPG)

The most interesting mucokinetic iodide product is this iodinated glycerol, which has been used since 1915.

Two studies have been carried out on IPG by the manufacturer. One, by Repsher et al. [105] compared IPG against placebo in chronic asthmatic patients, concluding that cough symptoms, bronchospasm and ability to expectorate were significantly improved by IPG. The second study was an evaluation, by Pavia et al. [106], of the changes in mucociliary clearance as demonstrated by a standard tracer radio-aerosol technique in chronic bronchitis. The patients as a group showed no significant improvement in mucus clearance, but a subgroup, characterised by the production of more copious sputum, did show a significant beneficial effect. This limited study suggests that, although some patients may show enhanced benefit after using iodopropylidene, current information does not allow the extrapolation of these findings to all patients with impaired mucokinesis.

Claims were made that the glycerol component could aid muscle relaxation; a similar claim has been made for glyceryl guaiacolate (guaiphenesin). It was also claimed that the drug was suitable for topical administration, since the glycerol helps to produce a stable aerosol [107].

DRUGS MODYFYING THE ADHESIVENESS OF THE GEL LAYER

BROMHEXINE (3,5-DIBROMO-2-AMINOBENZYLAMINE)

The pharmaceutical literature [108] reports the expectorant, antitussive, and, in some cases, bronchodilating properties of vasicine, an alkaloid obtained from *Adhatoda vasica Nees*.

Using this element as a starting point, over several years, a great number of vasicine derivatives have been synthesised by opening the quinazoline ring in the vasicine molecule to produce 2-amino-benzylamine derivatives. Compounds of the 3,5-dibromo-2-aminobenzylamine series (VI) were thus prepared in Germany, giving an effective preparation that reduces the viscosity of tenacious mucus, increases expectoration and has the secondary effect of facilitating respiration and alleviating cough.

Mucolytic Properties
Bromhexine plays a pharmacodynamic role in mucus production at the intracellular level. In various studies, quantitative as well as qualitative changes were noticed [109] in the secretory granules of the secreting epithelial cells. Such studies confirm the postulated site of each stage of synthesis and secretion in the preparation of epithelial mucin for secretion. Here, a low-molecular-weight secretion is produced, as a result of a different synthesis rate and enzymatic effects.

Response of the alveolar-capillary barrier
In addition to its specific effect on secretion, bromhexine apparently improves the permeability of the alveolar-capillary barrier, thus increasing the concentration of antibiotics in sputum.

Effects on the surfactant
Results are available to suggest that the action of bromhexine is not simply confined to the constituents of bronchial secretion. Morphometric studies of the changes occurring in the ultrastructure of type II alveolar cells in the lung of rats after bromhexine administration revealed a significant increase of such cells over controls. Moreover, within these cells, the lamellar bodies augmented significantly. Under administration of bromhexine, the naturally structurally unstable lamellar bodies in the lungs of animals were decidedly more stable than in control animals, which may indicate a change in the composition of the lamellae, perhaps in their phospholipidic part, leading to an increase in stability [109]. Bromhexine (more specifically its 8th metabolite, which will be reviewed later under the name of ambroxol) modifies the metabolism of type II alveolar cells [110]. The increased production can result in a higher secretion of phospholipids in alveolar spaces (particularly β-γ-dipalmitoyl-L-α-2-phophatidylcholine, the lecithin contained in surfactant that has maximum tensio-activity, i.e. capacity to lower surface tension in the alveolus to values close to zero dynes/cm), thus raising the quantity of surfactant available to spread over the interface. Tensio-active substances also have important anti-adhesive properties, modifying the adhesiveness of the gel layer of the mucus; in the case of bromhexine, other (mucoregulatory) mechanisms are also described.

Bromhexine has been used in the treatment of pathological conditions such as bronchitis, bronchiectasis, and asthma. Favourable effects were reported when giving bromhexine in bronchitis, particularly in less severe cases. Several double-blind studies [111, 112] demonstrated significant improvements in lung function tests (VC, FEV_1 and peak expiratory flow, PEF) in the bromhexine group *versus* placebo. Bromhexine was found to have an important effect on sputum viscosity and expectoration. These effects were demonstrated by many authors [113–115]. Also, in the presence of bronchiectasis, positive effects of bromhexine were seen in expectoration, amount, tenacity and colour of sputum, as well as the ease of breathing. Many investigators [116–118] reported a general decrease in sputum quantity and viscosity with auscultatory findings showing improvement when using bromhexine in the treatment of patients affected by bronchiectases. Acute bronchial asthma was considered to be a contraindication for bromhexine [119], and placebo-controlled studies failed to provide convincing evidence of the value of bromhexine in asthmatic patients. However, the intravenous administration of bromhexine was found to be beneficial in less severe asthmatic attacks [120]. Improvements were observed in sputum viscosity, facility of expectoration, cough, and dyspnoea. This agent is able to bring about an initial increase in sinus secretion with concurrent pronounced reduction in viscosity. There was a significant decrease in sinus pain while the patients' condition improved more rapidly than with antihistaminic drugs. In sinusitis as a result of infection, the efficacy of an antibiotic treatment was markedly improved by concurrent bromhexine administration [121].

Safety
Bromhexine has been widely used in all western European Countries, where, over many years, no severe side-effects have been recorded. No contraindications are known in pregnancy.

Ambroxol [trans-4-(2-amino-3,5-dibromobenzylamino)
cyclohexanol hydrochloride]
The benzylamine agent, ambroxol, is a derivative of vasicine, the active ingredient of the medical herb *Adhatoda vasica*, which has been used for centuries in India to manage respiratory tract disorders. As previously mentioned, it is the 8th metabolite of bromhexine. Originally developed as a mucolytic agent, ambroxol [trans-4-(2-amino-3,5-dibromonezy-lamino) cyclohexanol hydrochloride] was soon found to have effects on the secretory apparatus of the bronchial epithelium and pulmonary alveoli, which give the compound a unique pharmacological profile. *In vivo* and *ex vivo* experiments performed in humans [122, 123], moreover, demonstrate that ambroxol is able to act on altered mucus rheological properties, normalising the viscosity and reducing the adhesiveness of bronchial secretions to the bronchial wall. Such activity, however, does not originate from a direct action on the already secreted mucus [124], but from the 'regulating' and 'balancing' capacity of bronchial secretions at the glandular level.

Disse and Ziegler [125] showed that ambroxol is also able to stimulate the cilia of ciliated cells. Such stimulation was seen to be weaker than that of a β-adrenergic drug, such as salbutamol, used as a reference standard. An increased availability of surface-active phospholipid material may have reduced the viscosity and spinnability of mucus, as we will see later on [126]. A reduced viscosity may act synergistically with an increased ciliary activity [127] and thus result in a beneficial effect of ambroxol on the mucociliary transport velocity [127–129].

Mechanism of action of ambroxol
This is better explained by taking its activity on the surfactant system into consideration, this having been the topic of many research studies both from the morphological and biochemical viewpoints.

A significantly increased dimension of the lamellar bodies and pneumocytes in the treated group over controls was reported. The fact that ambroxol is able to selectively stimulate the development of the small organs linked with surfactant synthesis by phospholipid incorporation was investigated and confirmed by the autoradiographic model [130–132]. Furthermore, ambroxol not only accelerates the synthesis but also the secretion of surfactant from type II pneumocytes. The data that ambroxol inhibits phospholipase A from lung lysosomes and alveolar macrophages [133] suggest an alternative mechanism of action of the drug: the blocking of phospholipidic catabolism. Since the function of surfactant is to diminish the surface tension of the pulmonary parenchyma with a subsequent greater compliance of the organ, an improvement of respiratory function can be expected after ambroxol treatment.

Safety

Among the side-effects ascribed to ambroxol, nausea, vomiting and diarrhoea have been mentioned, which could have local or central origins. Complications have been described due to skin – and mucosal – hypersensitivity together with rashes, with or without itch and urticaria. The incidence of such complications is, however, very small.

MODIFICATIONS OF THE SOL LAYER AND HYDRATION OF MUCUS

Water

The sol layer that bathes the respiratory epithelium must demonstrate critical features for effective mucociliary clearance. It must be of appropriate depth (physiologically approx. $5\,\mu m$) and should just cover the extended cilia; the presence of this low viscosity fluid environment is essential if the cilia are to maintain their rapid, coordinated metachronal beat. A sol layer of inadequate depth results in slow ciliary beating or complete ciliostasis. In contrast, an inappropriately increased depth prevents the energy of the extended ciliary tips from engaging with the superficial gel layer (physiologically $\leq 5\,\mu m$), and the normal cephalad movement of this viscous layer is not promoted. Gross increases in the depth of the sol layer result in an encroachment on the lumen of the small airways, and this results in mucostasis; this in fact occurs with pulmonary oedema resulting from heart failure or from leaking of fluid across an impaired respiratory epithelium.

The sol layer must also maintain a suitable consistency. If it is hyperviscous, movement of the cilia is impeded. Its relationship with the gel layer should cause an abrupt change in viscosity at the boundary; if part of the gel layer becomes more similar to the sol layer, then clearance of the viscous component of the secretions up the mucociliary escalator is impaired. This undesired situation can paradoxically result from mucokinetic therapy if too much of a mucolytic agent is given and the gel layer is disrupted sufficiently to cause the airways to be 'drowned' in low-viscosity fluid. Surprisingly, in such cases, we can successfully refer to mucospissic agents (diuretics, corticosteroids and antibiotics when necessary). Conversely, in many cases of impaired mucokinesis, the problem appears to be related more to a deficiency in depth or increase in viscosity of the sol layer, and the objective of therapy is to restore this layer to its normal state. This can be accomplished by giving topical therapy that will act on both the sol and the gel layers, or by systemic therapy that causes the bronchial glands to secrete a low viscosity fluid that enters the sol layer. Such effects can be produced by drugs having direct or indirect actions on such bronchial gland secretion.

It is generally accepted that water is a valuable mucokinetic. However, it may surprise those who believe that water is the best expectorant or mucolytic to know that such claims are not based on clear evidence, but are generally the outcome of traditional clinical impressions. An overall problem is that clinical methods for studying mucokinesis remain relatively unsatisfactory, so the value of water in this specific sense is difficult to demonstrate quantitatively.

The average normal daily water requirement of an adult is approximately 2,500 ml. The equivalent losses include 1,500 ml in urine, 500 ml by insensible loss or by sweat through the skin and 100 ml in stool, the remaining 400 ml being lost through the respiratory tract.

A marked loss of free water is known as desiccation, whereas an accompanying loss of electrolytes results in dehydration, which usually produces more evidence of hypovolaemia such as tachycardia, hypotension and altered sensation.

In respiratory illnesses accompanied by desiccation and dehydration, there is a strong clinical impression that the mucus is adversely affected, resulting in decreased mucociliary clearance, hyperviscous secretions and possible inspissation or impaction of mucus in the distal airways. The results do not support the clinical practice of encouraging vigorous hydration for patients with chronic sputum production. This finding is in accordance with the opinion of Hirsch [134], who found only one report suggesting an objective decrease in sputum viscosity following systemic hydration. Wanner [135], in his extensive review, also concluded that there was no scientific basis to support the prescribing of increased hydration in the treatment of chronic syndromes associated with abnormal sputum.

In acute exacerbations of respiratory disease, as with any other disorder, it is appropriate to correct dessication or dehydration.

In vitro studies have shown that when 1 ml of water is added to 5 ml of sputum, it can reduce its viscosity by as much as 35%. Similarly, aerosolised water can be incorporated into sputum, leading to a gain in weight of up to 29% and a decrease in viscosity of up to 37%. These findings do not necessarily apply to the *in vivo* situation, since a very small proportion of an aerosol will be deposited in the lungs. Animal and human studies have shown that aerosolised water can be more effective than saline as a stimulant of sputum production and coughing since it can be more irritating to the mucosa. However, current textbooks on respiratory care demonstrate an awareness that simple aerosols of water and hypertonic saline solutions can no longer be recommended in mucokinetic therapy (except for the purpose of inducing the patient to cough), since they induce bronchoconstriction in broncho reactive patients.

Salts

Salts of sodium have played a major role in therapeutics throughout history. Most of the simple salts are electrolytes that continue to be used to provide specific ions for the maintenance of homeostasis or to correct deficits.

In therapeutics, sodium chloride is given mainly for intravascular rehydration and as a balanced, isotonic carrier fluid for introducing drugs into the venous system; under these circumstances, it is not thought to have any specific pharmacological effect.

Several sodium salts are used as electrolyte providers. There is a very slight chance of iodine hypersensitivity occurring with intravenous administration of sodium iodide, but when given as a slow infusion, the possibility of anaphylaxis is negligible. Hypertonic sodium bicarbonate, however, is considered to be one of the best mucokinetic agents for use by both aerosolisation and instillation. Sodium bicarbonate can be repeatedly nebulised or instilled into the airways, up to six times per day for several days. As is the case with saline, hypertonic concentrations can be irritating to the oropharyngeal mucosa and to the respiratory tree, and such solutions can induce coughing and bronchospasm. Potassium salts are not generally utilised as mucokinetic agents.

Numerous other salts have been used as expectorants, and many of the same salts are used as osmotic or irritant cathartics. They serve as non-specific gastric irritants, and can thereby stimulate expectoration through the gastro-pulmonary vagal reflex.

It is evident that the traditional belief in salts as respiratory drugs can be explained by a number of mucokinetic mechanisms. However, their comparative value cannot readily be established, and thus sodium chloride, sodium iodide and potassium iodide are likely to remain the favoured agents for loosening up abnormal mucus or for inducing expectoration.

VOLATILE INHALANTS AND BALSAMS

Many plants produce odorous volatile oils that are usually colourless when fresh, but slowly oxidise and resinify to coloured products on standing.

Guaiacol

Guaiacol is a volatile phenolic oil that can be derived from a number of sources, including beechwood, pine and guaiac wood. Guaiacol is usually obtained with creosote; each of these agents has been used for various purposes, including expectorant therapy, and each has been converted into a number of pharmaceutical products. Guaiacol has a burning taste and is irritating to the stomach, and it can readily induce nausea, vomiting and diarrhoea. The drug has been regarded as a general stimulant of secretions, and was thus believed to be an expectorant, but there is insufficient evidence for its effectiveness in humans. Among the numerous guaiacol products, its relatively soluble glyceryl ether has emerged as the most important, and it has gradually become the only valuable guaiacol, with generally accepted expectorant properties.

Guaiphenesin

Guaiphenesin was first synthesised in 1912 and was known as glycerol guaiacolate until the 1970s, when it was renamed. There is evidence that guaiphenesin does get into the sputum, but it is not clear whether it has any surface-active effects on the mucus within the airways. The drug may increase water content and its bonding in the gel, and lead to an increase in sputum nitrogen excretion, but this has not been substantiated. Other studies tend to suggest that guaiphenesin may improve symptoms in bronchitis and bronchiectases, but its effect on improving expectoration may be slight when conventional dosages are used. The overall conclusion is that adults who take large doses of guaiphenesin may experience subjective improvements in conditions characterised by abnormal sputum, but objective evidence of an effect cannot be clearly demonstrated.

Creosote

Currently, there is no enthusiasm for the use of creosote as an expectorant, and there are no studies to substantiate its effectiveness, although Boyd claims it may be effective in laboratory animals in toxic doses.

Terpenes

The volatile oils of odiferous plants are usually complex mixtures of chemicals, but many contain terpenes, made up of isoprene units. These units are linked together, forming complex molecules of two to six isoprene units.

Terebene has a rather agreeable, thyme-like odour and it has been used as an expectorant and for nasal congestion and cough as an inhalant (in hot water) or in pastilles. In these forms, it is probably little more than a harmless placebo.

Ipecacuanha

Few evaluations of the mucokinetic effectiveness of ipecacuanha have been carried out, and several older studies failed to show any benefit in chronic bronchitis.

CONCLUSION

Chronic bronchitis is characterised by mucociliary dysfunction resulting from structural defects of the cilia and alterations of the secretory apparatus (hypertrophy of submucosal glands, hyperplasia of goblet cells), accompanied by functional deficiencies of both components (ciliary dyskinesia and mucus chemical abnormalities inducing rheological deficiencies). The combination of ciliary impairment and rheologically impaired hypersecretion leads to a disruption of mucociliary interaction and hence the accumulation of secretions in the airways. Cigarette smoke appears to play a critical role in the pathogenesis of chronic bronchitis-associated mucociliary deficit. Whereas an excess of secretions as such may have minor effects on the natural course of airflow obstruction, this is not the case in the increased volume of secretions observed during acute exacerbations, where the disturbance could transiently (in less severe) or definitively (in most severe cases of chronic bronchitis) compromise airway function.

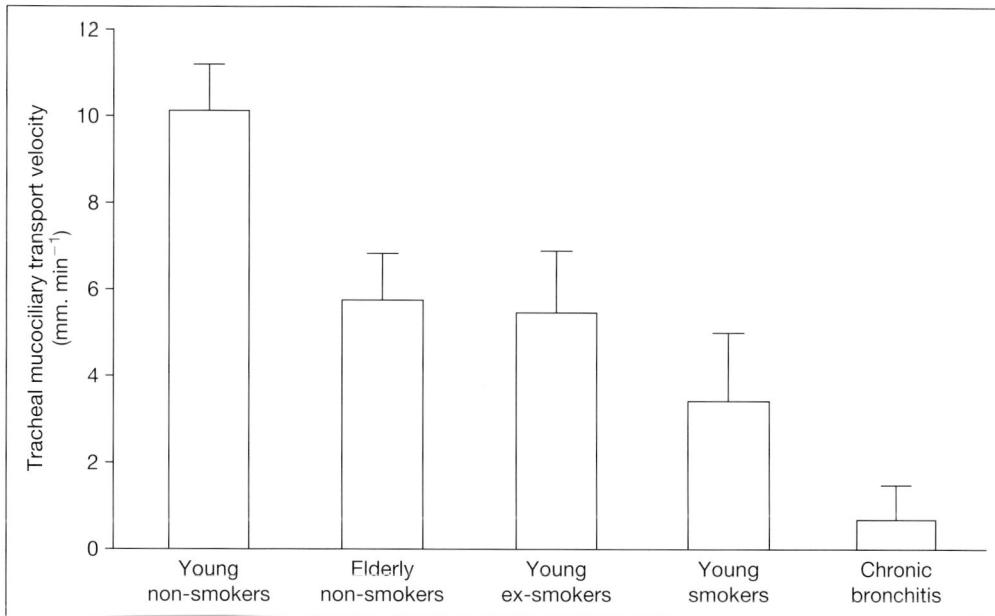

Figure 16.1 Mean (+ s.e.) tracheal mucociliary transport velocity in different classes of healthy subjects (n = 41) and in chronic bronchitics (n = 14). Note the independent effects of age, cigarette smoking and chronic bronchitis. Young non-smokers are the appropriate control of young ex-smokers and young smokers; elderly non-smokers are the appropriate control of chronic bronchitics [136].

Mucociliary clearance of inhaled aerosols and tracheal mucus velocity as assessed by surface markers are altered in patients with chronic bronchitis [136, 137]. Once a subject has developed chronic bronchitis, cessation of smoking does not reverse the slowing of mucociliary clearance: an analogous impairment of mucociliary transport has been reported in smokers and ex-smokers suffering from chronic bronchitis. Thus, chronic bronchitics and healthy smokers both exhibit impaired mucociliary function. However, the magnitude of impairment, although present in all of the above-mentioned conditions, is not the same [136, 138]: a greater deficiency of tracheal mucus transport has been observed in smokers and non-smokers with chronic bronchitis than in healthy smokers (Figure 16.1).

THE FUTURE

Although it is never possible to predict future developments in an area of active creative research, it is possible to establish certain reasonable expectations. In the field of bronchial mucology, it is likely that investigations currently in progress will yield important new insights into mucus structure and function, mucus composition, the regulation of mucus production and release and the role played by mucus in the biology of the airways. In addition, it is likely that the alterations that occur in mucus in disease will become better understood and defined. It is also likely that the ancient pharmacopoeia for modification of mucus will be placed on a firm scientific basis and be supplemented with newer agents. Finally, it seems likely that there will be an improved nosography and classification of the disorders characterised by quali/quantitative disturbances in the production of airway secretions [139].

Their properties include not only elasticity and viscosity, but also 'tackiness' (a measure of adhesiveness), 'spinnability' (a measure of the elongatability of the mucus thread), and the ability to contribute to the complex and composite function known as mucociliary clearance.

Nevertheless, the basic mucus structure consisting of a core protein with branched oligosaccharide side chains has been known for years. These side chains consist of sulphated and neutral sugars linked as O-glycosides to threonine and serine. The biochemical analysis of these molecules has been complicated by the high degree of substitution of the molecules with carbohydrates and of the largely degraded state of the peptide core obtained from the expectorated sputum. The availability of antibodies, together with molecular biological techniques, promises that the genes regulating the production of mucus core proteins will be identified.

It is becoming clear that respiratory tract mucus is a complex, heterogeneous material composed of glycoproteins, mucins, ions, water and lipids. Increasingly powerful biochemical techniques are permitting the characterisation of the individual sub-components of mucus.

Molecular biological techniques also offer unique opportunities for studying structure-function relationships. It is possible, for example, to introduce a specific type of mutation into an isolated gene. The effects of the mutation can then be studied by re-introducing the modified gene into an appropriate cell. Although the application of such techniques to a large, complex molecule such as a respiratory tract mucin is likely to be difficult, the general approach will probably become increasingly practicable. Years ago, bronchial epithelial cells and glandular epithelial cells were successfully cultured separately. These cells produce components of the respiratory tract mucus *in vitro* and are used as experimental systems in the following ways. Firstly, the availability of *in vitro* culture systems will greatly facilitate structural studies of respiratory tract mucins using molecular biological techniques so that, with such systems, it will be possible to characterise a variety of mucus components. Secondly, *in vitro* culture systems should permit detailed studies of the pathways of mucus biosynthesis from gene expansion to RNA translation and on to protein processing, so that it will be possible to determine the mechanisms that regulate the type and degree of carbohydrate substitution. Thirdly, it will be possible to determine if the various components present in mucus are regulated independently.

In a similar manner, both intact mucus and the components present within mucus can, for example, be analysed for their effects on inflammatory cells, airway progenitor cells, bacteria and inhaled substances including particles, gases, etc. It is likely that the many biologically active molecules present within mucus are involved in complex interactions with exogenous agents, inflammatory cells and the surrounding airway. The role mucus plays in such interactions will become increasingly defined in the near future.

There are a number of diseases characterised by the increased expectoration of (often abnormal) mucus. It is likely that both the physiological pathways leading to bronchial mucus production and expectoration and the biochemical basis for the abnormal quality of such material will become better defined.

Because of the high prevalence of respiratory tract disease, there are abundant 'traditional' as well as 'modern' agents thought to alter respiratory tract mucus [51]. However, it has been exceedingly difficult to document objective benefits in a large series of patients with several reasons to be hopeful that respiratory tract pharmacology will advance rapidly in the near future. Firstly, it is likely that the diseases characterised by altered respiratory tract mucus are heterogeneous. Thus, a given drug may only have a beneficial effect in some patients. A large series of patients, however, may include many individuals with different conditions that are unresponsive to the drug in question, and the beneficial effect may therefore be masked. The ability to subclassify airway diseases based on specific alterations in respiratory tract mucus should permit a more precise analysis of potential therapeutic agents. For example, it is readily conceivable that mucus characterised by either too little or too copious secretion of ions and water will have both abnormal physical properties and be characterised by cough and sputum production. An agent that stimulates the secretion of ions and water into respiratory tract mucus would be beneficial in one circumstance and harmful in another. Conversely, an agent with the opposite effects would also sometimes be beneficial and sometimes harmful, depending on the circumstances. It is likely that *in vitro* methods currently in development will permit both the production of such compounds and the rational selection for their use in specific, perhaps individualised, clinical conditions. Whereas a large number of diseases are characterised by alterations of respiratory tract mucus and consequent mucociliary disturbances, these conditions are considered together as relatively few syndromes. Specifically, it has been difficult to subclassify respiratory tract disorders based on either clinical parameters or macro-microscopic analysis of expectorated sputum [140]. It seems likely, however, that biochemical analysis of respiratory tract secretions should permit subclassification of respiratory disorders. Such subclassification would permit both a more accurate diagnosis and the development of more specific and targeted/tailored therapeutic interventions.

In addition, it should be possible to apply molecular biological techniques to the analysis of patients with respiratory tract disorders. It seems reasonable that the population will include individuals with different genetic variants of mucus components. cDNA probes, now available and becoming more widely used in various fields, will permit the description of variant forms of respiratory tract proteins. Moreover, it will be possible to determine whether or not variant forms are associated with specific disease states. So, such techniques will not only be able to define diseases, but potentially identify individuals who are at an increased risk of the development of specific airways disease following, for example, cigarette smoke inhalation, industrial exposure or urban pollution.

Finally, increasingly powerful biochemical and cellular techniques will permit increasingly precise clinical classification. Improved clinical classification should facilitate not only the development of specific therapeutic interventions, but also investigations into the aetiology of airway diseases [141].

REFERENCES

1. O'Sullivan DD, Bhaskar KR, O'Paskar-Hincman H, Reid LM. Proteo-glycans in airway secretions. *Eur J Respir Dis* 1987; 71(suppl 153):275–280.
2. Reid LM, O'Sullivan DD, Bhaskar KR. Pathophysiology of bronchial hyper-secretion. *Eur J Respir Dis* 1987; 71(suppl 153):19–25.
3. Sahu S, Lynn W. Hyaluronic acid in pulmonary secretions of patients with asthma. *Biochem J* 1978; 173:565–568.
4. Stockley RA. Proteolytic enzymes, their inhibitors and lung disease. *Clin Sci* 1983; 64:119–126.
5. Biajorklander J, Bake B, Hanson L. Primary hypo-gamma-globulinemia: impaired lung function and body growth with delayed diagnosis and inadequate treatment. *Eur J Respir Dis* 1984; 65:529–536.
6. Johnston RN, McNeill RS, Smith DH, Legge JS, Fletcher E. Chronic bronchitis: measurements and observations over 10 years. *Thorax* 1976: 31:25–29.
7. Widdicombe JG. The Sadoul Lecture: airway mucus. *Eur J Respir Dis* 1989; 2:107–115.
8. Niewoehner DE, Klienemann J, Rice DB. Pathological changes in the peripheral airways of young cigarette smokers. *New Engl J Med* 1974; 291:755–758.
9. Reid LM. Measurement of bronchial mucous gland layer. A diagnostic yardstick in chronic bronchitis. *Thorax* 1960; 15:132–141.
10. Higenbottam TW, Feyerabend C, Clark TJH. Cigarette smoking in asthma. *Br J Dis Chest* 1980; 74:279–284.
11. Pride NB. Epidemiology of bronchial hypersecretion, recent studies. *Eur J Respir Dis* 1987; 71(suppl 153):13–18.
12. Brumfitt W, Willoughby MLN, Bromley LL. An evaluation of sputum examination in chronic bronchitis. *Lancet* 1957; 2:1302–1309.
13. Lees AW, McNaught W. Bacteriology of lower-respiratory-tract secretions, sputum and upper-respiratory-tract secretions in 'normals' and chronic bronchitics. *Lancet* 1959; 2:1112–1114.
14. Kanner RE, Renzetti AD, Jr, Klauber MR, Smith CB, Golden CA. Variables associated with changes in spirometry in patients with obstructive lung disease. *Am J Med* 1979; 67:44–50.

15. Fletcher C, Peto R. The natural history of chronic airflow obstruction. *Br Med J* 1977; 1:1645–1648.
16. Johnston RN, McNeill RS, Smith DH, Dempster MB, Nair JR, Purvis MS, Watson JM, Ward FG. Five year winter chemo-prophylaxis for chronic bronchitis. *Br Med J* 1969; 4:265–269.
17. Wang EEL, Prober CG, Manson B, Corey M, Levison H. Association of respiratory viral infection with pulmonary deterioration in patients with cystic fibrosis. *New Engl J Med* 1984; 311:1653–1658.
18. Allegra L, Biasi F, de Bernardini B, Cosentini R, Tarsia P. Antibiotic treatment and baseline severity of disease in acute exacerbations of chronic bronchitis: a re-evaluation of previously published data of a placebo-controlled randomized study. *Pulm Pharmacol Ther* 2001; 14:149–55.
19. Castiglioni A. A History of Medicine. In: Krumbhaar EB (ed) Alfred A Knopf, New York, 1941.
20. Majno G. The Healing Hand. Man and Wound in the Ancient World. Harvard University Press, Cambridge, MA, 1975.
21. Cumston CG. An Introduction to the History of Medicine. Dorset Press, New York, 1987.
22. Mann RD. Modern Drug Use: An Enquiry on Historical Principles. MTP Press Ltd, Lancaster, UK, 1984.
23. Morris ET. Fragrance: the story of perfume from Cleopatra to Chanel. Charles Scribner's Sons, New York, 1984.
24. Moldenke HN, Moldenke AL. Plants of the Bible. Dover Publications Inc, New York, 1952.
25. Rosner F. Julius Preuss' Biblical and Talmudic Medicine. Sanhedrin Press, New York, 1978.
26. Adams F. The Genuine Works of Hippocrates, Vol I. William Wood & Company, New York, 1886.
27. Phillips ED. Aspects of Greek Medicine. St. Martin's Press, New York, 1973.
28. Gunther RT. The Greek Herbal of Dioscorides (illustrated and edited by a Byzantine). Hafner Publishing Co, New York, 1959.
29. Rohde ES. The Old English Herbals. Longman, Green & Co, London, 1922.
30. Dawson WR. A Leechbook or Collection of Medical Recipes of the Fifteenth Century. Macmillan & Co Ltd, London, 1934.
31. Hamarneh SK, Sonnedecker G. A Pharmaceutical view of Abucasis Al Zahrawi in Moorish Spain. EJ Brill, Leiden, Holland, 1963.
32. Hamarneh SK. Al Biruni's Book on Pharmacy and Materia Medica. Hamard National Foundation, Karachi, Pakistan, 1973.
33. Agarwal VS. Economic Plants of India. Kailash Prakashan, Calcutta, India, 1986.
34. Leake CD. An Historical Account of Pharmacology to the 20th Century. Charles C Thomas, Springfield, IL, 1975.
35. Cosman MP. A feast for Aesculapius: historical diets for asthma and sexual pleasure. *Annu Rev Nutr* 1983; 3:1–33.
36. Rosner F. Moses Maimonides' treatise on asthma. *Thorax* 1981; 36:245–251.
37. Saketkoo K, Januskiewicz A, Sackner MA: Effect of drinking hot water, cold water and chicken soup on nasal mucus velocity and nasal airflow resistance. *Chest* 1978; 74:408–410.
38. Guerra F. Aztec Medicine. *Med Hist* 1866; 10:315–338.
39. Salmon W. Pharmacopoeia Londinensis. Or, the New London Dispensatory. Thomas Dawks, London, 1678.
40. Culpepper N. Culpepper's Complete Herbal. W Foulsham, London, 1654.
41. Ziment I. Five thousand years of attacking athma: an overview. *Respir Care* 1986; 31:117–136.
42. Ziment I. The management of common respiratory diseases by traditional Chinese drugs. *Bull Orient Heal Arts Inst* 1988; 13:133–140.
43. Hsu HY, Peacher WG. Chen's history of Chinese medical science. *Bull Orient Heal Art Inst* 1980; 2:6.
44. Morse WR. Chinese Medicine. PB Hoeber, New York, 1938.
45. Li SC. Chinese Medicinal Herbs. In: Smith FP, Stuart GA (eds) Georgetown Press, San Francisco, 1973.
46. Xaio P. Recent developments on medical plants in China. *J Ethnopharmacol* 1983; 7:95–109.
47. Sharma PS. Ayurvedic medicine: past and present. *Prog Drug Res* 1979; 15:11–67.
48. Jaggi OP. All about Allopathy, Homeopathy, Ayurveda, Unani and Nature Cure. Orient Paperbacks, New Delhi, 1976.
49. Quisumbing E. Medicinal Plants of the Philippines. Manila Bureau of Printing, Manila, 1951.
50. Perry LM, Metzger J. Medicinal Plants of East and Southeast Asia: Attributed Properties and Uses. MIT Press, Cambridge, UK 1980.
51. Braga PC, Allegra L. Drugs in Bronchial Mucology. Raven Press, New York, 1989.
52. Sheffner AL. The reduction in vitro in viscosity of mucoprotein solutions by a new mucolytic agent, N-acetyl-L-cysteine. *Ann NY Acad Sci* 1963; 106:288–297.

53. Davis SS, Deverill LC. Rheological factors in mucociliary clearance. *Mod Probl Paediatr* 1976; 19:207–212.

54. Grandjean E, Berthet P, Ruffmann R *et al*. Efficacy of oral long term N-acetylcysteine in chronic bronchopulmonary disease: a meta-analysis of published double-blind placebo controlled trials. *Clin Ther* 2000; 22:209–221.

55. Poole P, Black P. Oral mucolytic drugs for exacerbation of chronic obstructive pulmonary disease: systematic review. *Br Med J* 2001; 322:1271–1274.

56. Stey C, Steurer J, Bachmann S *et al*. The effect of oral N-acetylcysteine in chronic bronchitis: a quantitative systematic review. *Eur Respir J* 2000; 16:253–262.

57. Gerrits C, Herings R, Leufkens H, Lammers J. N-acetylcysteine reduces the risk of re-hospitalisation in patients with COPD. *Eur Respir J* 2003; 21:795–798.

58. Allegra L, Blasi F, Capone P *et al*. Proprietà mucoattive ed antiossidanti della NAC ad alte dosi. *Giorn Ital Mal Tor* 2002; 56:193–202.

59. Behr J, Demedts M, Buhl R *et al*. IFIGENIA (Idiopathic Pulmonary Fibrosis International Group Exploring NAC I Annual): effects of N-acetylcysteine on lung function and gas exchange in IPF patients. *Eur Respir J* 2004; 24(suppl 48):668S (Abstract).

60. De Flora S, Grassi C, Carati L. Attenuation of influenza-like symptomatology and improvement of cell-mediated immunity with long term N-acetylcysteine treatment. *Eur Respir J* 1997; 10:1535–1541.

61. Santini M, Straface E, Ciprì A *et al*. Structural alteration of erythrocytes from patients with chronic obstructive pulmonary disease. *Haemostasis* 1997; 27:201–210.

62. Straface E, Matarrese P, Gambardella L *et al*. N-acetylcysteine counteracts erythrocyte alterations occurring in chronic obstructive pulmonary disease. *Biochem Biophys Res Comm* 2000; 279:552–556.

63. Rizzato G. Le Nuove Frontiere della Terapia con Antiossidanti. Effe Edizioni, Verona, Italy, 2001.

64. Hanly JG, Fitzgerald MX. Meconium ileus equivalent in older patients with cystic fibrosis. *Brit Med J.* 1983; 286:1411–1413.

65. Dechant KL, Noble S. Erdosteine. *Drugs* 1996; 52(6):875–881.

66. Braga PC, Del Sasso M, Sala MT, Giannelle V. Effects of erdosteine and its metabolites on bacterial adhesiveness. *Arzneim Forsch* 1999; 49:344–350.

67. Braga PC, del Sasso M, Zuccotti T. Assessment of the antioxidant activity on the SH metabolite I of erdosteine on human neutrophil oxidative burst. *Arzneim Forsch* 2000; 50:739.

68. Ziment I. Hydration, humidification and mucokinetic therapy. In: Weiss EB, Segal MS, Stein M (eds) Bronchial Asthma, Mechanism and Therapeutics, 2nd ed, chap 64. Little, Brown and Company, Boston, 1985.

69. Ziment I. Respiratory Pharmacology and Therapeutics. W.B. Saunders Co, Philadelphia, 1978.

70. Lieberman J. In vitro evaluation of the mucolytic action of urea. *JAMA* 1967; 202:694.

71. Yeager H. Tracheobronchial secretions. *Am J Med* 1971; 50:493–509.

72. Kordansky DW, Rosenthal RR, Norman PS. The effect of vitamin C on antigen-induced bronchospasm. *J Allergy Clin Immunol* 1979; 63:61–64.

73. Ogilvy CS, DuBois AB, Douglas JS. Effects of ascorbic acid and indomethacin on the airways of healthy male subjects with and without induced bronchocostriction. *J Allergy Clin Immunol* 1981; 67:363–369.

74. Richardson PS, Phipps RJ. The anatomy, physiology, pharmacology and pathology of tracheobronchial mucus secretion and the use of expectorant drugs in human disease. *Pharmacol Ther B* 1978; 3:441–479.

75. Zuskin E, Lewis AJ, Bouhuys A. Inhibition of histamine induced airway constriction by ascorbic acid. *J Allergy Clin Immunol* 1973; 51:218–226.

76. Palmer KNV. Sputum liquefiers. *Br J Dis Chest* 1966; 60:179–181.

77. Lieberman J. Measurement of sputum viscosity in a cone-plate viscometer. II. An evaluation of mucolytic agents in vitro. *Am Rev Respir Dis* 1968; 97:662–672.

78. Waring RI I, Mitchell SC, Shahh RR. The metabolism of S-carboxy-methyl-L-cysteine in man: isolation of an ester glucoronic acid conjugate from urine. *Xenobiotica* 1983; 13:311–317.

79. Havez R, Degand P, Roussel P, Randoux A. Mode d'action biochimique. *Poumon Coeur* 1970; 26:81–90.

80. Louisot P, Meister L. Information concerning the biochemical activity of SCMC. Report for the Italian Ministry of Health, 1970.

81. Rampoldi C, Caminiti G, Centanni C, Moavero NE, Abraham WM, Allegra L. I fenomeni ossidoriducenti e l'apparato respiratorio. *Giorn Ital Mal Tor* 1987; 41(suppl 6):385–408.

82. Allegra L, Della Torre F, Guadagni L, Guffanti E, Numeroso R. Caratteristiche funzionali respiratorie e reologia dell'escreato in bronchitici cronici trattati con S-carbossimetilcisteina per os. *Minerva Pneumol* 1979; 18(suppl 1):111–128.

83. Havez R, Degand P. Modifications biochimiques de l'expectoration sous traitment par la S-carboxy-methyl-cysteine. *Quad Ter Sper* 1972/73; 10:3–10.

84. Puchelle E, Aug F, Polu JM. Effect of the mucoregulator S-carboxy-methyl-cysteine in patients with chronic bronchitis. *Eur J Clin Pharmacol* 1978; 14:177–184.

85. Degand P. Etude biochimique du mode d'action de la S-carboxyméthylcystéine. *Bull Physiopathol Respir* 1973; 9:462–463.

86. Puchelle E, Zahm JM, Polu JM, Sadoul P. Drug effects on viscoelasticity of mucus. *Eur J Respir Dis* 1980; 10(suppl 61):195–207.

87. Clauzel M, Marty JP, Pélissier G. Notre experience du Viscotiol. Effects cliniques et biochimiques. *Lyon Medit Med* 1981; 17:1916–1919.

88. Girbino G, Bagnato C, Giacobbe G. La letosteina nella broncopatia cronica. *Arch Monaldi* 1983; 38:167–184.

89. Pannella G, Grimaldi U, Scaglione B, Zurlo M. Il 2-(alfa-tenoiltio)-propionil glicinato di lisina nella terapia delle broncopneumopatie ipercroniche. *Med Prax* 1982; 3:77–83.

90. Monteverde A, De Paoli F. Note terapeutiche sul 2-(alfa-tenoiltio)-propionil glicinato di lisina. *Med Prax* 1982; 3:85–90.

91. Olivieri D. Effetto della stepronina sale di lisina sulla clearance mucociliare. *Curr Ther Res* 1988.

92. Guslandi M, Barbieri P, Gaiani P, Nannini D. Noninvolvement of gastric mucus in the mucolytic effect of stronine lysine salt. *Int J Clin Pharmacol Res* 1988; 8:223–225.

93. Benvenuti C, Trezzi P. Valutazione clinica su 2569 pazienti della stepronina sale di lisina nella; patologia respiratoria con ipersecrezione mucosa. *Giorn Ital Ric Clin Ter* 1988; 9:53–60.

94. Allegra L, Abraham WM, Chapman GA, Wanner A. Disturbi del trasporto mucociliare nell'attacco d'asma e attività farmacologica di prevenzione. *Giorn Ital Mal Tor* 1982; 36:111–119.

95. Carratù L, Sofia M. Evaluation of mucociliary function using radioisotopes through a fibreoptic bronchoscope. *Int J Clin Pharmacol* 1986; 6:7–9.

96. Pozzi E, Luisetti M, Colombo ML, De Rose V, Nonis A. Sobrerol and chronic bronchitis: new elements suggesting unrecognized potential advantages. *Int J Clin Pharmacol Res* 1986; 6:11–17.

97. Allegra L, Bossi R, Braga PC. Action of sobrerol on mucociliary transport. *Respiration* 1981; 42:105–109.

98. Bisetti A, Fumagalli G, Mariani B. Studio policentrico sugli effetti del sobrerolo nel trattamento delle affezioni catarrali delle vie respiratorie. *Giorn Ital Mal Tor* 1982; 36(suppl 4):257–272.

99. Seidita F, Deiana M, Careddu P. Acute bronchial diseases in paediatrics. Therapeutic approach with sobrerol granules. *Giorn Ital Mal Tor* 1984; 38:191–194.

100. Balzano E, De Gaetani G. Il D-L-sobrerolo nel trattamento delle flogosi broncopolmonari acute e croniche. *Minerva Med* 1973; 64:1995–2003.

101. Gunella G, Del Bufalo C. Raffronto dell'azione mucolitica del sobrerolo e della N-acetilcisteina nele broncopneumopatie croniche. *Riv Pat Clin Tuberc Pneumol* 1982; 53:583–606.

102. Castiglioni CL, Gramolini C. Effect of long-term treatment with sobrerol on the exacerbations of chronic bronchitis. *Respiration* 1986; 50:202–217.

103. Reynolds JEF, Prasad AB. Martindale: The Extra Pharmacopeia. The Pharmaceutical Press, London, 1982.

104. Zanjanian MH. Expectorants and antitussive agents: are they helpful? *Ann Allergy* 1980; 44:290–295.

105. Repsher LH, Glassman JM, Soyka JP et al. Evaluation of iodopropylidene glycerol as adjunctive therapy in stable, chronic asthmatic patients on theophylline maitenance. *Today's Ther Trends* 1983; 1:77–89.

106. Pavia D, Agnew JE, Glassman JM et al. Effect of iodopropylidene glycerol on tracheobronchial clearance in stable, chronic bronchitic patients. *Eur J Respir Dis* 1985; 66:177–184.

107. Gordonoff T. Ueber den Standort der Expektoranten. *Ther Umsch* 1965; 22:309–316.

108. McIntosh D. A controlled evaluation of bromhexine and orciprenaline in the treatment of chronic bronchitis. *Br J Clin Pract* 1971; 25:547–554.

109. Gil J, Thurnheer U. Morphometric evaluation of ultrastructural changes in type II alveolar cells of rat lung produced by bromhexine. *Respiration* 1971; 28:438–456.

110. Renovanz HD, Merker HJ. Untersuchungen ueber die Lokalisation von 14C-Bromhexine in Respirationstrakt von Ratten. *Pneumologie* 1973; 148:125–133.

111. Christensen F, Kyer J, Ryskjaer S, Arseth-Hansen P. Bromhexine in chronic bronchitis. *Br Med J* 1970; 4:117–121.

112. Gent M, Knowlson PA, Prime SJ. Effect of bromhexine on ventilatory capacity in patients with a variety of chest diseases. *Lancet* 1969; 2:1094–1096.

113. Arold R, Schaetzle W. Histochemische Untersuchugen zur Sekretionsdynamik der Nasen- und Trachealschleimhaut von Meerschweinchen. *Arztnelm-Forsch* 1972; 26:121–129.
114. Clarke SW. Clinical trial of bromhexine in severe chronic bronchitics during winter. *Thorax* 1977; 27:429–432.
115. Hamilton WFD, Palmer KNW, Gent M. Expectorant action of bromhexine in chronic obstructive bronchitis. *Br Med J* 1970; 3:260–261.
116. Bamford TM. Effect of bisolvon. *Med J Aust* 1974; 61:943–946.
117. Mangold H. Clinical experimental experiences with a combination of berocillin and bromhexine in chronic bronchitis. *Therapiewoche* 1975; 25:1997–2002.
118. Vidal J, Decor Y. Interest of Bisolvon in pneumophthisiology. Gaz Hop (Paris).
119. Pecquer G. Action of Bisolvon during acute attacks of chronic bronchopathies. *J Med Nord Est* 1969; 6:57–58.
120. Sasaki H. Clinical experience with bromhexine injection against bronchial asthma attacks in children. *Pharmacol Ther B* 1979; 7:3159–3165.
121. Harris PG. A comparison of bisolvonmycin and oxytetracycline in the treatment of acute infective sinusitis. Scand Symp Bronchial Secretions, Stockholm, 1973 (Abstracts).
122. Morgenroth K, Schlake W. Unspezifische Begleitreaktion in der Bronchial Wand bei der Lungentuberkulose und ihre Behandlung mit Na872. Licht und Elektronen-Mikroskopische Untersuchungen an der Bronchial Wand bei Patienten mit Lungentuberkulose. *Wien Med Wochenschr* 1975; 125:34.
123. Allegra L, Bossi R, Braga PC. Rheology of bronchial fluids assessed by forced oscillations. In: Cosmi E, Scarpelli E (eds) Pulmonary Surfactant System Elsevier, Amsterdam, 1983, pp. 319–337.
124. Shimura S, Okubo T, Maeda S, Aoki T, Tomioka M. Effects of expectorants on relaxation behaviour of sputum viscoelasticity in vivo. *Biorheology*, 1983; 20:677–683.
125. Disse BG, Ziegler HW. Pharmacodynamic mechanism and therapeutic activity of ambroxol in animal experiments. *Respiration* 1987; 51(suppl 1):15–22.
126. Motta C, Touillon AM, Simon G, Dastugue B. Active lipid: a potential fluidifizer of cystic fibrosis mucus. In: Cystic Fibrosis: Horizons. Wiley, Chichester, 1984, p. 337.
127. Disse BG, Mason RJ, Voelker DR. Influence of ambroxol on surfactant lipids of rat alveolar type II cells in primary culture. *Eur J Respir Dis* 1987; 71(suppl 153):288–289.
128. Allegra L, Bossi R, Braga PC. Influence of surfactant on mucociliary transport. *Eur J Respir Dis* 1985; 67(suppl 142):71–76.
129. Bossi R, Braga PC, Allegra L. Ambroxol e trasporto mucociliare. *Monaldi Arch* 1984; 33:227–234.
130. Elmer G, Kapanci Y. Morphological approach to surfactant secretion in the lung with particular reference to ambroxol. *Prog Respir Res* 1981; 15:234–239.
131. Kapanci Y, Elmer G. Ambroxol and surfactant secretion. In: Cosmi E, Scarpelli E (eds) Pulmonary Surfactant System Elsevier, Amsterdam, 1983, pp. 263–272.
132. Stein O, Stein Y. Lipid synthesis, intracellular transport storage and secretion. Electron microscopic radioautographic study of liver after injection of tritiated palmitate or glycerol in fasted and ethanol-treated rats. *J Cell Biol* 1967; 33:319.
133. Heath MF, Jacobson W. The inhibition of lysosomal phospholipase A from rabbit lung by ambroxol and its consequences for pulmonary surfactant. *Lung* 1985; 163:337–344.
134. Hirsch SR. Mucociliary clearance: pathologic and clinical features. *Compr Ther* 1980; 6:56–61.
135. Wanner A. Clinical aspects of mucociliary transport. *Am Rev Respir Dis* 1977; 116:73–125.
136. Goodman RM, Yergin BM, Landa JF, Golinvaux MH, Sackner MA. Relationship of smoking history and pulmonary function tests to tracheal mucus velocity in nonsmokers, young smokers, ex smokers and patients with chronic bronchitis *Am Rev Respir Dis* 1978; 117:205–214.
137. Matthys H, Vastag E, Koehler K, Daikeler G, Fischer J. Mucociliary clearance in patients with chronic bronchitis and bronchial carcinoma. *Respiration* 1983; 44:329–337.
138. Santa Cruz R, Landa J, Hirsch J. Tracheal mucus velocity in normal man and patients with obstructive lung disease. *Am Rev Respir Dis* 1974; 109:458–463.
139. Allegra L, Braga PC. Bronchial Mucology and Related Diseases. Raven Press, New York, 1990.
140. Braga PC, Allegra L. Methods in Bronchial Mucology. Raven Press, New York, 1988.
141. Rennard SI, Robbins RA. Future directions in bronchial mucology. In: Allegra L, Braga PC (eds) Bronchial Mucology and Related Diseases Raven Press, New York, 1990.

Abbreviations

4-DAMP	4-diphenylacetoxy-N-methylpiperidine methobromide	eNANC	excitatory non-adrenergic non-cholinergic
AC	adenyl cyclase	EP	end point
Ach	acetylcholine	EPAC	exchanged protein activated by cAMP
AChE	acetylcholine esterase		
AKAP	AKinase anchor protein	EPP	equal pressure point
α AT	$\alpha1$ anti-trypsin	ERK	extracellular regulated kinases
AP-1	activator protein-1	ERS	European Respiratory Society
ATP	adenosine 5'-triphosphate	FEF_{50}	flow at 50% expired volume
ATS	American Thoracic Society	FEV_1	forced expiratory volume in one second
AUC	area under the curve		
BAL	bronchoalveolar lavage	FRC	functional residual capacity
β-ARs	β-adrenergic receptors	FVC	forced vital capacity
BTS	British Thoracic Society	G-CSF	granulocyte colony stimulating factor
cAMP	cyclic adenosine 3', 5'-monophosphate		
		GER	gastroesophageal reflux
CFC	chlorofluorocarbon	GM-CSF	granulocyte-macrophage colony stimulating factor
cGMP	cyclic guanosine monophosphate		
		GOLD	Global Initiative on Obstructive Lung Disease
ChAT	choline acetyl transferase		
CI	confidence interval	GRO-α	growth related oncogene α
CO	carbon monoxide	G_s	guanine nucleotide regulatory protein
COMT	catechol-O-methyltransferase		
COPD	chronic obstructive pulmonary disease	GSH	glutathione
		HARBS	high-affinity rolipram-binding site
CRDQ	Chronic Respiratory Disease Questionnaire		
		HDAC	histone deacetylase
CRQ	chronic respiratory quality of life questionnaire	HFA	hydrofluoroalkane
		HO-1	heme oxygenase-1
CTGF factor	connective tissue growth	HRQOL	health-related quality of life
		IC	inspiratory capacity
DLCO	lung diffusion capacity of carbon monoxide	IFN-γ	interferon-γ
		IL	interleukin
ECG	electrocardiogram	IP-10	interferon-γ-inducible protein
EELV	end expiratory lung volume	I-TAC	interferon-inducible T-cell α-chemoattractant
eGPx	extracellular glutathione peroxidase		
		LABA	long-acting $\beta2$-agonist
ENA	epithelial neutrophil activating protein	LARBS	low-affinity rolipram-binding site

LTB$_4$	leukotriene B$_4$	PEF	peak expiratory flow
mAChR	muscarinic acetylcholine receptors	PKA	protein kinase A
		PLCβ	phospholipase Cβ
MAO	monoamine oxidase	Ppl	pleural pressure
MAP	mitogen-activated protein	PTP	protein tyrosine phosphatase
MBP	major basic protein	RCT	randomised clinical trial
MCP1	macrophage chemotactic protein-1	ROS	reactive oxygen species
		RV	residual volume
MDI	metered dose inhaler	SGRQ	St George's Respiratory Questionnaire
Mig	monokine induced by interferon-γ		
		SLPI	secretory leukoprotease inhibitor
MIGET	multiple inert gas expiratory technique		
		SpO$_2$	pulse oximetry
MMP	matrix metalloproteinase	SVC	slow vital capacity
MPO	myeloperoxidase	TDI	Transition Dyspnoea Index
NE	neutrophil elastase	TGF	transforming growth factor
NAC	N-acetyl-L-cysteine	TGV	thoracic gas volume
NEP	negative expiratory pressure	TIMP	tissue inhibitors of MMPs
NF-κB	nuclear factor-kappa B	TLC	total lung capacity
NK	natural killer	TLC	total lung capacity
NO	nitric oxide	TMV	tracheal mucus velocity
PaO$_2$	oxygen partial pressure	TNF-α	tumour necrosis factor-α
PCNA	proliferative cell nuclear antigen	VC	vital capacity
PDE	phosphodiesterase	VEGF	vascular endothelial growth factor
Pdi	transdiaphragmatic pressure		
PEEPi	intrinsic positive end-expiratory pressure	VEGFR	vascular endothelial growth factor receptor

Index